Caring for Your School-Age Child

This invaluable volume was prepared under the editorial direction of distinguished pediatrician Edward L. Schor, M.D., and draws on the contributions and practical wisdom of more than 60 pediatric specialists and a seven-member AAP editorial review board. Written in a warm, accessible style and illustrated with more than 100 helpful drawings and diagrams, this book gives you the information you need to safeguard your child's most precious asset: his or her health.

In *Caring for Your School-Age Child* you'll find:

- A guide to your child's personal and social development, including the stages of puberty
- Guidance on being involved in your child's schooling, from starting school to developing good homework habits and reinforcing learning
- Practical suggestions for dealing with sibling rivalry, bed-wetting, and temper tantrums
- The best ways to encourage good nutrition and physical fitness
- Advice on effective discipline and optimal nurturing

Plus reliable information on:

- Choosing childcare and when your child wants to babysit
- Safety and injury prevention, plus handling emergency situations
- Learning disabilities, attention deficit hyperactivity disorder, and stuttering
- Common medical problems, from colds to swimmer's ear
- Chronic conditions and diseases, including asthma and diabetes

Child Care Books from
the American Academy of Pediatrics

Caring for Your Baby and Young Child
Birth to Age 5

Caring for Your School-Age Child
Ages 5 to 12

Caring for Your Adolescent
Ages 12 to 21

Guide to Your Child's Symptoms
Birth Through Adolescence

Guide to Your Child's Nutrition

Your Baby's First Year

CARING FOR YOUR SCHOOL-AGE CHILD

Ages 5 to 12

Editor-in-Chief:

Edward L. Schor, M.D.
Medical Director
Division of Family and Community
  Health
Iowa Department of Public Health
Des Moines, Iowa

Editorial Board:

William Lord Coleman, M.D.
Associate Professor of Pediatrics
Clinical Center for the Study of
  Development and Learning
University of North Carolina School of
  Medicine
Chapel Hill, North Carolina
Psychosocial Development and Child
  Behavior
Children in School

Paula Duncan, M.D.
Associate Clinical Professor of
  Pediatrics
University of Vermont Medical School
Coordinator of Health Services,
  Burlington School District
Burlington, Vermont
Children in School

Lawrence D. Hammer, M.D.
Associate Professor of Pediatrics
Stanford University School of
  Medicine
Stanford, California
Nutrition

Maurice E. Keenan, M.D.
Pediatrician, Massachusetts General
  Hospital
Assistant Professor of Pediatrics,
  Harvard Medical School,
  Boston, Massachusetts

Lucy M. Osborn, M.D.
Professor of Pediatrics and Family and
  Preventive Medicine
University of Utah Health Science
  Center
Salt Lake City, Utah
Promoting Health and Normal
  Development

Michael L. Weitzman, M.D.
Professor and Associate Chairman of
  Pediatrics
University of Rochester School of
  Medicine
Rochester, New York
Chronic Health Problems

David W. Willis, M.D.
Clinical Assistant Professor of
  Pediatrics and Psychiatry
Oregon Health Science University
Consultant in Behavioral and
  Developmental Pediatrics, Emanuel
  Children's Healthcare Center
Portland, Oregon
Psychosocial Development and Child
  Behavior

BANTAM BOOKS

New York   Toronto   London   Sydney   Auckland

CARING FOR YOUR SCHOOL-AGE CHILD: AGES 5 TO 12
A Bantam Book

PUBLISHING HISTORY
Bantam hardcover edition published December 1995
Bantam trade paperback edition / October 1996
Revised trade paperback edition / July 1999

A note about revisions:
Every effort is made to keep CARING FOR YOUR SCHOOL-AGE CHILD
consistent with the most recent advice and information available
from the American Academy of Pediatrics. In addition to major
revisions identified as "Revised Editions," the text has been
updated as necessary for the additional reprinting listed above.

The charts that appear on pages 5–8 are used with permission of
Ross Products Division, Abbott Laboratories, Columbus, Ohio
43216, from *NCHS Growth Charts*. Copyright © 1982 Ross Products
Division, Abbott Laboratories.

Library of Congress Cataloging-in-Publication Data

Caring for your school-age child : ages 5 to 12 /
editor-in-chief, Edward L. Schor . . . [et al.].
p.   cm.
ISBN 0-553-37992-5
1. Child care. 2. Child rearing.   3. School
children.   4. Child development.
I. Schor, Edward L.
[HQ772.C354   1999]
649'.124—dc21   99-12639
CIP

premium hardcover ISBN 0-553-80124-4

Published simultaneously in the United States and Canada

Bantam Books are published by Bantam Books, a division of Ran-
dom House, Inc. Its trademark, consisting of the words "Bantam
Books" and the portrayal of a rooster, is Registered in U.S. Patent
and Trademark Office and in other countries. Marca Registrada.
Bantam Books, 1540 Broadway, New York, New York 10036.

PRINTED IN THE UNITED STATES OF AMERICA

RRH   10 9 8 7 6 5 4 3 2 1 (hc)
RRH   10 9 8 7 6 5 4 3 2 1 (pbk)

Reviewers and Contributors

Barbara Howard, M.D.
David Jaffe, M.D.
Tom Jaksic, M.D.
Michael Jellinek, M.D.
Jerri Ann Jennista, M.D.
Steve Kohl, M.D.
Leonard Krilov, M.D.
Susan Levitsky, M.D.
Moise Levy, M.D.
Stephen Ludwig, M.D.
Kathleen Mahon, M.D.
Robert Mendelson, M.D.
Bruce Meyer, M.D.
Sylvia Micik, M.D.
David Mininberg, M.D.
George Nankervis, M.D.
Michael Nelson, M.D.
Jay Noffsinger, M.D.
Ellen Perrin, M.D.
James Perrin, M.D.
John Poncher, M.D.
Peter Rappo, M.D.
Anthony Richtsmeier, M.D.
Hugh Sampson, M.D.
Lawrence Schachner, M.D.
Sanford Schneider, M.D.
Alfred Smith, M.D.
Gary Smith, M.D.
Howard Spivak, M.D.
Martin Stein, M.D.
George Sterne, M.D.
J. Lane Tanner, M.D.
David Tinkelman, M.D.
Deborah Tolchin, M.D.
Hyman Tolmas, M.D.
Thomas Tonniges, M.D.
John Udall, M.D.
Martin Ushkow, M.D.
Joe Weinberg, M.D.
Lani Wheeler, M.D.
Robert Wiebe, M.D.
Mark Wolraich, M.D.

Illustrations

Jeanne Brunnick

Writer

Richard Trubo

Additional Assistance

Debbie Carney

This book is dedicated to
all the people who recognize that children
are our greatest inspiration in the present
and our greatest hope for the future.

PLEASE NOTE

The information contained in this book is intended to complement, not substitute for, the advice of your child's pediatrician. Before starting any medical treatment or medical program, you should consult with your own physician, who can discuss your individual needs with you and counsel you about symptoms and treatment.

The information and advice in this book apply equally to children of both sexes (except where noted). To indicate this, we have chosen to alternate between masculine and feminine pronouns throughout the book.

The American Academy of Pediatrics constantly monitors new scientific evidence and makes appropriate adjustments in its recommendations. For example, future research and the development of new childhood vaccines may alter the regimen for the administration of existing vaccines. Therefore, the schedule for immunizations outlined in this book is subject to change. These and other potential situations serve to emphasize the importance of always checking with your pediatrician for the latest information concerning the health of your child.

Contents

RESOURCES FROM THE AMERICAN ACADEMY OF PEDIATRICS

The American Academy of Pediatrics develops and produces a wide variety of public education materials that teach parents and children the importance of preventive and therapeutic medical care. These materials include books, magazines, videos, brochures, and other educational resources. Examples of these materials include:

- Brochures and fact sheets on allergies, child-care issues, divorce and single parenting, growth and development, immunizations, learning disabilities, nutrition and fitness, sleep problems, substance abuse, and television

- Videos on immunizations, newborn care, nutrition education, and asthma

- First-aid and growth charts, child health records, and books for parents

- A web site at www.aap.org

- *Healthy Kids* magazine (call 800-759-7076 to subscribe)

For a copy of the Academy's *Parent Resource Guide,* send a self-addressed, stamped #10 envelope to:

> American Academy of Pediatrics
> Department PRG
> P.O. Box 927
> Elk Grove Village, IL 60009–0927

For help in finding a qualified pediatrician or pediatric subspecialist, contact the "Pediatrician Referral Source" of the American Academy of Pediatrics by sending the name of your town (or those nearby) and a self-addressed, stamped envelope to:

> American Academy of Pediatrics
> Pediatrician Referral
> P.O. Box 927
> Elk Grove Village, IL 60009–0927

FOREWORD

Caring for Your School-Age Child: Ages 5 to 12 is the second in a three-volume series of child-care books developed by the American Academy of Pediatrics. The other books in this series include *Caring for Your Baby and Young Child: Birth to Age 5* and *Caring for Your Adolescent: Ages 12 to 21.*

The American Academy of Pediatrics is an organization of 55,000 primary care pediatricians, pediatric medical subspecialists, and pediatric surgical specialists committed to the attainment of optimal physical, mental, and social health for all infants, children, adolescents, and young adults. This book is part of the Academy's ongoing education efforts to provide parents and caregivers with quality information on a broad spectrum of children's health issues.

What distinguishes this book on the middle years of childhood from others in bookstores and on library shelves is that it has been written and extensively reviewed by members of the American Academy of Pediatrics. An eight-member editorial board developed the initial material with the assistance of over sixty contributors and reviewers. The final draft was then reviewed by countless numbers of pediatricians. Because medical information on children's health is constantly changing, every effort has been made to ensure that this book contains the most up-to-date information available.

A special feature of this book is the "Where We Stand" boxes that are found throughout. These boxes highlight health issues that are of special importance to the Academy in its role as a child-health advocacy organization.

It is the Academy's hope that this book will become an invaluable resource and reference guide for parents. We believe it is the best source of information on matters of children's health and well-being. We are confident that readers will find the book extremely valuable, and we encourage readers to use it in concert with the advice and counsel of their own pediatrician, who will provide individual guidance and help on issues related to the health of their children.

Joe M. Sanders, Jr., M.D.
Executive Director

Introduction: Preparing Your Child for the World Outside Home

When their youngsters reach the middle years of childhood, many parents breathe a sigh of relief. Finally, the period of their offspring's infancy, toddlerhood, and preschool years—a time when children grow so dramatically and require constant attention—is behind them. At the same time, adolescence and its perceived turmoil seem far off in the future. At least for the moment, these parents reason, they can relax a little. The middle years, they say, is a time when nothing much happens.

But, in fact, that is hardly the case. Families remain extremely important, and parenting can become even more challenging.

The middle years of childhood are years of enormous social growth. Between the ages of five and twelve, children's intellectual competence develops dramatically, and they become noticeably better at logical thinking, reasoning, and problem-solving. With these skills in hand, they begin to try out what they have learned at home in the outside world. These years offer children opportunities

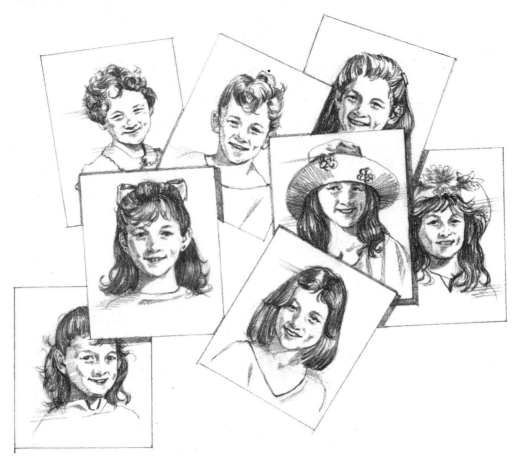

to see how the skills, behavior, beliefs, and values that serve them at home can work in the company of new friends and strangers.

The middle years are complex years, when children's self-esteem is tested and (it is to be hoped) is reinforced daily. Children must "find themselves" and become more independent while simultaneously gaining acceptance among their friends and retaining a secure place within their families. Most children find excitement and personal gratification during these years; some do not. Some children spend these years trying to manage or avoid problems—problems with friends, feelings, school, or within the family; they may not have the opportunity or the energy to succeed with the developmental tasks of this period of their lives.

The habits and behavior patterns that children develop during these years will strongly influence their later health and well-being, their successes at school and work, and their relationships. This book is written to assist par-

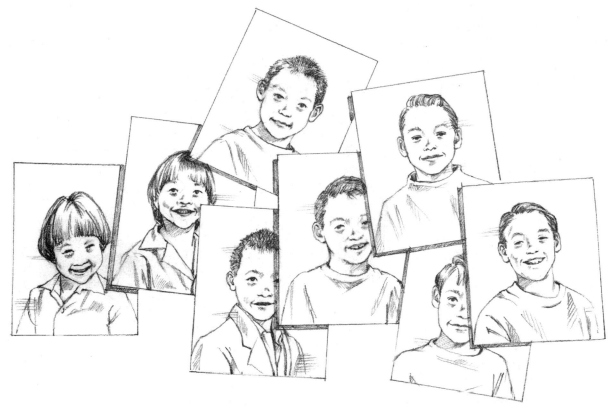

ents, teachers, and others to help children take advantage of the experiences these years provide—to build a firm foundation of healthy behavior, emotional well-being, and academic and social skills for their adolescence and their adult lives.

Since you have chosen to read this book, you already have some of the characteristics—namely, awareness and interest—necessary to guide a child through the middle years. Children seem to have an innate desire to explore, to learn, to grow, and to do their best, whatever the situation. Parents have that same determination as they go about raising their children, but sometimes, just like their children, parents need information, advice, and encouragement in order to succeed. It is one of the great myths of our time that parents should be self-sufficient and have the correct instincts and wisdom to solve all the problems that arise during childhood. Trial and error, learning from experience, is how most parenting takes place.

Still, there is a role for the advice of experts and of those who previously have traveled the parental path. The information in this book is provided by pediatricians, members of the American Academy of Pediatrics, who are national experts in their fields. They have studied child health and development, watched and learned from the tens of thousands of families for whom they have cared, and are parents themselves.

FAMILIES TODAY

Everyone knows that a child's experience within his or her family today is different from what it was a generation ago. Grandparents, cousins, uncles, and aunts are as likely to be many miles away as they are to be living around the corner. Today, fewer children live with both of their parents, many live with only their mothers, and some live in households with stepparents. Moreover, the number of siblings in the home has decreased. Daily routines are dictated as much by the work schedule of the parents as by the needs and wishes of the family, and there seems to be less time just to be a family—spending time together simply to enjoy each other's company.

Growing Up in a Family

The changes and complexities in family life demand that we pay attention to families, for they remain the place where children grow up. During the preschool years families are like incubators, providing children with a safe place where they can feel loved and cared about and discover who they are. In the middle years families provide a working model in which children can observe and practice relationships with other people. Families also provide a supportive environment in which children can find help in understanding, coping with, and finding their place in the world around them. This is quite a task to accomplish for a social institution like the family, which is barraged by outside pressures, many beyond their control.

Children's relationships with their parents change forever during these years. You and your youngster will spend much fewer of your waking hours together now. Monitoring your child's activities and behavior, and teaching him new skills, will become more of a hands-off process for you, and your child must struggle to develop strategies for controlling and managing his own behavior.

A BRAVE NEW WORLD

During the middle years, children first venture into the world alone, physically unaccompanied by their families. Schools become of great importance in the lives of children. They are the site of new social contacts with both adults and other children, as well as new expectations for the child. By participating in school activities and organizations, children develop friendships unrelated to their families for the first time. In so doing they face a confusing array of unfamiliar and sometimes unfathomable social behaviors.

Children will discover that other adults do not communicate directly with them and are not as easily understood as are their parents. Sometimes children have difficulty understanding the meaning and intention of what adults say. They will observe and be confused by the differences between spoken values and adult behavior. School will challenge the way they use their time, control their impulses, and measure their self-worth. Middle-years children develop their first intimate friendships and learn the essential skill of working things out to accommodate others. While friendships are extraordinarily important, they also can be marred by rivalry and jealousy.

To succeed and grow amid shifting interests and allegiances, children must learn about themselves as players in a social game and must discover how best to get along in this new arena. Their expanding self-awareness becomes increasingly stable and comprehensive. They develop standards and expectations for their own behavior, and become more independent and self-sufficient. While they try on new roles and attitudes in order to learn about themselves, they still will need to be able to turn to their families, especially to their parents, for guidance and stability.

RECURRING THEMES

There is no magic formula parents can apply to guarantee that their children will have a happy and successful life during the middle years. There is, though, much that parents can do and say that will be helpful. First and foremost, parents will need to model the values and behavior they wish their children to adopt, and direct their children into situations that reinforce and reward them. Whether it is responding to people less fortunate than themselves or choosing what foods to eat, children's behavior is in part an imitation of behavior they have observed.

Second, parents need to learn how to communicate with their children and to find opportunities to practice these skills. Simply listening is a fundamental communication skill. Parents must listen to their children, actively trying to hear what messages they are attempting to convey. The better that parents understand their children, the better able they will be to work together to meet challenges and solve problems when they arise. Good parents are those who have made the effort to know their children well, and have succeeded. Children whose parents know and understand them will have fewer personal and social problems.

In addition to active listening, successful communication is based on mutual respect, shared experiences, and open expression of thoughts and feelings. By paying attention to each child's personal skills and uniquely individual character, parents will find much to admire and respect.

Third, parents must support their children and be an advocate for them in many settings. Parents should not ignore or deny their child's problems; good parents are actively involved in their child's world, interpreting, guiding, coaching, and cheerleading.

Throughout this book, we offer advice on how these parenting skills can be acquired and applied.

HOW TO USE THIS BOOK

Sometimes you simply want to understand your child (or someone else's child) better, or to feel reassured that you are doing all right. At other times you want to help with a specific problem. Of course, the better you understand your child, and the development and the world of children, the better equipped you will be to work on a problem, and the less likely you are to be bothered by uncertainty, sadness, guilt, or anger over the way things are going.

This book has two kinds of chapters to meet these different needs. Some chapters provide background information about school-age children, their development, behavior, health, schools, and the social issues they confront. These chapters take a little longer to read, but the information they contain is basic and can be applied to many situations. By reading them, you also will learn the boundaries of normal growth, development, and behavior. Other chapters address specific problems that commonly occur during a child's middle years. You can turn to these for advice about a problem you and your child (or you and your student) are facing.

Being a parent at this time in our society is perhaps more difficult than it has ever been. But parenting is a natural process that can be enhanced by learning about your child and understanding your own feelings and inclinations. We hope that the advice contained in this book, when added to your own desire to act in your youngster's best interests, will contribute to the health and happiness of your child and of the next generation of children.

PART I

PROMOTING HEALTH AND NORMAL DEVELOPMENT

1

PHYSICAL DEVELOPMENT THROUGH PUBERTY

Most parents believe that their youngster's childhood passes much too quickly. Only yesterday, it seemed, you sang lullabies over your child's crib, or watched her crawl for the first time or take her first steps. Now she is bigger, more coordinated, more independent—and moving toward the much more dramatic changes of puberty that lie ahead.

The steady physical development that occurred during the preschool years will continue during middle childhood, although it will not proceed at nearly as rapid a rate as the growth that will follow in adolescence. The present changes tend to be more gradual and steady, all part of the evolution toward adulthood.

Most children have a slimmer appearance during middle childhood than they did during the preschool years, due to shifts in the accumulation and location of body fat. As a youngster's entire body size increases, the amount of body fat stays relatively stable, giving her a thinner look. Also, during this stage of life a child's legs are longer in proportion to her body than they were before.

On average, the steady growth of middle childhood results in an increase in height of a little over 2 inches a year in both boys and girls. Weight gain averages about 6.5 pounds a year. But these are only averages. A number of factors, including how close the child is to puberty, will determine when and how much your child grows. In general, there tends to be a period of a slightly increased growth rate between ages 6 and 8 years, which may be accompanied by the appearance of a small amount of pubic hair.

Perhaps more than any other factor, your youngster's pattern of growth and ultimate height will be influenced by heredity. Your son, for example, may want to be one of the tallest boys in his class, and he may aspire to play professional basketball. However, if both you and your spouse have below-average stature, his height as an adult will be more like yours than like his favorite sports idol's. While there are exceptions, tall parents usually have tall children, and short parents usually have short children. Those are the realities of genetics.

Even so, if your child seems *unusually* short or tall relative to her friends of the same age, talk with your pediatrician. The doctor may recommend X-rays to determine your child's bone growth. A true growth disorder can sometimes

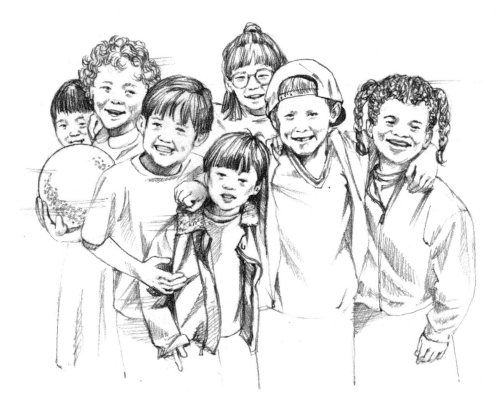

GIRLS: 2 TO 18 YEARS
PHYSICAL GROWTH
NCHS PERCENTILES*

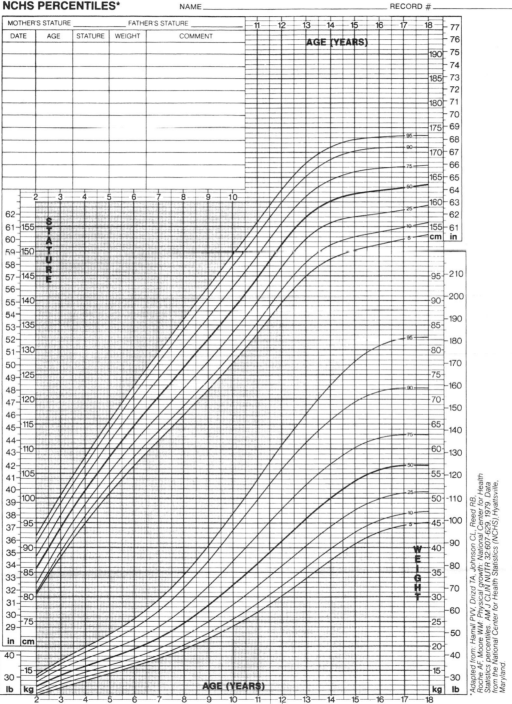

*Adapted from: Hamill PVV, Drizd TA, Johnson CL, Reed RB, Roche AF, Moore WM. Physical growth: National Center for Health Statistics percentiles. AM J CLIN NUTR 32:607-629, 1979. Data from the National Center for Health Statistics (NCHS), Hyattsville, Maryland.

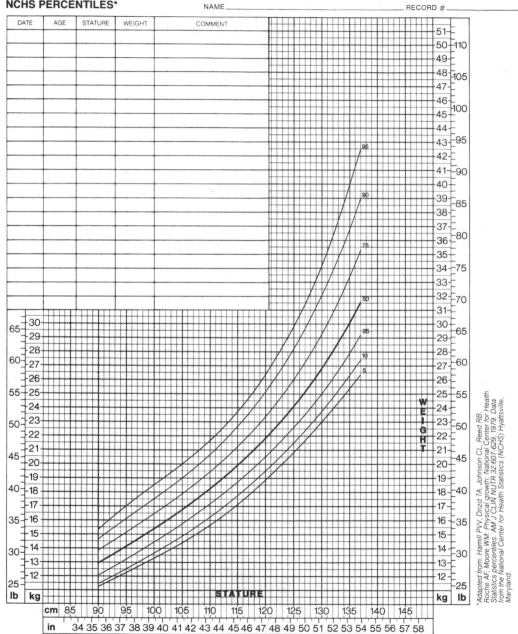

**GIRLS: PREPUBESCENT
PHYSICAL GROWTH
NCHS PERCENTILES***

NAME _____ RECORD # _____

Reprinted with permission
of Ross Laboratories

*Adapted from: Hamill PVV, Drizd TA, Johnson CL, Reed RB,
Roche AF, Moore WM: Physical growth: National Center for Health
Statistics percentiles. AM J CLIN NUTR 32:607-629, 1979. Data
from the National Center for Health Statistics (NCHS) Hyattsville,
Maryland.

© 1982 Ross Laboratories

BOYS: 2 TO 18 YEARS
PHYSICAL GROWTH
NCHS PERCENTILES*

NAME _____ RECORD # _____

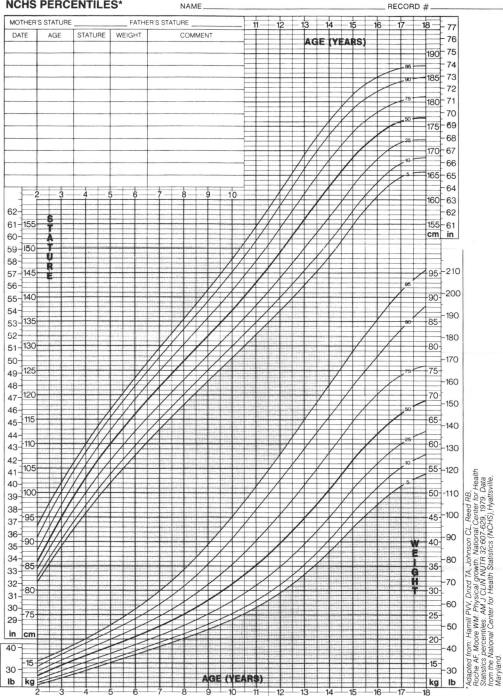

*Adapted from: Hamill PVV, Drizd TA, Johnson CL, Reed RB, Roche AF, Moore WM: Physical growth: National Center for Health Statistics percentiles. AM J CLIN NUTR 32:607-629, 1979. Data from the National Center for Health Statistics (NCHS), Hyattsville, Maryland

© 1982 Ross Laboratories

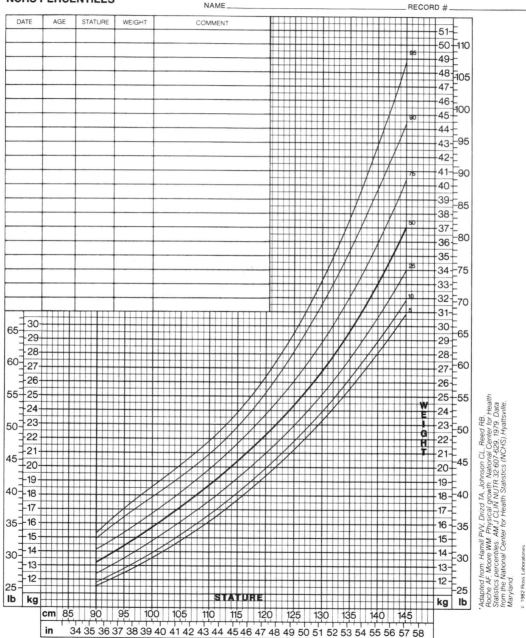

BOYS: PREPUBESCENT PHYSICAL GROWTH NCHS PERCENTILES*

Reprinted with permission of Ross Laboratories

NAME _____ RECORD # _____

*Adapted from: Hamill PVV, Drizd TA, Johnson CL, Reed RB, Roche AF, Moore WM. Physical growth: National Center for Health Statistics percentiles. AM J CLIN NUTR 32:607-629, 1979. Data from the National Center for Health Statistics (NCHS), Hyattsville, Maryland

© 1982 Ross Laboratories

be treated by administering growth hormones; however, this therapy is reserved for youngsters whose own glands cannot produce this hormone, thus interfering with normal growth. Physicians do not recommend this treatment for healthy boys and girls who may want (or whose parents may want them) to grow to be 6 feet tall instead of 5 feet 8.

Just as height can vary from youngster to youngster, so can the timing of a child's growth. Despite the averages mentioned above, many youngsters in middle childhood often experience clear growth spurts, followed by periods in which they grow very little. Some children grow as much as three times faster during a particular season of the year, compared with their "slow" seasons. These individual variations in timing—along with hereditary factors—are largely responsible for the wide variations in size among youngsters of the same age. Height differences among children in a typical elementary school classroom range from 4 to 5 inches.

A number of other factors—so-called environmental influences—can affect physical development as well. Nutrition is important to normal growth processes, and thus you should make an effort to ensure that your child consumes a well-balanced diet. Your youngster's need for calories rises during times of rapid growth, gradually increasing as she moves through middle childhood into puberty. However, if the calories consumed exceed those expended, your child may develop a weight problem. (See Chapter 6, "Special Diets, Special Needs.")

Some parents worry that their child is not eating as much as she should. However, even with what seems to be relatively low food intake, children can grow at normal rates. Even if your school-age child is a picky eater, you do not usually have to worry that this frustrating behavior is impairing her growth. During these picky-eater phases, do not fall into the trap of feeling she will starve and thus give in to her desire for junk food. Her fluctuating eating habits may be due to normal slow-growth periods. Or she may simply have uniquely personal, unpredictable preferences or distastes for certain foods. In general, youngsters outgrow these food preferences without any harm to their physical well-being. As long as your child is gaining weight appropriately (4 to 7 pounds per year) and is eating a healthy variety of foods, you can feel comfortable that her nutritional needs are being met.

In our relatively affluent society severe malnutrition is uncommon. Nevertheless, when a child's caloric intake is severely restricted—as in a disorder such as anorexia nervosa, or during a chronic illness—then her development and her overall health can be seriously harmed. Certainly if your child is losing weight, discuss this situation with your doctor. (For more information about anorexia nervosa, see Chapter 27, "Eating Disorders.")

Your child also needs to exercise regularly to ensure normal physical development. Youngsters who spend their free time watching TV or engaging in other sedentary pursuits rather than playing outdoors may have impaired

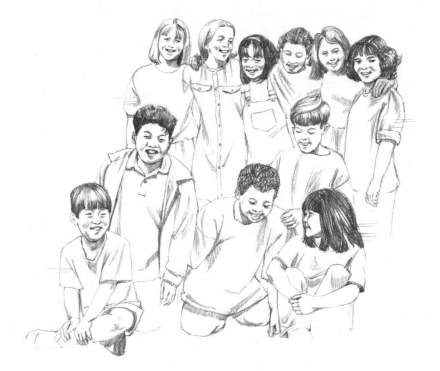

bone growth. Recent studies have shown that when physical activity is increased, bones are denser and stronger. Even so, there is no evidence that a very strenuous exercise program will help your child grow faster or bigger; running marathons, for example, will not stimulate her physical growth.

During middle childhood, you will probably notice a number of other prepubertal changes. Your child will become stronger as her muscle mass increases. Her motor skills—in both strength and coordination—will improve, too, reflected in gradual improvements in tasks ranging from tying her shoes to throwing a baseball accurately. At five years old, a typical youngster can skip, walk on her tiptoes, and broad-jump. She is capable of lacing her own shoes, cutting and pasting, and drawing a person with a head, body, arms, and legs. By age six, a child can bounce a ball four to six times, skate, ride a bicycle, skip with both feet, and dress herself completely without help. While a seven-year-old may not be able to catch a fly ball, a ten-year-old probably can. While a nine-year-old can build a model or learn to sew, most six-year-olds cannot.

A school-age child's hair may become a little darker. The texture and appearance of her skin will gradually change as well, becoming more like that of an adult.

Puberty often begins earlier than parents think. Breast budding in girls—their first sign of puberty—starts at age ten on average, with some girls starting as early as eight and others not starting until thirteen. The peak growth period (in height, weight, muscle mass, and the like) in girls occurs about one year after puberty has begun. Menstruation usually starts about two years after the onset of puberty; on average, the first menses occurs just before girls turn thirteen.

Boys enter puberty about one year later than girls. The first sign is enlargement of the testes and a thinning and reddening of the scrotum, which happens at an average age of eleven but may occur anytime between nine to fourteen years. For boys, the peak growth period occurs about two years after the beginning of puberty. Puberty is made up of a clear sequence of stages, affecting the skeletal, muscular, reproductive, and nearly all other bodily systems. (See the chart on page 12 for more information on the progression of puberty.)

Although boys and girls are generally of similar height during middle childhood, that changes with the beginning of puberty. Particularly in junior high school, girls are often taller than their male classmates, but within a year or two, boys catch up and usually surpass their female classmates. About 25 percent of human growth in height occurs during puberty.

There are many opportunities during this time of life for you to talk to your child about what she's experiencing. Your child needs to understand the physical changes that will occur in her body during puberty. You should emphasize that these changes are part of the natural process of growing into adulthood, stimulated by hormones (chemicals that are produced within the body).

Also, while fully respecting her desire for privacy, keep track of your child's bodily changes. As the age ranges above indicate, there are wide variations of "normal" in the time when puberty begins; remind your youngster that while she and her friends will grow at different rates, they will eventually catch up with one another.

On occasion, youngsters start puberty either very early or very late. There is no need to overreact to this phenomenon. Even so, girls should be checked by their physician if they begin pubertal changes before age eight, while boys should be evaluated if they enter puberty before age nine. Likewise, see a doctor if there are no pubertal changes in a girl by age thirteen or a boy by age fourteen.

Also, contact your physician if your child's pubertal development does not follow the pattern on the adjacent chart—for example, if your daughter begins menstruation *before* she experiences breast development. Your child can still continue seeing her pediatrician throughout these times of dramatic physical changes, and adolescence.

Stages of Puberty

As children approach and move through adolescence, they proceed through the following five stages of puberty:

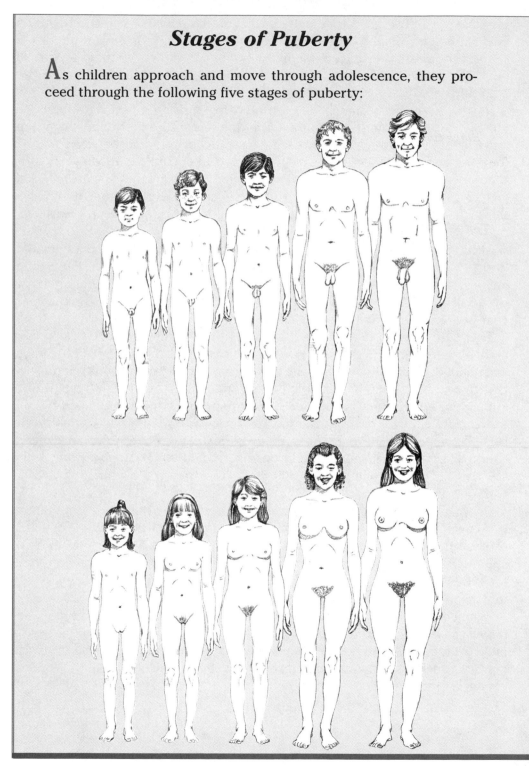

	Boys	Girls
Stage one	Prepubertal No sexual development	Prepubertal No sexual development
Stage two	Testes enlarge Body odor	Breast budding First pubic hair Body odor Height spurt
Stage three	Penis enlarges Pubic hair starts growing Ejaculation (wet dreams)	Breasts enlarge Pubic hair darkens, becomes curlier Vaginal discharge
Stage four	Continued enlargement of testes and penis Penis and scrotal sac deepen in color Pubic hair curlier and coarser Height spurt Male breast development	Onset of menstruation Nipple is distinct from areola
Stage five	Fully mature adult Pubic hair extends to inner thighs Increases in height slow, then stop	Fully mature adult Pubic hair extends to inner thighs Increases in height slow, then stop

CONCERNS OF GIRLS ABOUT PUBERTY

Menstruation. Many concerns about puberty center on menstruation. Spend time helping your daughter prepare for her first period. There is no reason for a girl to be surprised by her menarche, not knowing what is happening or why.

Remember, menstruation may begin sooner than you expect. Certainly, once your daughter's breast development has started, the two of you should fully discuss this topic. If you do not have adequate knowledge, ask your pediatrician to refer you to some informational sources. Some pediatricians schedule special educational visits at the time of puberty.

Discuss the biology of menstruation, describing it as a normal bodily process. Mention that her periods may be irregular, particularly in the beginning as her body adapts to rapid physiological changes. Also, let her know that several months before her first period, fluid may be secreted by glands within her vagina. This substance may be clear or white in color, and watery to thick in consistency. Tell her not to worry, and that this so-called physiologic leukorrhea is normal.

Explain that she may experience some cramping before or during her periods. If the cramps become severe, her doctor may have some suggestions for alleviating them, perhaps with physical exercises or medication.

Of course, discuss hygiene related to menstrual cycles. Be certain your daughter has the supplies she will need for her first period. Since she may be away from home when that first period begins, discuss how to use pads or tampons. She should understand the need to change pads or tampons several times a day, and that tampons should not be worn overnight. Of course, girls can shower or bathe while menstruating.

Many girls will ask if they can participate in activities such as swimming, horseback riding, or physical education classes. Reassure your daughter that she can take part in normal activities while menstruating. Exercise can sometimes even ease the cramps associated with periods.

Breast Development. Some girls also have anxieties about breast development. For example, one breast usually begins to develop before the other. Explain to your daughter that as her breasts develop, it is quite normal for one to be somewhat larger than the other, and that breast size is seldom symmetrical. Also, when a girl first notices the lump beneath one nipple, she may worry that this is cancer; reassure her that one breast is beginning to develop before the other, but if questions persist, consult your doctor.

If a girl's breasts start to develop relatively early, she often feels embarrassed and self-conscious. To help your daughter feel more comfortable in a situation like this, she may prefer to wear loose-fitting clothing that disguises her early breast development. Also, be willing to buy her a "training bra" when she requests one.

CONCERNS OF BOYS ABOUT PUBERTY

Boys have pubertal concerns and worries, too, including:

Voice Change. As their larynx (or voice box) enlarges and the muscles or vocal cords grow, their voice may "crack" as they speak. While this can be embarrassing and annoying, it's a normal part of the growth process.

Wet Dreams. Boys may awaken in the morning with damp pajamas and sheets. These "wet dreams," or nocturnal emissions, are caused by an ejaculation, not urination, that occurs during sleep; they are *not* an indication that the boy was having a sexual dream. Explain this phenomenon to your son, and reassure him that you understand that he cannot prevent it from happening. Wet dreams are just part of growing up.

Involuntary Erections. During puberty, boys get erections spontaneously, without touching their penis and without having sexual thoughts. These unexpected erections can be quite embarrassing, especially if they occur in public—at school, for example. Inform your son that these unexpected erections are normal and are a sign that his body is maturing. Explain that they happen to all boys during puberty, and that with the passage of time they will become less frequent.

Breast Enlargement. Many boys experience swelling of the breasts during the early years of puberty. Most often, your son may feel a flat, buttonlike bump under one or both nipples. His breasts may also feel tender or even painful. After a few months—sometimes longer—the swelling will disappear; these boys will not develop true breasts.

One Testicle Lower than the Other. Uneven testicles, although they may be embarrassing in the boys' locker room, are both normal and common.

As your child approaches and enters puberty, be sensitive to his or her need for privacy. Preteenagers will tend to become more modest while they bathe, for example, or change their clothes. Respect this desire for privacy, not only as it relates to their bodies but in other aspects of life as well, such as not reading their mail and remembering to knock before entering their rooms.

Children also become more sensitive about their body image during this time. Their interest in grooming increases, and they are more likely to be self-conscious about their appearance, thanks largely to the influence of their peers and the media. Watch for signs of a child who has a distorted body image, which can contribute to eating disorders in some cases. (See also Chapter 27, "Eating Disorders.")

Also, avoid even good-natured teasing of your child about his or her pubertal development. Because most youngsters feel self-conscious during this time, they will become embarrassed if they are kidded about the changing shape of their bodies or their deepening voices.

2

KEEPING YOUR CHILD HEALTHY

W hen a child's health is threatened by an illness or an injury, parents know to seek medical care, and they value the services that are available. But both you and your doctor have an equally important role to play in *maintaining* your youngster's good health, preventing illness and injury during childhood, and helping establish habits that will promote health and well-being for a lifetime.

CHOOSING A PEDIATRICIAN

When seeking the best medical care for your children, where should you turn? Most parents rely on a pediatrician, a medical doctor (M.D., D.O.) who specializes in the care of children. Pediatricians have special training in the health and illnesses of youngsters

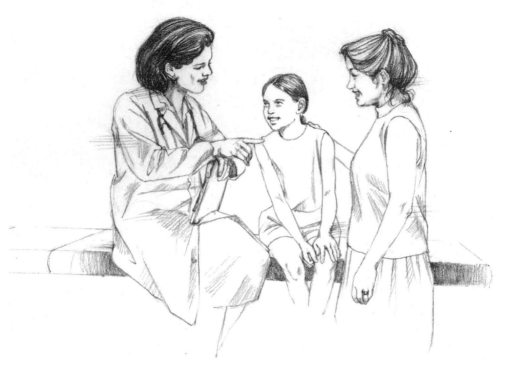

Choose a pediatrician who communicates effectively with both you and your child.

through the age of adolescence, and most are certified by the American Board of Pediatrics after passing a comprehensive examination covering all areas of health related to infants, children, and young adults.

By your child's middle years, you probably have already found a pediatrician with whom you are happy. However, the occasion may arise where you need to find a new doctor—perhaps you have moved to a new city or your pediatrician has retired.

In circumstances like these, try to obtain a referral from your present pediatrician. He or she may know a colleague in the city where you are moving, or one who is taking over the retiree's practice. Friends and family members might also recommend one or more pediatricians for you to consider.

There are other good sources of names of qualified pediatricians:

- The American Academy of Pediatrics can supply you with names of board-certified pediatricians in your community. For assistance, send the name of the desired area and a self-addressed, stamped envelope to: American Academy of Pediatrics, Pediatrician Referral Source, P.O. Box 927, Elk Grove Village, Il 60009–0927.

- Most local/county medical societies provide referral services to pediatricians in their area who are taking new patients.

- If you are located near a major medical center, community hospital, or teaching hospital, contact its department of pediatrics for the names of doctors in your area.

Interviewing Pediatricians

With a list of doctors in hand, call the office of each. Explain that you are looking for a pediatrician for your child, and inquire about the doctor's background and training, as well as general office procedures. If you are impressed with what you hear, arrange for an interview during which you can meet the doctor and ask some additional questions. It may be more convenient to do this interview by telephone. Here is some key information you might inquire about and consider during this first meeting:

- What medical school did the pediatrician attend, and where did he or she undergo postgraduate and residency training? (Medical directories in many public libraries—such as the *Directory of Medical Specialists* and the *American Medical Directory*—can also help answer these questions.)

- What are the doctor's present hospital appointments? If it becomes necessary for your youngster to be hospitalized, where would he be admitted?

- Is the pediatrician's office conveniently located? Is it easily accessible by automobile or public transportation?

- Are the office hours convenient for your own schedule? If you are a working parent, you may desire evening or weekend hours.

- What is the doctor's policy on taking and returning phone calls? Is there a nurse in the office who can answer routine questions?

- Is the doctor in a group practice with other physicians? Does another physician cover for the doctor at times? Who handles phone calls when the office is closed or during vacations?

- Do you sense a genuine interest by the doctor in the problems of *your* child, including particular health disorders he may have?

- Do both the physician and the office staff appear amicable and courteous? Do they demonstrate compassion and patience? Or do you feel rushed in the office, as though the doctor is eager to move on to the next patient?

RECOMMENDATIONS FOR PREVENTIVE PEDIATRIC HEALTH CARE

Committee on Practice and Ambulatory Medicine

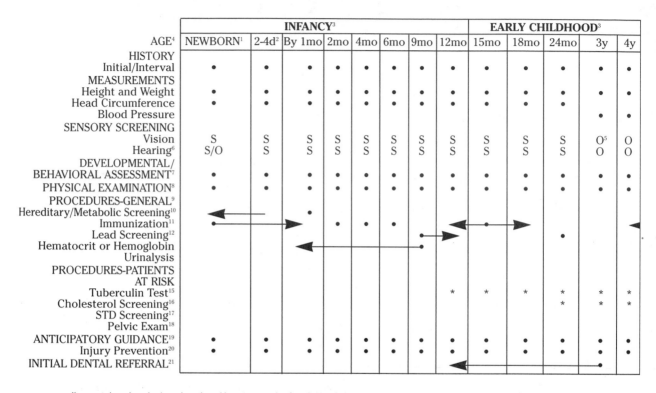

	INFANCY[3]								EARLY CHILDHOOD[3]				
AGE[4]	NEWBORN[1]	2-4d[2]	By 1mo	2mo	4mo	6mo	9mo	12mo	15mo	18mo	24mo	3y	4y
HISTORY Initial/Interval	•	•	•	•	•	•	•	•	•	•	•	•	•
MEASUREMENTS Height and Weight	•	•	•	•	•	•	•	•	•	•	•	•	•
Head Circumference	•	•	•	•	•	•	•	•	•	•	•		
Blood Pressure												•	•
SENSORY SCREENING Vision	S	S	S	S	S	S	S	S	S	S	S	O[5]	O
Hearing[6]	S/O	S	S	S	S	S	S	S	S	S	S	O	O
DEVELOPMENTAL/ BEHAVIORAL ASSESSMENT[7]	•	•	•	•	•	•	•	•	•	•	•	•	•
PHYSICAL EXAMINATION[8]	•	•	•	•	•	•	•	•	•	•	•	•	•
PROCEDURES-GENERAL[9]													
Hereditary/Metabolic Screening[10]	◄—————		•										
Immunization[11]	•————►			•	•			◄—•—►					◄
Lead Screening[12]								•———►			•		
Hematocrit or Hemoglobin			◄—————				•						
Urinalysis													
PROCEDURES-PATIENTS AT RISK													
Tuberculin Test[15]								*	*	*	*	*	*
Cholesterol Screening[16]											*	*	*
STD Screening[17]													
Pelvic Exam[18]													
ANTICIPATORY GUIDANCE[19]	•	•	•	•	•	•	•	•	•	•	•	•	•
Injury Prevention[20]	•	•	•	•	•	•	•	•	•	•	•	•	•
INITIAL DENTAL REFERRAL[21]								◄—————			•		

Key: • = to be performed   * = to be performed for patients at risk   S = subjective, by history   O = objective, by standard testing method ◄————► = the range during which a service may be provided, with the dot indicating the preferred age.

NB: Special chemical, immunologic, and endocrine testing is usually carried out upon specific indications. Testing other than newborn (e.g., inborn errors of metabolism, sickle disease, etc.) is discretionary with the physician.

The recommendations in this publication do not indicate an exclusive course of treatment or serve as a standard of medical care. Variations, taking into account individual circumstances, may be appropriate.

Each child and family is unique: therefore, these **Recommendations for Preventive Pediatric Health Care** are designed for the care of children who are receiving competent parenting, have no manifestations of any important health problems, and are growing and developing in satisfactory fashion. **Additional visits may become necessary** if circumstances suggest variations from normal. These guidelines represent a consensus by the Committee on Practice and Ambulatory Medicine in consultation with national committees and sections of the American Academy of Pediatrics. The Committee emphasizes the great importance of **continuity of care** in comprehensive health supervision and the need to avoid **fragmentation of care**.

A **prenatal visit** is recommended for parents who are at high risk, for first-time parents, and for those who request a conference. The prenatal visit should include anticipatory guidance and pertinent medical history. Every infant should have a newborn evaluation after birth.

1. Breastfeeding encouraged and instruction and support offered.
2. For newborns discharged in less than 48 hours after delivery.
3. Developmental, psychological, and chronic disease issues for children and adolescents may require frequent counseling and treatment visits separate from preventive care visits.
4. If a child comes under care for the first time at any point on the schedule, or if any items are not accomplished at the suggested age, the schedule should be brought up to date at the earliest possible time.
5. If the patient is uncooperative, rescreen within six months.
6. Some experts recommend objective appraisal of hearing in the newborn period. The Joint Committee on Infant Hearing has identified

MIDDLE CHILDHOOD[3]				ADOLESCENCE[3]										
5y	6y	8y	10y	11y	12y	13y	14y	15y	16y	17y	18y	19y	20y	21y
•	•	•	•	•	•	•	•	•	•	•	•	•	•	•
•	•	•	•	•	•	•	•	•	•	•	•	•	•	•
•	•	•	•	•	•	•	•	•	•	•	•	•	•	•
O	S	S	O	S	O	S	S	O	S	S	O	S	S	S
O	S	S	O	S	O	S	S	O	S	S	O	S	S	S
•	•	•	•	•	•	•	•	•	•	•	•	•	•	•
•	•	•	•	•	•	•	•	•	•	•	•	•	•	•
←—•—→				•←————————→										
				←————— 13 —————→										
				•←————— 14 —————→										
•														
*	*	*	*	*	*	*	*	*	*	*	*	*	*	*
*	*	*	*	*	*	*	*	*	*	*	*	*	*	*
					*	*	*	*	*	*	*	*	*	*
					*	*	*	*	*	*	←— * — 18 — * —→			*
•	•	•	•	•	•	•	•	•	•	•	•	•	•	•
•	•	•	•	•	•	•	•	•	•	•	•	•	•	•

patients at significant risk for hearing loss. All children meeting these criteria should be objectively screened. See the Joint Committee on Infant Hearing 1994 Position Statement.

7. By history and appropriate physical examination: if suspicious, by specific objective developmental testing.

8. At each visit, a complete physical examination is essential, with infant totally unclothed, older child undressed and suitably draped.

9. These may be modified, depending upon entry point into schedule and individual need.

10. Metabolic screening (e.g., thyroid, hemoglobinopathies, PKU, galactosemia) should be done according to state law.

11. Schedule(s) per the Committee on Infectious Diseases, published periodically in *Pediatrics*. Every visit should be an opportunity to update and complete a child's immunizations.

12. Blood lead screen per AAP statement "Lead Poisoning: From Screening to Primary Prevention" (1993).

13. All menstruating adolescents should be screened.

14. Conduct dipstick urinalysis for leukocytes for male and female adolescents.

15. TB testing per AAP statement "Screening for Tuberculosis in Infants and Children" (1994). Testing should be done upon recognition of high risk factors. If results are negative but high risk situation continues, testing should be repeated on an annual basis.

16. Cholesterol screening for high risk patients per AAP "Statement on Cholesterol" (1992). If family history cannot be ascertained and other risk factors are present, screening should be at the discretion of the physician.

17. All sexually active patients should be screened for sexually transmitted diseases (STDs).

18. All sexually active females should have a pelvic examination. A pelvic examination and routine Pap smear should be offered as part of preventive health maintenance between the ages of 18 and 21 years.

19. Appropriate discussion and counseling should be an integral part of each visit for care.

20. From birth to age 12, refer to AAP's injury prevention program (TIPP)® as described in "A Guide to Safety Counseling in Office Practice" (1994).

21. Earlier initial dental evaluations may be appropriate for some children. Subsequent examinations as prescribed by dentist.

- How are visits for acute illnesses handled? Can you make an appointment on short notice if your child needs to see the pediatrician because of a sore throat or an infection, for example?

- Does the doctor communicate clearly, using layman's language (not medical jargon) to explain illnesses and treatments, and does the doctor make an effort to ensure that all your questions are answered?

- What are the doctor's usual fees for sick visits, routine examinations, and immunizations? What is the office policy regarding the processing of insurance forms?

- In what managed-care programs does the doctor participate?

- If your child should ever develop a complex illness that necessitates the care of one or more specialists, will your pediatrician coordinate care among all the doctors providing treatment?

Keeping Medical Records

Because you might change pediatricians from time to time, it's useful to keep accurate medical records of your child's health. Your records should include the following information:

- **Physicians** (including the name and address of your child's previous pediatrician)

- **Hospitalizations** (dates, illnesses, and treatments)

- **Immunizations,** including the dates on which they were administered

- **Your child's height and weight** at each pediatrician's visit

- **Special care** that your child has received: the particular disease or condition, the age at which it began, and what therapy was used

- **Screening tests** to evaluate your child's vision, hearing, lead levels, and other aspects of your child's health

- **Family history,** the diseases that run in your extended family—including allergies, asthma, diabetes, heart disease, and high blood pressure—and that might be important for your pediatrician to know about.

Managed Care

Traditionally, families paid for health care each time a service was provided. This "fee-for-service" was paid directly by patients or by their insurance plan. Under fee-for-service, parents selected their child's primary doctor, decided which specialists to see, and even chose their hospital. Insurance plans that paid these fees, called indemnity insurance plans, spelled out what health care benefits were covered, and different plans' benefits varied greatly.

Today, many families' health insurance purchases health care services through a managed-care organization (MCO). An MCO normally contracts with a network or group of health care providers—doctors, hospitals, therapists, home health agencies, and others—to provide health services. Most MCOs pay only for services provided through their networks. If you join a managed-care plan whose network does not include your child's doctors, you may have to choose new physicians. An MCO usually will pay your child's health care provider a monthly or yearly rate for all the services your child uses, no matter how often he receives care. This capitation rate determines the doctor's salary. Often the doctor has a financial incentive to limit patients' use of services, including consultation with specialists and other health care providers, medication, hospital services, laboratory tests, and other aspects of care. On the other hand, a managed-care system may provide better access to care and better coordination among health care providers. Before you sign up for any insurance plan or managed-care program, be sure you understand your child's health care needs and how well the health care benefits that are offered will meet those needs.

Resolving Problems

Your child can continue to be treated by a pediatrician through adolescence. But no matter how carefully you have made your choice of a pediatrician, sometimes the chemistry between doctor and patient or between doctor and parent may become less than ideal. After several office visits you may decide that your expectations are not being met. In these instances, make an effort to discuss the problem with the pediatrician. Most difficulties can be smoothed out and resolved. On occasion, you might make a decision to switch physicians if the relationship continues to be unsatisfactory.

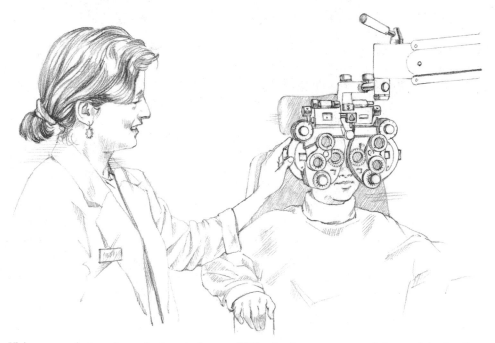

Vision screening, an important part of your child's checkups, may reveal the need for further vision testing.

WHEN TO SEE YOUR PEDIATRICIAN

The American Academy of Pediatrics recommends that your middle-years child have a routine well-child examination at least every two years, with annual checkups advised at ages 5, 6, 8, 10, 11, and 12 years old. During these doctor's visits, your physician will conduct a number of evaluations, such as measurement of height, weight, and blood pressure, a check of vital functions, a vision and hearing screening, and a complete physical examination. The doctor will ensure that your youngster's immunizations are up to date, and ask about your child's diet, exercise habits, and sleep patterns. He or she can also refer you to other health professionals: For example, children should receive regular dental checkups beginning at age three; if a pediatrician detects eye problems during routine screening, he or she may refer your child to an ophthalmologist for further evaluation and care.

Your pediatrician is interested not only in your child's physical health, but also in his or her mental and emotional well-being. It is appropriate to discuss such concerns as your youngster's school experiences, relationships with peers, family difficulties, and daily stresses.

During these middle years, also encourage your child to adopt good personal hygiene habits: bathing regularly; routinely washing hands before eating and after going to the bathroom, as a way of preventing the spread of infectious diseases; brushing teeth at least twice a day, and flossing once.

The following chapter will discuss a variety of important ways in which your child can stay healthy. Through these preventive measures you can reduce your child's risk of illness and injury—and keep down your medical expenses in the process.

IMMUNIZATIONS

Now that your youngster is in the middle years of childhood, she should already have received most of the immunizations generally recommended by pediatricians. Recent epidemics of preventable diseases have prompted the American Academy of Pediatrics to change its immunization recommendations so that additional shots are now advised between ages four and twelve. Before middle childhood—during infancy and through the preschool years—she should have already been protected against measles, mumps, and rubella (MMR); diphtheria, pertussis (whooping cough), and tetanus (DTaP or DTP); polio; hepatitis B and *Haemophilus influenzae B* (Hib) infections; varicella (chicken pox); and rotavirus. In most parts of the country, states and/or school districts require children to have completed these inoculations before they can enter kindergarten.

The success of modern vaccines is one of the truly extraordinary accomplishments of medical science. In earlier generations many school-age children contracted communicable diseases like polio and whooping cough, frequently with devastating consequences. Some children died; others were left with permanent impairments, perhaps dependent on a wheelchair. But the development of vaccines has made many of these childhood illnesses relatively rare and has thus improved the lifetime health and well-being of millions of people. These immunizations help children build their own defenses against infectious diseases by forming infection-fighting substances called antibodies, which kill the invading bacteria or viruses.

Unfortunately, some parents have become complacent about their children's immunizations. They have erroneously presumed that these serious diseases have disappeared or have been eradicated. Some parents have been frightened away by reports of possible side effects associated with certain vaccines.

However, the risks of *not* receiving immunizations are immense. (In some states, parents are legally accountable to obtain appropriate care for their children.) As a responsible parent, *you need to ensure that your child receives all of the currently recommended vaccines*. Today's vaccines are safe and generally produce only mild side effects (such as fever or localized redness). Severe adverse reactions are extremely rare.

Recommended Childhood Immunization Schedule
United States, January – December 1999

Vaccines[1] are listed under routinely recommended ages. ⬚ Bars indicate range of recommended ages for immunization. Any dose not given at the recommended age should be given as a "catch-up" immunization at any subsequent visit when indicated and feasible. ⬭ Ovals indicate vaccines to be given if previously recommended doses were missed or given earlier than the recommended minimum age.

Age ▶ Vaccine ▼	Birth	1 mo	2 mos	4 mos	6 mos	12 mos	15 mos	18 mos	4-6 yrs	11-12 yrs	14-16 yrs
Hepatitis B[2]	Hep B										
		Hep B			Hep B					Hep B	
Diphtheria, Tetanus, Pertussis[3]			DTaP	DTaP	DTaP		DTaP[3]		DTaP	Td	
H. influenzae type b[4]			Hib	Hib	Hib	Hib					
Polio[5]			IPV	IPV		Polio[5]			Polio		
Rotavirus[6]			Rv[6]	Rv[6]	Rv[6]						
Measles, Mumps, Rubella[7]						MMR			MMR[7]	MMR[7]	
Varicella[8]						Var				Var[8]	

Approved by the Advisory Committee on Immunization Practices (ACIP), the American Academy of Pediatrics (AAP), and the American Academy of Family Physicians (AAFP).

1 This schedule indicates the recommended ages for routine administration of currently licensed childhood vaccines. Combination vaccines may be used whenever any components of the combination are indicated and its other components are not contraindicated. Providers should consult the manufacturers' package inserts for detailed recommendations.

2 *Infants born to HBsAg-negative mothers* should receive the 2nd dose of hepatitis B vaccine at least 1 month after the 1st dose. The 3rd dose should be administered at least 4 months after the 1st dose and at least 2 months after the 2nd dose, but not before 6 months of age for infants.

Infants born to HBsAg-positive mothers should receive hepatitis B vaccine and 0.5 mL hepatitis B immune globulin (HBIG) within 12 hours of birth at separate sites. The 2nd dose is recommended at 1–2 months of age and the 3rd dose at 6 months of age.

Infants born to mothers whose HBsAg status is unknown should receive hepatitis B vaccine within 12 hours of birth. Maternal blood should be drawn at the time of delivery to determine the mother's HBsAg status; if the HBsAg test is positive, the infant should receive HBIG as soon as possible (no later than 1 week of age).

All children and adolescents (through 18 years of age) who have not been immunized against hepatitis B may begin the series during any visit. Special efforts should be made to immunize children who were born in or whose parents were born in areas of the world with moderate or high endemicity of HBV infection.

3 DTaP (diphtheria and tetanus toxoids and acellular pertussis vaccine) is the preferred vaccine for all doses in the immunization series, including completion of the series in children who have received 1 or more doses of whole-cell DTP vaccine. Whole-cell DTP is an acceptable alternative to DTaP. The 4th dose (DTP or DTaP) may be administered as early as 12 months of age, provided 6 months have elapsed since the 3rd dose and if the child is unlikely to return at age 15–18 months. Td (tetanus and diphtheria toxoids) is recommended at 11–12 years of age if at least 5 years have elapsed since the last dose of DTP, DTaP, or DT. Subsequent routine Td boosters are recommended every 10 years.

4 Three *H. influenzae* type b (Hib) conjugate vaccines are licensed for infant use. If PRP-OMP (PedvaxHIB and COMVAX [Merck]) is administered at 2 and 4 months of age, a dose at 6 months is not required. Because clinical studies in infants have demonstrated that using some combination products may induce a lower immune response to the Hib vaccine component, DTaP/Hib combination products should not be used for primary immunization in infants at 2, 4, or 6 months of age, unless FDA-approved for these ages.

5 Two poliovirus vaccines currently are licensed in the United States: inactivated poliovirus vaccine (IPV) and oral poliovirus vaccine (OPV). The ACIP, AAP, and AAFP now recommend that the first two doses of poliovirus vaccine should be IPV. The ACIP continues to recommend a sequential schedule of two doses of IPV administered at ages 2 and 4 months, followed by two doses of OPV at 12–18 months and 4–6 years. Use of IPV for all doses also is acceptable and is recommended for immunocompromised persons and their household contacts.

OPV is no longer recommended for the first two doses of the schedule and is acceptable only for special circumstances such as: children of parents who do not accept the recommended number of injections, late initiation of immunization which would require an unacceptable number of injections, and imminent travel to polio-endemic areas. OPV remains the vaccine of choice for mass immunization campaigns to control outbreaks due to wild poliovirus.

6 Rotavirus (Rv) vaccine is shaded and italicized to indicate: 1) health care providers may require time and resources to incorporate this new vaccine into practice; and 2) the AAFP feels that the decision to use rotavirus vaccine should be made by the parent or guardian in consultation with their physician or other health care provider. The first dose of Rv vaccine should not be administered before 6 weeks of age, and the minimum interval between doses is 3 weeks. The Rv vaccine series should not be initiated at 7 months of age or older, and all doses should be completed by the first birthday.

7 The 2nd dose of measles, mumps, and rubella vaccine (MMR) is recommended routinely at 4–6 years of age but may be administered during any visit, provided at least 4 weeks have elapsed since receipt of the 1st dose and that both doses are administered beginning at or after 12 months of age. Those who have not previously received the second dose should complete the schedule by the 11- to 12-year-old visit.

8 Varicella vaccine is recommended by any visit on or after the first birthday for susceptible children, i.e., those who lack a reliable history of chicken pox (as judged by a health care provider) and who have not been immunized. Susceptible persons 13 years of age or older should receive 2 doses, given at least 4 weeks apart.

For maximum effectiveness and protection, immunizations should be administered at particular ages. Based on recommendations from the American Academy of Pediatrics, your pediatrician can advise you as to when your child should receive immunizations.

Most children will have received all of their recommended immunizations prior to starting school. Children ages four through six should receive booster doses of diphtheria, tetanus and pertussis (DTaP), polio, and measles, mumps, and rubella (MMR) vaccines prior to entering school. If your school-age child has not received these booster immunizations, they should be given promptly. Sometimes the booster MMR is given between ages 11–12 years. An additional Td (tetanus and diphtheria) booster is recommended at age 11–12, and then every 10 years.

Because research is ongoing into developing new and improved ways to protect children from serious diseases, immunization guidelines change frequently. Talk with your pediatrician about his or her recommendations for your child. Here are some of the current recommendations for middle childhood:

- **MMR Booster**—Each child should receive a second MMR vaccine. This booster dose is recommended to be given at 4 to 6 years of age. If this dose was not given earlier, it should be given at 11 to 12 years of age. In recent years physicians have become particularly concerned about outbreaks of measles, with more than half of the affected children having received only one MMR inoculation.

- **Pneumococcal Vaccine**—A vaccine is available that can prevent meningitis and pneumonia caused by *Streptococcus pneumoniae* bacteria. Healthy children sometimes develop a serious illness from these bacteria. Youngsters with certain conditions or diseases are more vulnerable and thus should be vaccinated. These high-risk children include those with chronic lung disease or sickle-cell disease, or those who have had their spleens removed (either because of accidents or as part of the treatment for certain illnesses). This pneumococcal inoculation also is advised for children whose immune system is suppressed, perhaps because of cancer or medications that have weakened their immunity.

- **Influenza Vaccination**—An annual flu shot each fall is especially important for certain children. These youngsters, for whom an infection by the influenza virus would be severe or even fatal, include those with heart disease, an impaired immune system, chronic lung disease (including asthma and cystic fibrosis), and abnormalities of hemoglobin, the substance that carries oxygen in the blood. The siblings and parents of these children also should be vaccinated. The vaccine may be administered to any healthy child or adolescent. Influenza can cause serious illness in healthy children. However, currently it is not feasible to recommend routine vaccination for all children.

- **Chicken Pox Vaccination**—A vaccine to protect against chicken pox is recommended for all healthy children between 12 and 18 months of age who have never had the disease. Children under 13 who have not had chicken pox and were never vaccinated also should receive a single dose of the vaccine. Although chicken pox will not cause complications in most healthy children, certain groups are at a higher risk of developing more severe problems. These include children who are under one year of age, have weak immune systems, have eczema and other skin conditions, or are adolescents. Children over age 13 who have not had varicella (chicken pox) should receive two doses of the vaccine, one month apart.

- **Hepatitis B Vaccine**—A vaccine to prevent hepatitis B is recommended as part of the basic series of immunizations to be given to children during their first year of life. Hepatitis B is a viral illness that affects the liver. Infected children can have no symptoms or a mild illness; however, hepatitis B can progress to severe liver disease, and can lead to the development of liver cancer. The virus can be passed from mother to infant at the time of birth or from one household member to another. It can be spread through contact with infected blood from contaminated needles or contaminated surgical or dental instruments. Teenagers can also contract this disease through sexual intercourse.

Most children in their middle years will have received hepatitis B immunization during infancy. Children who have not been vaccinated may begin the three-dose series during any childhood visit to their pediatrician. Because adolescence is a time of increased risk of contracting hepatitis B, it is important that children are completely immunized by age thirteen. The second dose is ordinarily given at least one month after the first, and the third dose is administered at least four months after the first dose and at least two months after the second.

WHERE WE STAND

The American Academy of Pediatrics believes that the benefits of immunization far outweigh the risks incurred by childhood diseases, as well as any risks of the vaccines themselves. Despite highly publicized cases of severe adverse effects associated with the vaccines—particularly the pertussis component of the DTP immunization—these unfortunate outcomes are very rare. The AAP believes that immunizations are the safest and most cost-effective way of preventing disease, disability, and death, and it urges parents to ensure that their children are immunized against dangerous childhood diseases.

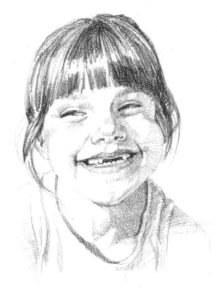

YOUR CHILD'S TEETH

A child in the middle years who ignores the day-to-day care of his teeth—including brushing them at least twice a day and flossing once a day—runs the risk of tooth decay, toothaches, and lost teeth.

Your child may need some help brushing until he is between ages seven and ten. Even if his intentions are good, he may not have the dexterity to clean his teeth well. Ideally, the teeth should be brushed within five to ten minutes after eating. Also, for long-term dental health, your child needs to care for his gums as well; he should be taught to floss regularly, preferably once a day, in order to help prevent gum (or periodontal) disease in adulthood.

A tartar-control toothpaste can help keep plaque from adhering to your child's teeth. Also, fluoride in the toothpaste can strengthen the exposed outer enamel of the youngster's teeth and help prevent cavities. Fluoride also has been added to the water supply in many cities. If your own tap water has less than the recommended levels of this nutrient, your pediatrician may suggest that you add fluoride to your child's diet beginning at age six months, often as part of a vitamin supplement. Fluoride treatment should continue until age sixteen. Ask your doctor or dentist for guidance.

Your dentist may also suggest placing sealants on your child's molars. These thin plastic coatings prevent plaque from accumulating and becoming trapped in the pits and fissures of the teeth. They are appropriate for all rear teeth that have grooves in them, and because they are extremely successful in preventing cavities, they are cost-effective too. Sealants may need to be reapplied during adolescence. With a combination of sealants and fluoride treatment, the incidence of cavities can be reduced by 90 percent.

Diet can also play a role in healthy teeth. In particular, minimize your child's contact with high-sugar and sticky sweets and other carbohydrates. Cut back on snacking on sweets between meals, when these foods are more likely to linger in the mouth without brushing.

Make sure your youngster has dental checkups twice a year for cleaning, as well as for X-rays as recommended by your dentist. Parents may choose to utilize a pedodontist, a dentist with special interest and expertise in children's dentistry. Regular preventive appointments will significantly decrease your child's chances of ever having to undergo major dental treatment. Also, contact your dentist whenever your child complains of a toothache. This pain could be a sign of a decayed tooth. Until the dentist can see your child, treat the pain with acetaminophen by mouth.

Care of the baby teeth is as important as looking after the permanent teeth. If your child loses his baby teeth by decay or accident too early, his permanent teeth can erupt prematurely and come in crooked because of limited space. According to orthodontists, 30 percent of their cases have their origins in the premature loss of baby teeth.

Erupting permanent teeth cause the roots of baby teeth to be reabsorbed so that by the time they are loose there is little holding them in place besides a small amount of tissue. Baby teeth ordinarily are shed first at about age six when the incisors, the middle teeth in front, become loose. Molars, in the back, are usually shed between ages ten and twelve, and are replaced with permanent teeth by about age thirteen. Children usually wiggle their teeth loose with their tongues or fingers, eager to hide them under their pillow for the "tooth fairy." If your child wants you to pull out the already loose tooth, grasp it firmly with a piece of tissue or gauze and remove it with a quick twist. Occasionally, if a primary tooth is not loosening sufficiently on its own, your child's dentist may suggest extracting it.

Around the time of puberty, parents begin to worry about whether their youngsters have a perfect bite and whether their teeth are symmetrical. At this age, many children are fitted with retainers (a removable appliance) and other pre-orthodontia devices, aimed at correcting misaligned teeth by gradually moving them into a proper position. Your dentist is an excellent source of information about when this apparatus is appropriate, and whether a consultation with an orthodontist is advisable.

3

SAFETY AND INJURY PREVENTION

Between ages six and twelve, 51 percent of all deaths are caused by unintentional injuries. Each year thousands of children are involved in automobile crashes as passengers or pedestrians. Thousands more drown, suffer severe burns, or are victims of gunfire or other accidents—most of which are preventable. While some of these injuries result in death, many more damage children, leaving them with lifelong impairments.

Keep in mind that while youngsters in middle childhood are seeking more independence, they often are not able to handle every challenge. When riding their bicycles, for instance, they may not have the capacity to judge their own speed, or the speed of an oncoming car and how long it will take that car to reach them and/or stop. Or they might be coerced into playing with matches or play with a handgun found in a bedroom closet.

The following guidelines will help to prevent some of the most common injuries of middle childhood:

INJURIES

Car Safety

In middle childhood, automobile crashes are responsible for more deaths than any other cause. In 1997, 1,791 U.S. children younger than 15 years were killed and 282,000 were injured as occupants in motor vehicles.

Yet most of these fatalities and injuries could be avoided with the use of seat belts. For children under 40 pounds, a forward-facing safety seat should be used as long as the child fits well (ears below the top of the back of the seat and shoulders below the harness slots of the seat). A belt-positioning booster seat should be used when the child has outgrown the safety seat but is too small to fit properly in a vehicle safety belt. Belt-positioning boosters are always used with a lap/shoulder belt.* They raise children up so that the seat belt fits correctly. Shield boosters do not provide as much upper body protection and are not intended for children over 40 pounds. In addition, shield

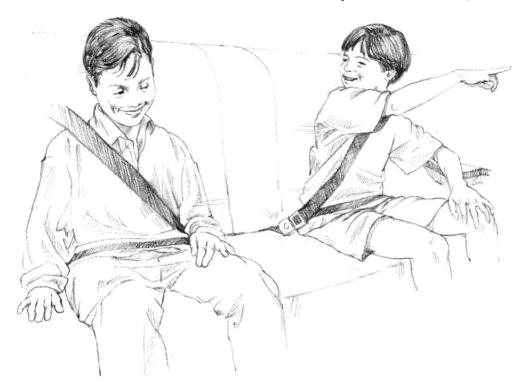

Teach your children to take personal responsibility for buckling their seat belts.

* American cars and many foreign cars made before 1990 do not have the shoulder harness portion of the seat belt in their back seats. If your car has only lap belts, take it to your dealer, who will properly install the shoulder harnesses at a small cost.

boosters should not be used for children under 40 pounds, even if they are labeled for use at a lower weight. Shield boosters should only be used without their shields as belt-positioning boosters. Studies show that if children were properly restrained, the number of fatalities would decline by 70 to 85 percent, and serious injuries would decrease by 50 to 60 percent.

For children who have outgrown their booster seats, be sure their seat belt fits properly. The shoulder belt should fit across the shoulder and upper chest, not the face or neck. The lap belt should be buckled low and flat across the pelvis (not the abdomen) and fit snugly. (In a crash, a child can be injured if propelled against a loose-fitting belt—as well as against a dashboard or a seatback.) The shoulder belt should never be positioned under the child's arm. Keep in mind that lap/shoulder belts do not fit children properly until they are 54 inches tall, have a sitting height of 30 inches, and weigh 80 pounds. A child cannot ride comfortably and remain properly restrained until he is tall enough for his knees to bend over the edge of the seat when his back is resting firmly against the seat back.

Whenever possible, children should sit in the back seat. Front seats expose children to serious injury from air bags, which are not placed to protect children or short individuals. Also, in automobile crashes, severe injury can result from being thrown into the windshield glass. Children should not sit in the front seat.

Despite educational programs aimed at improving car safety, a large number of school-age children are not properly restrained. As a driver, before starting the engine of your car, check to make certain that all children in your vehicle are buckled in place, and then buckle your own belt. Children must be appropriately restrained, even if the distance traveled is just a block; the majority of crashes occur within a five-mile radius of home.

Car safety habits should be established as early in life as possible, and they are among the most important gifts you can give your youngster. Children who always use car seats, booster seats, and seat belts have developed this safety habit. It is important to teach your children to take personal responsibility for buckling their own belts, whether riding with you or another adult. Remember, children learn by example, so to reinforce seat-belt use, buckle your own belt whenever you are in the car, whether you are the driver or a passenger. Never begin a car trip until all occupants are safely restrained.

Here are some other car safety tips:

- Prohibit your children and other passengers from extending their heads or limbs out the car window.

- Keep all doors locked while the car is in motion.

- Pick up and drop off children at the curb or driveway.

- Use power window locks if they are available on your car.

WHERE WE STAND

About one thousand children and adolescents are injured each year while riding in the back of pickup trucks; another hundred or more are killed. These young people are often ejected from the back of the truck during a collision or a rollover. Their deaths or injuries, however, could have been prevented.

The American Academy of Pediatrics believes that passengers should be prohibited from riding in truck beds or in any other area of a vehicle that does not have a seat and a seat belt. Only a few states presently have such bans. We also urge you to educate your children about the dangers of riding in open truck beds, and never allow them to do so.

- Equip each car with a fire extinguisher and first aid kit.

- Loose objects—particularly heavy ones, such as luggage or bicycles— should be placed in the car trunk or on the roof rack rather than inside the car. Not only can these unsecured items obstruct the driver's view, but they can be tossed about the car in a crash—as can an unbuckled driver or passenger—striking and injuring the occupants.

- Never leave young children alone in the car.

As your children become more involved in extracurricular activities, you'll be driving them back and forth more, and car pooling will probably make sense. When you drive children in a car pool, you must be as responsible for every child in the car as you are for your own.

Be clear about your expectations of your child riders: everyone must buckle up and safety rules must be obeyed. Children in groups can get unruly, so pull over if any child gets out of control; don't drive if you are distracted by misbehavior. And never transport more children than your car can safely accommodate.

Not only does car pooling save time, it is also an opportunity to observe how your child interacts with peers and find out what children talk about and what pressures they place on one another.

Other Motorized Vehicles

Although children in the middle years cannot drive automobiles, some of them (usually with their parents' blessings) are still being allowed into the driver's seat of other types of motorized vehicles. Most commonly, these youngsters are driving tractors, lawn mowers, personal watercraft, mopeds, minibikes, trail bikes, all-terrain vehicles (ATVs), and snowmobiles. Some of these vehicles are designed and advertised to be used primarily by school-age youngsters.

While children in this age group are physically able to turn the steering wheel and reach the gas pedal of these motorized vehicles, they lack the co-ordination, the reflexes, and the judgment to avoid crashes. For that reason youngsters should *not* be allowed to drive them.

In addition, these vehicles achieve high speeds but provide no protective covering. Therefore, when a crash does occur, there is a high risk of serious injury. Minibikes (two-wheeled vehicles that resemble small motorcycles) have a crash rate 400 percent higher than that of bicycles, with most injuries occurring from falls or collisions. There are more than thirty thousand crashes per year on trail bikes, with about one third of them occurring in youngsters under the age of fourteen.

ATVs have received considerable attention in recent years—much of it negative because of their high crash rates. These off-road vehicles can achieve speeds as high as 30 to 50 miles per hour, and they enjoyed a surge in popularity in the 1980s. But the three-wheel models in particular are prone to overturning on hills and slopes. Many children have died, often after suffering serious head injuries. Head injuries also are responsible for deaths on snowmobiles, which can achieve high rates of speed and are prone to rollovers. Tractors, riding mowers, and personal watercraft also tend to roll over, causing serious injuries. None of these vehicles are appropriate for children to drive.

Bicycle Safety

Mastering the art of riding a two-wheel bicycle gives most children a feeling of pride and newfound independence. Overnight they acquire a means of transportation to school or the playground.

Learning to ride a bicycle is like other motor skills—some children are ready earlier than others. Starting with training wheels is helpful but not always necessary to learn to coordinate watching, listening, pedaling, steering, and balancing. Younger children may depend on training wheels until they are five or six, and sometimes older. Use a bicycle helmet from the first time your child climbs on a bicycle. When your child feels ready to ride without training wheels (and he will let you know), add protective pads to cushion the falls that are inevitably part of the learning process.

However, riding a bicycle poses serious risks. Each year, about 400 children and adolescents die in the United States in bicycle accidents; another 400,000 end up in emergency rooms because of bicycle injuries.

The majority of bicycle-related deaths involve collisions between a bicycle and an automobile, often when the child darts out of a driveway or alley and strikes, or is struck by, a car. Or the bicyclist may be riding on the street *against* rather than *with* the flow of traffic. Most of these collisions are preventable if both parents and children learn the rules of the road, wear helmets, and never ride at night.

Many more injuries happen when a child falls off a bicycle, which can cause everything from serious contusions to a broken arm to a severe head injury. These events often occur when the youngster rides too fast and loses control of the bike, rides on a rough surface, or is double riding or stunt riding. Some injuries are caused when the child's clothes become entangled in the bicycle mechanism.

To keep your youngster from ending up in an emergency room or a wheelchair, do not let her ride on the street or in traffic until she can ride confidently and adhere to the basic rules of the road. Make sure she understands and abides by safety guidelines like these:

- **Wear a bicycle helmet at all times.**

    This first point is particularly important. Buy a helmet at the same time you purchase your child's first bicycle. Also encourage your child to use the same helmet for other types of play like roller-skating and skateboarding. The helmet should adhere to the safety standards of the American National Standards Institute (ANSI) or the Snell Memorial Foundation. (Look for a sticker affixed to the helmet that says "Snell Approved" or "Meets ANSI Z90.4 Standard.") These helmets can absorb most of the impact of a crash, thus protecting the head from serious injury. (Studies show that helmets can reduce the risk of brain injury by up to 85 percent.) Remind your child to use the helmet's chin strap to keep it in place at all times. Make helmet use a firm rule; your child should not be riding a bike without using a helmet.

- Stop at all points where a driveway, sidewalk, alley, or side street intersects with a street. Look both ways before proceeding.

- Obey all traffic lights and signs. They are there for bicycles as well as automobiles.

- When cycling with friends, ride in single file instead of riding abreast of one another and perhaps extending out into traffic. Use bicycle paths if at all possible.

- Avoid all trick and double riding, such as a second child riding on the handlebars.

- Do not ride at dusk or after dark.

- Ride in the same direction as traffic.

- Do not wear loose-fitting pants or other clothing that could become caught in the bicycle chain or other mechanism. Wear shoes and tie the laces.

- Do not wear earphones while riding. Listening to music muffles the traffic sounds that help you ride safely.

- If objects need to be carried, they should be placed in a backpack or a basket, allowing both hands to remain on the handlebars at all times. The backpack should not be so heavy that it affects the balance of the rider.

Choose your child's bicycle carefully. If her bike is the wrong size for her, she is more likely to lose control and be injured. Although some parents tend

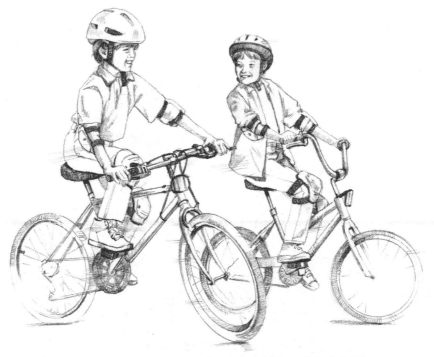

Helmets should be worn every time your children ride their bikes.

to buy a bike that their youngster can "grow into," an oversized bike is dangerous.

When shopping for a bike with your child, first have her sit on the seat; while gripping the handlebars she should be able to put the balls of both feet on the ground. For a boy, make sure that he can place both of his feet flat on the ground when straddling the center bar, with about a one-inch clearance

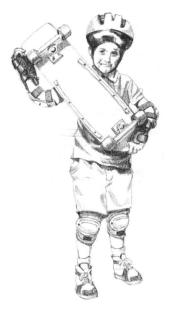

between the bar and his crotch. Girls' bikes should be similarly sized. Although coaster brakes are more appropriate for a younger child, an older youngster who prefers hand brakes should try them out, making sure she can grasp them comfortably and apply enough pressure to bring the bike to a halt.

Teach your child to keep her bicycle in good condition. Have her check the seat and handlebar height, the brakes, and the tire inflation regularly.

Skateboard Safety

The use of skateboards by middle-years children has increased significantly in recent years. Not only do these young skateboarders have a high center of gravity, but they do poorly at breaking their falls. As a result, there has been a rise in the number of skateboard-related injuries, including those to the arms, legs, head, and neck. In one study of five- to nine-year-olds who received medical treatment, only one third of skateboard injuries were classified as minor; the remaining two thirds were labeled moderate or severe.

If your child rides a skateboard, she should wear a helmet and protective padding and wrist guards to minimize the chances of injury. Also, she should never ride the skateboard in or near traffic. Homemade ramps have proven particularly dangerous for youngsters.

In-Line Skating

Traditional roller skates have all but been replaced by in-line skates. This low impact sport uses more muscles than running, yet can provide good aerobic exercise. Skates differ widely in price and construction. Children's feet should feel comfortable in the boot, and their ankles should be well supported by a snugly buckled or strapped top. In general, children should be able to properly put on and remove their skates.

Skate wheels vary in size and hardness. Smaller wheels provide a lower center of gravity that may help beginning skaters feel more stable. Large wheels are faster and last longer. Softer wheels absorb bumps from small irregularities better than hard wheels, and provide better traction on smooth surfaces. In-line skates also come with a brake that drags along the ground when the child shifts weight.

Safe in-line skating takes both practice and precaution. Helmets, knee and elbow pads, and wrist guards should be standard equipment for skaters. Children should learn to skate on flat, open paved surfaces free from traffic. Basic technique should be learned and practiced slowly; speed and technique should progress together. Parents should set clear rules for when and where skating is permissible.

Here are some safety guidelines for your middle-years child:

- Always wear protective gear.

- Skate under control and leave plenty of room to stop.

- Always skate on the right side of paths and sidewalks, and pass on the left.

- Avoid uneven pavement and areas with heavy traffic.

- Observe traffic regulations, and yield to pedestrians.

Too often, children venture into streets and try out stunts before they are fully able to control their skating.

Water Safety

Drownings rank behind only motor-vehicle accidents as the leading cause of death among youngsters in middle childhood. Most often, these tragedies occur when children swim without adequate adult supervision. In most cases, these children (and their parents) have overestimated their swimming ability and their knowledge of water-survival skills.

Here are some guidelines to keep your middle-years child safe in and near the water:

- Make sure your youngster learns how to swim from an experienced and qualified instructor. Check for available lessons at local recreation centers, YMCAs, and summer camps.

- Never allow your child to swim alone or play by or in water away from the watchful eye of an adult. Ideally, this adult should be trained in cardiopulmonary resuscitation (CPR). Also, teach your child to use the buddy system even when swimming with large groups of friends.

- Do not allow your child to engage in horseplay that might result in injury.

- Prohibit your child from diving unless someone has already determined the depth of the water and checked for underwater hazards.

- Do not allow your child to swim in areas where there are boats or fishermen. Nor should she swim at beaches where there are large waves, a powerful undertow, or no lifeguards. Make sure she understands that swimming in one body of water (e.g., a backyard pool) may be different from swimming in another (a river or ocean).

- While riding in a boat, you and your child should always wear a personal flotation device.

WHERE WE STAND

The American Academy of Pediatrics feels strongly that parents should never—even for a moment—leave children alone near open bodies of water, such as lakes or swimming pools, nor near water in homes (bathtubs, spas). For backyard pools, rigid, motorized pool covers are not a substitute for four-sided fencing, since pool covers are not likely to be used appropriately and consistently. Parents should learn CPR and keep a telephone and emergency equipment (such as life preservers) at poolside.

- Do not permit your child to rely on an air mattress, inner tube, or inflatable toy as a life preserver. If these devices deflate, or your child slips off them, she could be in serious trouble.

- Your child should never be permitted to swim during a lightning storm.

- If you have a backyard swimming pool, it should be enclosed with high and locked fences on all four sides, especially the side that separates the house from the pool.

- When your youngster is old enough—usually by her high school years—she should learn life-saving skills such as CPR, taught in most cities through community agencies or the American Red Cross.

FIRE AND BURN PREVENTION

Burns are one of the leading causes of death among children, with most of these fatalities occurring in home fires. Even more often, deaths in fires are caused by smoke inhalation.

Your family's best protection against fire-related injuries is to equip your home with smoke detectors. Thousands of lives could be saved every year if detectors were in place, awakening families in time to allow them to escape their burning homes. Install the detectors throughout the house, mounting them on the ceiling or on the wall 6 to 12 inches below the ceiling. They should be placed in halls adjacent to the bedrooms, as well as in the living room, garage, and other parts of the home where they can awaken the family if a fire has broken out. Test battery-operated detectors every six months to ensure that the batteries are still fresh. In general, batteries need to be changed once a year. (Many units emit a beeping sound when the batteries become weak.)

Home fire extinguishers are another good idea. Keep extinguishers in the parts of the house where a fire is most likely to start (the kitchen and the workroom, for example). However, use the extinguisher only for a small fire; if the fire is large, everyone should leave the dwelling *immediately,* and you should call the fire department from a neighbor's home. If children are home alone, instruct them to evacuate the house at once in case of a fire, even if it is a small one. Your child should learn to call 911, but he should understand that his own safety comes first, and he should make the call from another home.

Hold regular fire drills with everyone in the family participating. During these drills, plan and rehearse all possible escape routes for fires occurring in various parts of the house, as well as a place for family members to meet once they are outside. Since many fires—including most fatal ones—occur at night, conduct some of your drills after dark. A flashlight should be available at the bedside of every family member. Also, teach your children to "stop, drop, and roll" if their clothing should catch fire.

Of course, discourage your children from playing with matches, lighted candles, cigarette lighters, or other flammable devices. Also, keep in mind that most fatal home fires are caused by adults and their cigarettes; typically, a cigarette or its ashes fall on a bed or a couch, smolder for several hours, and then burst into flames, often after the family is asleep. Do not smoke in your house. Portable heaters also are responsible for many home fires and burns, and if their use is necessary, they should be used only with great caution.

Most burns that are not fatal are *not* related to fires. Most often, these are scalds from hot liquids—for example, when a child turns over a cooking pot upon himself, or turns the knobs on a bathtub faucet so that hot water flows on him. Children also sometimes suffer burns by touching a hot iron, a coil on an electric stove, a curling iron, hot barbecue charcoal, or fireworks.

To avoid scalding burns, reduce the temperature of your water heater so the water is never hotter than 120 degrees Fahrenheit. Keep hot irons out of children's reach and keep children away from the stove when food is cooking. Also, keep hot-steam vaporizers away from a child's reach, and keep portable heaters away from children and from flammable materials, such as curtains, as well. Teach your child not to play with matches.

In recent years, nearly 12,000 people in the United States were treated for fireworks-related injuries in emergency departments; more than half were children. Every type of legally available firework has caused serious injury or death. Fireworks should never be used by children or other family members. Rather than risk your child's health, families should attend public fireworks displays conducted by professionals.

STAYING SAFE AT HOME: LATCHKEY KIDS

Until about the age of eleven or twelve, most children are not able to handle stressful or emergency situations that require mature decision making on their own. Therefore it is best for parents to arrange for an adult or a responsible older adolescent to be at home when they are not present or for some other structured supervision.

However, your child may be an exception and be sufficiently mature at the age of eight to ten years to be home alone after school. Before her first day on her own, however, you need to make sure she feels safe and secure, and that she is prepared for dealing with knocks on the door, emergencies, and injuries. Some communities offer courses in babysitting that can also serve as good

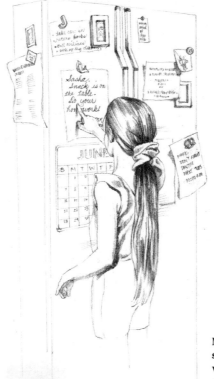

Make sure your child feels safe and secure and is well prepared to deal with emergencies if she will be home alone after school.

preparation for self-care. Nevertheless, your child should not be home alone until she is comfortable with that arrangement. Here are some issues that you should discuss with her:

- Does she know her full name, address, and phone number? Does she know your full name as well, and the address and phone number of your workplace, or other ways to reach you at work? (You might call every day to be sure your child has arrived home safely and that nothing at home is out of the ordinary; children appreciate the sense of security this form of supervision provides.)

- Does she have an established routine to follow so she knows what she is supposed to do and where she is supposed to be?

- Can your child use the telephone correctly, particularly when calling you, a neighbor, or emergency services (911)?

- When she returns home from school every day, does your child know how to lock the door behind her? Can she remember to call you and/or a neighbor as soon as she arrives home, and then check in again at designated times?

- Have you instructed your child never to enter your home if a door is ajar, or if a window is open or broken?

- Have you talked about what to do if someone knocks at the front door while she is home alone? (The best advice: She should not open the door and should tell the person knocking that you are home but are busy and unable to answer the door.)

- Have you and your child discussed how she should exit your home quickly in case of a fire? Does she know which exits are safest, depending on the location of the fire? Does she know what to do in case of an emergency or an earthquake, and is she familiar with basic first aid (e.g., applying pressure to a cut)?

GUN SAFETY

Firearm violence has become a public health crisis in the United States. Guns are widely available in our society and are kept in millions of American homes. According to the Center to Prevent Handgun Violence, almost 8.7 million children and adolescents have access to handguns, and many are either unaware of or ignore the possible consequences of handling these lethal weapons. Their mere presence poses a very real danger to children.

School-age children are curious about and often attracted to guns. They sometimes see guns as symbols of power. So do many adolescents and adults.

The availability of handguns in settings where children live and play has led to a devastating toll in human lives, reflected in some sobering and almost unthinkable statistics: Every two hours, someone's child is killed with a gun, either in a homicide, a suicide, or as a result of an unintentional injury. In addition, an unknown but large number of children are seriously injured—often irreversibly disabled—by guns but survive. Major urban trauma centers are reporting an increase of 300 percent in the number of children treated for gunshot wounds; in fact, one in every twenty-five admissions to pediatric trauma centers in the United States is due to gunshot wounds.

Parents should realize that a gun in the home is forty-three times more likely to be used to kill a friend or family member than a burglar or other criminal. To compound this problem, depressed preteenagers and teenagers commit suicide with guns more frequently than by any other means.

The best preventive measure against firearm injuries and deaths is not to own a gun. However, if you choose to have firearms in your home, adhere to these rules for gun safety:

- Never allow your child access to your gun(s). No matter how much instruction you may give him or her, a youngster in the middle years is not mature and responsible enough to handle a potentially lethal weapon.

- Never keep a loaded gun in the house or the car.

- Guns and ammunition should be locked away safely in separate locations in the house; make sure children don't have access to the keys.

- Guns should be equipped with trigger locks.

- When using a gun for hunting or target practice, learn how to operate it before ever loading it. Never point the gun at another person, and keep the safety catch in place until you are ready to fire it. Before setting the gun down, always unload it. Do not use alcohol or drugs while you are shooting.

Even if you don't have guns in your own home, that won't eliminate your child's risks. Half of the homes in the United States contain firearms, and more than a third of all accidental shootings of children take place in the homes of their friends, neighbors, or relatives. A Center to Prevent Handgun Violence survey estimated that about 135,000 students carried handguns to school each day, and another 270,000 brought handguns to school at least once; that figure may be even higher today.

Here is some important information you need to communicate to your youngsters:

- Let them know that risks of gun injuries may exist in places they visit and play.

- Tell them that if they see or encounter a gun in a friend's home or elsewhere, they must steer clear of it, and tell you about it.

WHERE WE STAND

The American Academy of Pediatrics strongly supports gun control legislation. We believe that handguns, deadly air guns, and assault weapons should be banned.

Until handguns are banned, we recommend that handgun ammunition be regulated, that restrictions be placed on handgun ownership, and that the number of privately owned handguns be reduced. Handguns must be removed from the environments in which children live and play.

- Talk with the parents of your child's friends, and find out if they have firearms in their home. If they do, insist that they keep them unloaded, locked up, and inaccessible to children.

- Make sure your children understand that violence on TV and in the movies is not real. They need to be told—and probably reminded again and again—that in real life, children are killed and hurt badly by guns. Although the popular media often romanticize gun use, youngsters must learn that these weapons can be extremely dangerous.

CRIME, VIOLENCE, AND YOUR CHILD

We live in a violent society. As the statistics in the previous section on guns point out, children are not immune to the growing dangers of modern life.

At some point during their childhood, many youngsters experience or witness a crime or other traumatic event. Some events are unintentional—perhaps a traffic accident, a household or schoolyard injury, or a natural disaster such as an earthquake or a hurricane. Others are perpetrated crimes or other acts of violence; it seems as though children everywhere have seen not only fights on neighborhood playgrounds but also sometimes muggings, shootings, and even murders and terrorists' attacks. During middle childhood, too many youngsters are exposed to gang and drug-related violence, drive-by shootings, and physical assaults, frequently resulting in serious injuries, occasionally even in death.

Then there are the dozens of crimes and violent acts on TV and in the movies that children may view each week. This ever-present violence in the media, along with the brutal acts that children may see and sometimes personally experience, can have many adverse consequences for them. Some youngsters learn to resolve their own conflicts in a violent manner. Others become seemingly desensitized to violence and the pain and distress of others. Some retreat into a shell, avoiding people and the world around them.

When your child is exposed to an actual traumatic event, including a violent crime, his response may vary. Some youngsters become fearful. They may avoid leaving home, and they may have difficulty concentrating in school. Even minor changes in their daily routines can upset them terribly. Their appetites often change, too, and they may complain of headaches, stomachaches, and other vague symptoms. They might have trouble sleeping.

Post-traumatic stress disorder, a condition widely discussed as it applies to Vietnam war veterans, can occur in childhood as well. Like soldiers who have experienced the turmoil of battle, children exposed to violence often feel emotional and physical "aftershocks" for months or even years. Some of these

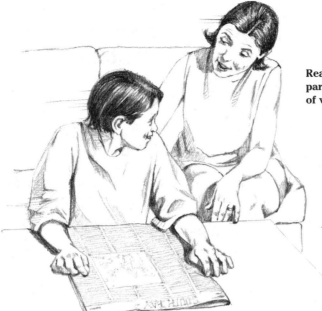

Reassurance should be a part of every discussion of violence.

symptoms—from fear to physical disorders—have already been described. Children often relive the event again and again in their minds, frequently making it harder for them to function normally in their day-to-day lives. And their own behavior may become more aggressive, violent, and even self-destructive.

If your own child finds himself in this situation, consider how it is affecting not only him but the entire family. Are your family members interacting with one another and with the outside world differently? Have your routines and activities changed?

Be sure to encourage your child to discuss the violence. Allow him to express what he is feeling, whether it be fear, anxiety, or anger. Talk about it, again and again if necessary. Remember, if he has been exposed to or has witnessed a violent occurrence, he will need a great deal of support and often will need counseling in order to handle his feelings. There are many experienced mental-health professionals who can assist in treating your child for the stress he feels in the aftermath of a violent experience.

In the weeks and months after the violent or traumatic episode, do everything you can to make sure that your child feels secure, and that a sense of normalcy returns to his life. Make certain that he is adequately supervised and protected throughout the day and night. Discuss with him the potentially dangerous situations that may exist and how to avoid them in the future. Encourage him to express his fears, and reassure him that he will be all right. Explain to him the steps that have been taken to ensure that he is protected and safe.

Also, get involved in your community to address the issue of violence. By

What If Your Child Is Being Bullied?

Whether on the school playground or in the neighborhood park, children in the middle years sometimes find themselves the target of bullies. When that happens, these bullies can not only frighten a youngster, shaking his confidence and spoiling his play, but they can also cause bodily injury.

Avoiding a bully is one reason your child may be reluctant to go to school. Perhaps he is being forced to relinquish his lunch money to this bully. Or he might be fearful of physical harm. If you suspect a problem like this, you need to take action to ensure your child's safety and well-being. Here are some strategies he can adopt with your help, and which will help make him safer:

- Tell your child not to react to the bully, particularly by giving in to demands. A bully relishes intimidating others and likes nothing better than to see his victim cry or become visibly upset in other ways. Getting that response reinforces the bullying behavior. Your child should try to keep his composure and simply walk away.

- If your child's attempts at disregarding a bully's taunts aren't effective, he should become assertive with his harasser. While standing tall and looking his tormentor in the eyes, he should clearly and loudly make a statement like, "Stop doing that now.

joining with other parents, as well as with schools, community organizations, businesses, and law enforcement agencies, you can help provide your child with a more secure environment and reduce the risk of violence in the lives of all children, including your own.

Finally, one other type of violence deserves mention here—namely, the fear of war. Thanks to vivid depictions of war on television, many children in the middle years are not only anxious about war-related death and injury to themselves and their families but also are afraid of separation and abandonment if a parent or older sibling goes off to war. These youngsters might be afraid to go to school. Or they may have nightmares and disrupted sleep.

In cases like this, reassure your child that you and your family are safe, and that a war thousands of miles away is not going to affect your family and your city directly. It is much harder, of course, to convince your youngster that the

If you keep on, I'm going to report you to the principal." Or, "I'll talk to you, but I'm not going to fight. So put your fists down now." Sometimes, a strong statement will defuse the situation, and the bully will try to find another, weaker target. Drawing the attention of peers to the bullying situation can embarrass the bully. If your child isn't used to reacting assertively, help him rehearse what he will say if he is confronted.

- Encourage your child to form strong friendships. A youngster who has loyal friends is less likely to be singled out by a bully, or at least he'll have some allies if he does become a target of harassment.

- Talk to your son's teacher or to the principal of his school if the situation with the bully persists. You might be reluctant to intervene, perhaps because your child is embarrassed to have you do so, or because you believe he needs to learn to deal with these situations on his own. On the other hand, you don't want your child's self-confidence to weaken, or his physical well-being to be jeopardized. Your youngster deserves to attend school in a safe environment, even if it means both you and the school staff need to become involved.

Let the principal or teacher talk to the bully when he or she sees the inappropriate behavior taking place on the school grounds. This is generally a more effective approach than having you speak with the child or his parents.

people he sees on TV in the war zone are going to be all right. Talk with him about war, about how sad it is, and tell him that you hope the fighting is over soon and that as few people get hurt as possible. Remind him that wars have occurred throughout history, and that life and the world will go on, despite this particular war.

Some families find that their child is not only unafraid of war but actually becomes preoccupied with military matters and fantasies about going off to foreign lands and fighting distant enemies. This is a sign of identifying with the values of the larger society. If this occurs with your youngster and it disturbs you, sit down with him and discuss the differences between the myths and the realities of war.

SEXUAL ABUSE

Sexual abuse is a difficult subject for most people to discuss. But as frightening and offensive as the topic may be, sexual abuse is a serious and, unfortunately, not infrequent problem. Literally millions of children are victims of this form of abuse. According to studies, 25 percent of adult women and 10 percent of adult men can remember being sexually abused as children or adolescents. Most of this victimization occurs between eight and twelve years of age.

Sexual abuse includes any kind of sexual act or behavior with a child. It includes not only intercourse but also fondling the youngster's genitals, forcing the child to fondle an adult's genitals, mouth-to-genital contact, or rubbing the adult's genitals on the youngster. Other types of sexual abuse may also take place, even though they may not involve physical contact—for instance, an adult exposing his genitals to a child, showing pornographic pictures or videotapes to a youngster, or taking pictures of the child for obscene purposes.

Strangers do molest children. But in at least 80 percent of cases, the perpetrators of sexual abuse are known to the child, and are often authority figures whom the child trusts. He or she might be a parent, a stepparent, an adult relative (uncle, grandfather), a family friend, a neighbor, a babysitter, a teacher, a coach or Scout leader, or an older sibling or cousin. While children usually understand who a "stranger" is, they may be caught off guard by the advances of someone they know and respect. The offender usually manipulates the child into engaging in sexual activity, using threats, bribes, or aggressive persuasion, and convinces the child that she has no choice but to participate. The children most susceptible to these assaults have obedient, compliant, and respectful personalities.

In many cases the sexual abuse involves more than just a single incident. Often it is a pattern of ongoing sexual contacts, frequently beginning in the early years of middle childhood and persisting into adolescence. Sometimes the abuse stops only when the maturing child is capable of extricating herself from this terrible situation, often by reporting the incident to another adult. Even after the abuse has stopped, the psychological repercussions of the abuse can last a lifetime.

Preventing Sexual Abuse

Without alarming your middle-years child, you need to alert her that sexual abuse exists, while reassuring her that it probably never will happen to her. Teach her that no matter who may threaten her sexually—even if it is a trusted adult—she must be willing to clearly and forcefully say "No" or "Stop" and walk (or run) away. She also must know that she should always come to you if

Signs of Sexual Abuse

Here are some symptoms that could indicate that a child has been sexually abused:

- She seems to be afraid of a particular person or place and being left alone with that individual.

- She overreacts to a question about someone's touching her.

- She suddenly seems more aware of and preoccupied with sexual conduct, words, and parts of the body.

- Her behavior changes dramatically in any number of ways. A younger child may regress to bed-wetting or soiling her underwear. Or her eating habits might change. She may relate to peers differently, either by withdrawing or by becoming more aggressive. She might act up in school, her motivation and concentration may suffer, and her grades may fall. She may appear fearful, frequently crying and clinging to her parent(s), or alternatively, she may avoid normal family intimacy.

- She has unreasonable anxiety over a doctor's physical examination.

- She has inexplicable physical complaints, such as headaches, stomachaches, or genital itching or pain.

- She draws unusually frightening or sad pictures, using a lot of black and red colors.

- She masturbates excessively and tries to get other children to perform sexual acts.

a sexual incident ever happens to her, no matter who the perpetrator is and no matter what kind of warning the offender has given her ("Don't tell anyone or I'll hurt you"). Make sure she understands that she won't get into trouble if she tells you about such an incident. Also remember that while girls are the usual victims of sexual abuse, about 10 percent of victims are boys.

Here are some other recommendations from the American Academy of Pediatrics that can minimize your child's risk of molestation:

- Teach your child about the privacy of body parts, and that no one has the right to touch her if she tells the individual not to do so. She should understand that some touching is "good" but some is "bad": Explain that an adult's giving a loving hug is different from his putting a hand on her buttocks or inner thigh. She has the right to say no to *anyone* who tries to touch her in the parts of her body that are normally covered by a bathing suit. Naturally, your child should respect the right to privacy of other people too.

- Sit down with your child and explain various situations that might indicate that a possible child molester is making advances. For example, a molester might offer a child candy or toys. (If your child has acquired any unexplained toys or gifts, ask who gave them to her.) He may offer the child money to run an errand or do a short-term job (raking leaves, shoveling snow). He might dress as a clown, Santa Claus, or another trusted or heroic figure to lure the youngster. He might claim that an emergency situation has arisen ("Your mother was in an automobile accident—come with me, and I'll take you to the hospital to see her"). Or he may ask the child for assistance: directions to a particular street or landmark, or help in finding a missing dog or cat. Make sure your child understands that if she encounters a potentially dangerous situation like these, she should run away.

- Tell a child that a molester or abductor may offer her alcohol or drugs to reduce her inhibitions.

- Tell your child that threats from a molester or anyone else are against the law—"If you tell your mother what we did, I'm going to hurt/kill her"—and to tell you immediately about them.

- If your youngster is in a position to do door-to-door solicitation—perhaps selling Girl Scout cookies or collecting money for a newspaper route—have an adult go with her. Warn your child that she should *never* enter someone else's home unless an adult accompanies her.

- Investigate whether your youngster's school has an abuse-prevention program. If not, encourage the school board to institute one. In recent years there has been a dramatic increase in preventive programs to educate children about the disclosure of sexual abuse.

- Monitor the activities at your child's child-care facility or summer camp. Participate in these activities whenever possible. Listen carefully when your child tries to tell you something of a sexual nature, particularly if she seems to have difficulty talking about it. As much as possible, create an environment at home in which sexual topics can be discussed comfortably. (See Chapter 4, "Children, Parents, and Sexuality," for additional information on this issue.)

- Spend enough time with your child that she does not feel the need to seek the attention of other adults. Children from unhappy or broken homes tend to be the easiest targets for molesters, since these youngsters may be eager for attention and affection.

- If you do not already know whom your child spends time with, find out. If your youngster spends time in isolated or remote places with adults or older children, investigate what might be going on there. Question the motives of adults who want to spend large amounts of time alone with your child.

When Sexual Abuse Occurs

Most victims of sexual abuse remain silent. Often feeling guilty and helpless, they do not run to tell their mother or another trusted adult. Sometimes, when the perpetrator is a family member, they believe that by telling someone, they may split their family apart. Or they may feel embarrassed by what has happened, or they may have been warned by the offender to remain quiet. All the while, however, they may be emotionally devastated. They may withdraw from family and friends, stop participating in school activities, experience chronic anxiety and insomnia, and exhibit aggressive and self-destructive behavior.

Sometimes a sexually abused child may eventually tell her friends what has occurred. Or she may say something sketchy to a parent that hints at the abuse without describing it clearly.

When a child is examined by a doctor, the physician may detect physical signs of sexual abuse, such as genital or anal changes. The physician might also find evidence of sexually transmitted diseases such as gonorrhea or herpes. However, often the doctor is unable to find physical evidence of sexual abuse, even though the abuse occurred.

If your youngster comes to you and reveals that she has been sexually abused, take it seriously. *Too often, children are not believed, particularly if they implicate a family member as the perpetrator.* You need to listen to your child, gently and sensitively ask questions to obtain more information, and then take active steps to protect her. Contact a pediatrician, the local child-protection service agency or social welfare bureau, or the police (sexual abuse is a violation of the law). If you don't intervene in this way, the abuse might continue for many more months and even years; at the same time, the child will come to believe, correctly, that home is not safe and that you are not available to help.

In the days and weeks ahead, make sure your abused child understands that she is not responsible for the abuse, and let her know how brave she was to tell you what happened. Reassure her that this abuse will not occur again. Offer plenty of love and support. If you are dealing with anger of your own, she might think that some of it is directed toward her, so continually reassure her that you are *not* upset with her and are proud of her for telling you what has happened.

Your child should be treated for any physical injuries, either internal or external, related to the abuse. Your youngster also needs to be examined by a physician if charges are going to be brought. Most children and their families will also need professional counseling to help them through this ordeal.

A number of factors will influence the psychological impact of sexual abuse upon a child, including:

- *The nature of the sexual activity, the frequency, and the use of force.* The more intrusive the abusive experience, the more difficult and confusing it will be for the youngster. Sexual victimization that happens over a long period is much more damaging than a one-time episode. It can lead to runaway behavior and sexual promiscuity and interfere with relationships and intimacy later in life. Perhaps most significantly, the use (or threatened use) of force or bodily harm upon the child or her family members can significantly intensify the youngster's psychological trauma. She may react with feelings ranging from anxiety and fear to guilt and depression.

- *The age and developmental status of the child.* A younger child may have less difficulty with a brief sexual experience than an older one. This younger child may not fully comprehend what has happened to her, and more often, she may have been subjected to less force and coercion from the perpetrator. By contrast, an older youngster may understand more about the abusive experience and may feel more guilt, fear, and other emotions.

- *The relationship of the child and the abuser.* Although victimization by someone unknown to a child is upsetting, it may not be as bewildering as when incest occurs—that is, when a relative abuses a child sexually. With incest, the youngster may feel confusion about her relationship with the perpetrator and whether she can trust this individual again. The child also may feel more pressure *not* to disclose the abuse if a family member is involved.

- *The family's reaction.* If you are supportive of your child and convince her that she is not at fault and that she will be protected, the trauma can be minimized. If family members fail to act on the information they are given by the child, the abuse will likely persist, and the child's sense of trust and intimacy will be damaged.

To repeat, without expert guidance your youngster could suffer some serious, lasting psychological effects from the abuse. Your pediatrician can give you a referral to a counselor, as can the local child-protection agency. In many communities there are sexual-abuse support networks, treatment groups, and therapists who specialize in sexual victimization. All sexually abused children need an evaluation by a professional who is knowledgeable about the psychological consequences of abuse, and who can recommend treatment if it is needed. Families, too, can benefit from support and counseling to help them deal with their own feelings and more effectively provide emotional support for their child.

For additional information about sexual and other types of child abuse, contact the National Committee for Prevention of Child Abuse, P.O. Box 2866, Chicago, Illinois 60690.

SUBSTANCE USE AND ABUSE

Parents are well aware of the tremendous problem of substance abuse in childhood and adolescence. The use of tobacco, alcohol, and other drugs by young people has grown significantly and has become nearly an epidemic. While the statistics change each year, recent findings are disturbing; some are frightening. Approximately one hundred thousand American children under the age of thirteen smoke. Tobacco use by girls is increasing at a faster rate than use by boys. Of adults who smoke regularly, the average age at which they started was twelve and a half, and most were regular smokers by age fourteen. Thirty-five percent of twelve- to seventeen-year-olds have tried marijuana, with many first exposed to this drug in the late elementary grades. Problem drinking often begins in the elementary school years. Before their high school graduation, over 90 percent of adolescents have consumed alcohol. In one study, 22 percent of fifth-graders, 14 percent of fourth-graders, and 8 percent of third-graders reported drinking to the point of intoxication.

Leading authorities feel that most efforts aimed at the prevention of substance abuse must begin *before* adolescence, during the middle years of childhood. Prevention, including raising awareness of risks, the communication of values, and providing the example of desirable behavior, must occur in all arenas of the child's life—home, school, and community. The degree and effectiveness of this education can influence what behavior will occur during adolescence.

The use of tobacco, alcohol, or other drugs always begins with experimentation and casual usage. The use of these substances starts in a social setting, usually under very strong peer pressure. But what begins as a social event may turn into drug dependency. The longer one of these substances is utilized,

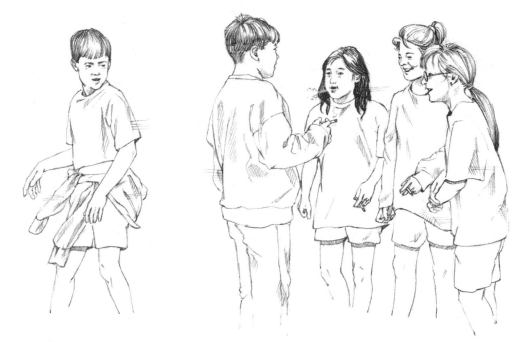

Substance use often begins as a result of peer influence.

the more habitual its use becomes, and the greater the risk of both psychological and physiological addiction.

When a young person starts experimenting with drugs, he often has the illusion that he can control its use, denying that the substance is potentially addictive. Also, children are notoriously unable to base present behavior on future consequences, and they feel immune to bad outcomes. Nevertheless, as habitual use gradually becomes established and dependence upon the substance grows, the youngster increasingly loses control of the drug use.

Some parents say that they are actually relieved that their youngster is smoking cigarettes rather than using an illegal substance like marijuana. However, they are feeling a false sense of comfort. Tobacco use is the leading cause of preventable death. Researchers believe that an individual's use of drugs progresses along what is called a *substance use hierarchy*. Thus, the entrance or "gateway" drug for many young people is tobacco, but they then move on to alcohol. They then may experiment with marijuana, cocaine, and other types of illegal drugs. However, it is known that adolescents who engage in one type of risky behavior, like smoking, are more likely to be involved in others, such as drug use and sexual activity. They are also more likely to have academic problems. Fortunately, this is not an inevitable chain of events.

How susceptible is your own child to the temptations of substance abuse? Many factors contribute to his potential vulnerability, from his own emotional

Secondhand Smoke and Children

If you smoke and are having difficulty motivating yourself to stop, bear in mind that the research is conclusive: Parental smoking is a serious health hazard for children. Youngsters who live in the same households as smokers inhale cigarette smoke. As a result, they run a higher risk of developing asthma, bronchitis, pneumonia, and middle-ear disease. These children also have more difficulty getting over colds.

Of the 4,000-plus chemicals that have been identified in environmental tobacco smoke, at least forty are known to cause cancer.

Here is what the American Academy of Pediatrics suggests:

- If you would like to quit smoking but have been unable to, contact your physician; there are many low-cost programs available to help.

- If your spouse or another member of your household is a smoker, provide him or her with support to quit.

- If you or other members of your household are not able to give up cigarettes, do not smoke inside the house. And by no means should anyone smoke in an automobile in which children ride.

needs and existing behavioral problems to family and community values. But your own attitude toward substance use is probably *the* major factor determining whether your child will use drugs. If you smoke, that is the example you are setting for your child. It will become harder for you to persuade him not to use cigarettes when he sees you smoking. And when you bring cigarettes into the home or leave incompletely smoked cigarettes in ashtrays, they become too easily available if your child or his friends decide they want to try one.

Thus, if you want to spare your child the added health risks caused by smoking, you must first start by refraining from using cigarettes yourself. Chil-

WHERE WE STAND

Alcohol is the drug most often abused by the largest number of children and adolescents. The American Academy of Pediatrics is strongly opposed to the use of alcohol by children and adolescents and supports a ban on alcohol advertising and promotion.

dren whose parents smoke are more than twice as likely to use cigarettes eventually than are the children of nonsmokers.

In the same way, if either parent is a heavy alcohol or drug user, a child is much more likely to become involved in their use, due to both exposure and availability. He will have considerable difficulty understanding why he should not use these substances as he longs to feel more grown-up.

The media play another influential role in substance abuse. Athletes and entertainers who appear in the media with a drink in their hand or a cigarette in their mouth can influence children. Advertisers are targeting children and adolescents, especially girls, in efforts to encourage future use of tobacco products and alcohol. Tobacco companies play on girls' desire to be attractive and thin in their efforts to promote smoking. Advertising is also intended to "normalize" the use of alcohol and tobacco—conveying the impression that "everyone is doing it."

But perhaps even more important are the peer influences. A youngster's friends can affect his decisions regarding substance use. All children and adolescents desire the approval of peers as they become increasingly independent of their families and develop their own identities. If your child's friends have drugs available, he will be encouraged and perhaps coerced into trying them. Although your family's values can help strengthen your youngster's convictions and resistance against substance use, the social pressures he faces may be overwhelming. It is extremely important that you know your child's friends; ideally, you should know their families as well. In this way, you can guide your youngster's choice of friends and help him make his own decisions when facing peer pressure.

Some children are much more vulnerable to these peer influences than others. Children with a poor self-concept or a strong need for acceptance will tend to try harder to win approval from their peers and will more readily conform to their friends' behavior. These same children may have conduct problems, depression, anxiety, or family stresses, and they may also find a numbing relief and excitement in the use of illicit and self-destructive substances. Drug use also may give them a sense of pleasure, freedom, and independence, and a chance to rebel and assert themselves in a world that otherwise seems to give them little control or autonomy.

How to Help Your Child Be Substance-Free

A child with healthy self-esteem has much less need to abuse drugs and other substances. A number of factors can contribute to a child's feeling good about himself, many of which come from positive interactions within the family and from his successful performance at school and in other social settings. The section "Self-Esteem," page 132, discusses this topic more thoroughly, but here are a few ways you can strengthen your child's self-concept.

- Raise your youngster to feel that he is important in your life and to believe that his feelings and thoughts really matter. Be respectful of his wishes, and try to understand his perspective and instill in him a sense of self-worth. Show an interest in his schoolwork. Participate in his hobbies and other activities. Spend time reading books together or playing games of his choice.

- Be honest with your child in all aspects of your relationship with him. Parents who lie or break promises give their child reasons to distrust them; he will lose the desire to please his mother and father, including in areas like substance abuse.

- Acknowledge and celebrate your child's successes and achievements, which can help him build a sense of personal confidence and power in the world. Cheer his successes in school and with peers, and when he demonstrates responsibility at home.

- Clearly articulate your own attitudes about substance abuse. At the same time, examine your own use of substances and what kind of model you are presenting to him.

There are other strategies you can use to encourage your child to avoid tobacco, alcohol, and other drugs. For instance, answer all his questions about these substances honestly. Formal antidrug programs at schools and commu-

WHERE WE STAND

The American Academy of Pediatrics opposes the use of tobacco in any form. Smoking should be prohibited in all public places, and children should not be exposed to tobacco smoke at home or school. We also support a complete ban on tobacco advertising, the use of harsher warning labels on cigarette packages, and an increase in the cigarette excise tax.

Currently 43 percent of children aged 2 months to 11 years live in a home with at least one smoker. If you smoke, quit. If you can't quit, don't smoke around children (especially indoors or in the car). Children of parents who smoke have more respiratory infections, bronchitis, pneumonia, and reduced pulmonary function than children of nonsmokers.

nity organizations are most effective when they include a component that teaches children social skills for dealing with peer pressure. These types of efforts address self-esteem, and offer opportunities to practice techniques to use when encountering negative peer influences.

An important part of this educational process is to remind your child of the health hazards associated with tobacco use. Smokers run ten times the risk of death from lung cancer that nonsmokers do. Cigarettes double the risk of heart disease and are the most common cause of lung diseases like chronic bronchitis and emphysema. Even though these are chronic diseases that may take many years—even decades—to develop, let your youngsters know that the earlier they start smoking, the greater their chance of eventually developing these conditions. For example, smokers who start before age fifteen have cancer rates nineteen times higher than nonsmokers.

Children are not particularly motivated by long-term consequences, so remind your child of the more immediate drawbacks to smoking. Young people often believe that kids who smoke are "cool" and sophisticated. Cigarette advertising, for example, stresses the social desirability of smoking. But in fact, smoking stains teeth. It causes bad breath and a hacking cough, plus leaves a strong tobacco odor on clothes. The habit also costs quite a lot. And for children who like sports, the use of cigarettes can keep them from running and swimming as well as they could if they didn't smoke; high school coaches now routinely demand that their young athletes do not smoke.

What About Chewing Tobacco?

A growing number of young people are using chewing or smokeless tobacco as an alternative to cigarettes. The potential for its use is particularly high among young boys who imitate some adult professional athletes. This is a dangerous and unhealthy option. The nicotine in smokeless tobacco is as addicting as the nicotine in cigarettes. Smokeless tobacco also can cause sores and white patches in the mouth and throat, and cracking and bleeding of the lips and gums. It can interfere with a youngster's sense of taste and smell too. Even worse, it can lead ultimately to the development of cancer of the throat, mouth, and gums. You should discourage your child's use of these products as strongly as you resist his use of cigarettes.

WHAT TO DO IF YOUR CHILD IS USING ILLEGAL SUBSTANCES

Most children involved in using illicit substances are not receiving adequate parental supervision of their activities. And if their peers are smoking, they are probably doing so too. If you discover your school-age child experimenting with cigarettes or alcohol, do not overreact. Punishment on a first offense will probably not be very helpful, nor will threats and a power struggle. Instead, use your parental influence and take this opportunity to again communicate your own attitudes about smoking and drinking. At the same time, learn from your child why she has smoked or used alcohol. Discuss the peer pressure she may be experiencing, and together consider how to deal with it effectively. Talk about how the values of her friends and their families may conflict with your own. Be clear about what you believe is right and wrong, healthy and unhealthy, safe and unsafe. Also, teach your child to use her conscience as a guide; this will encourage her to be responsible for herself and it will show that you trust her to show good judgment.

When children in the middle years use substances like tobacco, alcohol, and other drugs repeatedly, it is no longer experimentation but a problem. Children who engage in this type of risky behavior are more likely to engage in other high-risk activities. You should take the same steps as you would with a child who is experimenting with illicit substances, but you also need to consider what might be motivating your child to jeopardize her health in this way. Look at this drug abuse in the context of what else is happening in her life. It signals a serious problem, including her association with peers who are supplying her with the illicit substance.

In the middle childhood years, it is not too late to help your child pick and choose good friends, ones who you feel are good influences upon her. Discuss with her what she values in a friendship, and how to meet and make friends with children whose values are similar to hers and those of your family. Set limits on her association with children who appear to lead her away from your own values, thus protecting and teaching her to make good judgments.

Your pediatrician can recommend evaluation by a child psychiatrist or psychologist, or participation in an alcohol or drug-abuse program, which are critical before the pressures of adolescence begin.

4

CHILDREN, PARENTS, AND SEXUALITY

Sexuality is part of every person's life, no matter what his or her age.

Children in their middle years have great curiosity about sex. They may giggle with one another about their "private parts," share dirty jokes, and scan through dictionaries looking up taboo words.

The process of learning about sex actually began years earlier, as soon as they were able to observe, listen to, and sense the world around them. Initially, most of their learning took place at home, but now, as they move through middle childhood, many messages about sexuality come from the outside environment—not only from their peers but also from the media, including movies, television, and advertisements.

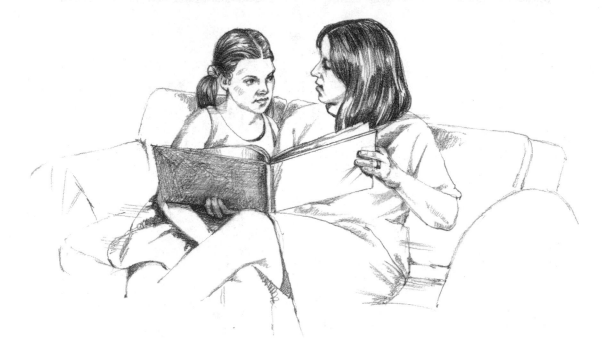

Discussing issues of sexuality with your child is one of the most important parenting responsibilities.

TALKING TO YOUR CHILD ABOUT SEX

Discussing issues of sexuality with your child is one of the most important parenting responsibilities. However, many mothers and fathers feel uncomfortable with the subject of sex. The stereotype of nervous parents anxiously trying to explain the birds and the bees to their youngsters is all too real in many households. For some parents, it is easier simply to avoid talking about the subject altogether.

If that sounds familiar, you need to overcome your hesitancy about discussing sexually related issues. Perhaps you have difficulty picturing your own child as sexually curious, asking for detailed information about sexual matters, and someday having a sexual relationship. Although studies show that four of five parents believe they have an obligation to provide sex education for their offspring, fewer than half of mothers supply their daughters with any information; fathers participate in sex education even less often.

While many school systems offer sexuality education in middle school or high school, there is no better place for children to learn about sexuality than from their parents. It is one of your most important parenting responsibilities.

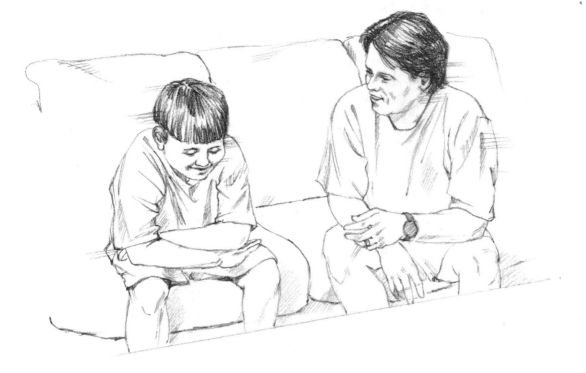

If you relinquish that role, your child will still learn about sex, but from other children, television, popular songs, magazines, and other sources. Much of this information will be inaccurate. At the same time, you will lose an important opportunity to discuss with your youngster the values you associate with sex. In a one-on-one conversation, you can personalize the issues with your child, discuss your child's fears and worries, and make sure sexuality education is offered before pressures for sexual behavior increase.

Even if you find it difficult to talk frankly about some aspects of sexuality, children are entitled to a more factual perspective than they get from TV or from friends. Make an extra effort to become your youngster's primary source of sexual information.

Not only do children learn about sexuality from what parents say, but also from parents' behavior. A large part of children's sex education comes from observing the behaviors and interactions of those they love. Keep in mind that for a child, sexual interest is not synonymous with sexual activity. When youngsters in middle childhood pose questions about sex, they are not interested in having sexual intercourse themselves but may be fascinated with the subject because they sense that it is taboo or secret. Puberty in girls starts at an average age of ten years, and in boys it begins a little later. The physical changes your child is experiencing or witnessing among friends will trigger a lot of questions. While these questions should be answered directly, proper education about sexuality also encompasses topics like sexual roles, sexual orientation, and establishing relationships in the future.

How Do I Start?

The earlier you begin the process of sex education, the better. Sex education for children does not center on the act of sex, but rather includes the broader concept of sexuality—the physical, emotional, and social aspects of being a boy or girl, man or woman in our culture, and the roles and relationships that are part of being male or female. Ideally, you have had continuing conversations about sexual issues since your youngster's earliest years. If you wait until he or she reaches puberty or adolescence to start communicating on these important matters, parent-child dialogue will be much more difficult. You need to become comfortable with these discussions as early as possible, so that you can lay a firm educational foundation and establish a pattern of openness and easy dialogue before puberty.

Many adults had very little sex education when they were growing up. They may have learned about sex from the movies or from friends and thus may not have accurate information themselves about human anatomy and the biology of sex. They may be uncertain what is appropriate and understandable during various stages of their child's development. These parents need to obtain accurate information—from books or from their pediatrician—that they can pass on to their youngster. Some schools include parents in their health-education courses for children, and some pediatricians offer family sex-education talks in the evenings. In addition to increasing their own knowledge, parents also may find a book or two they can share with their child—books that reflect their own values.

Some parents are afraid they will not know the answers to all their children's questions. If that situation arises, offer to find out the information and discuss it later. Over time, as you answer their questions, both you and your children will become more comfortable with talking about sexuality.

The information that parents give can be guided primarily by the questions a child asks. Some children, however, may not ask directly for specific information, particularly if they believe their parents are uncomfortable with the topic. Other youngsters may test their parents by asking "embarrassing" questions.

As a general rule, when your child asks questions, answer her with clear, short, straightforward explanations. Do not overwhelm your youngster with more information than she asked for; instead, follow up your responses with an inquiry of your own, such as "Does that answer your question?" A few days later you might ask your child: "Is there anything else you're wondering about related to the discussion we had last week?"

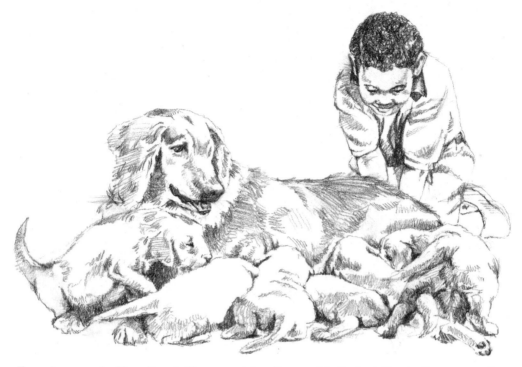

Everyday opportunities—"teachable moments"—often provide the best time to discuss sexually related topics.

Even when questions are not posed, take the initiative and use everyday opportunities—so-called teachable moments—to discuss appropriate, sexually related topics. For example, you can bring up sexual issues when

- a pregnancy or a birth occurs in the family

- issues arise during television viewing, like news stories about AIDS, rape, sexual harassment, or homosexuality

- children mention words with sexual overtones that they have heard in the schoolyard or the playground

- your older child helps change the diaper of a brother and notices that the baby has an erection. (Describe this bodily process matter-of-factly as a natural part of life.)

- you and your child observe the sexual behavior of pets or animals in zoos or on farms, allowing you to discuss mating and reproduction

To build your own confidence, you might try talking over these issues first with another adult—perhaps your spouse or a friend. This will give you an op-

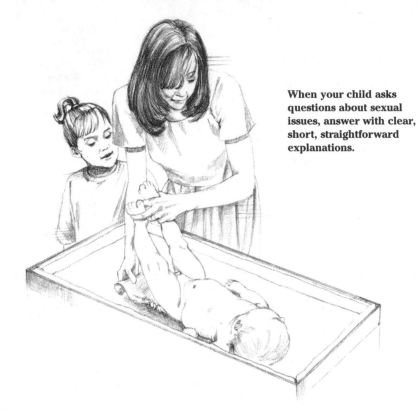

When your child asks questions about sexual issues, answer with clear, short, straightforward explanations.

portunity to think about what questions may arise and help you to clarify your responses. Also, find out what your child is learning in school about sexuality so you can build upon it.

If you are finding it difficult to communicate with your child about sex, perhaps because of your own inhibitions and anxieties, ask for help from another adult in this educational process. Perhaps a relative or a close family friend or your pediatrician can convey the information about sexuality that your child needs during this important time in her life. Your clergyman might also help. In cases like this, however, you should make a special effort to convey your value system to your youngster; *no one* can do this better than you.

There are also books available for youngsters that you can read before giving them to your child. If there's anything in them you don't agree with, you can discuss it with your child.

What Are Your Child's Interests in Sexuality?

"How are the bodies of boys and girls different?"

"How old do girls have to be before they can have a baby?"

"Do you have to get married to have a baby?"

"Why do boys get erections?"

"What is a period?"

"How do people have sexual intercourse?"

"Why do some men like other men?"

These are the kinds of questions that school-age children ask. Each of them deserves a straightforward answer, perhaps beginning with a question of your own ("What do you know already?") to get the dialogue flowing and give you the opportunity to correct any misinformation. If you have a sense of your child's existing level of knowledge, you will have a point of reference from which to introduce new facts. Some children, however, will play dumb and deny knowing things in an effort to get their parents to repeat and confirm what the children have heard in the past.

In the first years of life youngsters are curious primarily about anatomical differences between males and females. Later, they may also pose questions about sexually related phenomena: "Where do babies come from?" or "How are babies made?" By age eight or nine they may have acquired many of these facts but have not yet tied them together in a way that makes sense to them.

Middle childhood encompasses years in which your child will experience considerable growth and development; in your discussions with your child, take into account your youngster's age, experience, knowledge, physical development, and emotional maturity. Here are the basic facts that your child needs to know as he or she moves toward puberty:

- What are the body parts related to sexuality, including their actual names and their functions? (If you use euphemisms for parts of the sexual anatomy, you will give the impression that there is something offensive about them.) Your child may already be curious about her own body, examining it and becoming familiar with her own physical sensations. You can use this natural curiosity to provide information about male and female sexual anatomy.

- How are babies conceived and born?

- What is puberty? How will your child's body change as she goes through this stage of life? (See Chapter 1, "Physical Development Through Puberty.")

- What is menstruation? Both boys and girls can benefit from this information.

- What is sexual intercourse?

- What is masturbation? Emphasize that masturbation and self-exploration are aspects of sexuality. Help your child approach this subject (and all other parts of sexuality) without a sense of guilt. It is important to dispel the myths about masturbation. (See page 71.)

- What is the function of birth control? Explain that if a man and a woman want to have sexual intercourse but do not want to have a baby, they need to use some type of contraceptive. You can even explain the basic types of birth control methods and how they prevent ovulation or fertilization.

- What are sexually transmitted diseases and how are they contracted? Potentially deadly sexually transmitted diseases like AIDS cannot be ignored; the more information your child has about them, the better.

- What is homosexuality? Children become increasingly aware of relationships between people of the same sex. They may sense a social unacceptability that they misconstrue as disapproval of having feelings toward a good friend. In responding to this question, use the opportunity to discuss your family's attitudes about homosexual relationships, and also to reassure your child that liking and loving people does not depend on their gender and is different from liking someone sexually.

- What ethical guidelines should be part of your child's sexual behavior later in life? A value system is critical, helping youngsters place sexual issues in a context that is thoughtful, considerate, and healthy and that will encourage meaningful adult relationships.

At different stages of development your child will ask the same questions, but will be seeking different answers. For instance, questions like "Where do babies come from?" may arise several times during middle childhood, but as your child matures he or she will be able to understand more sophisticated responses.

COMMON SEXUAL CONCERNS

Parent and child alike experience certain sexual anxieties as the youngster enters and moves through puberty.

Some parents worry that when it comes to sex, all their child is thinking about is sexual intercourse. That belief is erroneous, and it interferes with communication between the generations. As your youngster begins puberty, he or she will be much more interested in looking attractive to the opposite sex, and finding and keeping a boyfriend or girlfriend, than in the act of making love.

Another misconception is also quite common among adults: Many parents are convinced that if they teach their child about sex, they will be encouraging him or her to become sexually active at an early age. They feel that by talking about sex, they are sanctioning it. But in fact the opposite is true. As children enter and pass through adolescence those who are the best informed about sexuality are the most likely to postpone intercourse. School-based sexuality education that promotes abstinence but also teaches birth control methods has achieved both delays in sexual activity and increased use of contraception by those who become sexually active. By contrast, when children do not get information from their parents, they turn to friends or other sources from whom they are more apt to receive *mis*information; that ignorance—and the inability to discuss sexuality with their parents—may lead them to earlier sexual intercourse, and a greater vulnerability to sexually transmitted diseases and unwanted pregnancies. To repeat, it is *mis*information or a lack of communication that gets youngsters into trouble.

As mentioned earlier, when you talk about sexuality, do not overlook discussing values. Perhaps your own value system seems old-fashioned by current standards—which can cause you to become anxious. Even so, do not feel pressured to change. If you openly explain your beliefs—and the reasons for them—to your child, you may give your youngster the strength to resist peer pressure to have sexual intercourse before he or she is ready.

MASTURBATION

Masturbation is an aspect of childhood sexuality that parents find hard to respond to comfortably and appropriately. Part of the difficulty may be the need to acknowledge that children are sexual beings. The misunderstandings and secrecy about masturbation add to parent and child discomfort.

By definition, masturbation is self-stimulation of the genitals. It is done by both boys and girls and is normal behavior.

Just how common is masturbation during the various stages of childhood? Up to the age of five or six years, masturbation is quite common. Young children are very curious about their bodies and find masturbation pleasurable and comforting. Youngsters also are curious about the differences between girls and boys, and thus in the preschool and kindergarten years they may occasionally explore each other's body, including their genitals.

From age six on, the incidence of masturbation in public tends to subside, largely because children's social awareness increases and social mores assume greater importance. Masturbation in private will continue to some extent and remains normal.

When pubertal development begins—accompanied by an increase of sexual hormones, thoughts, and curiosity—body awareness and sexual tensions rise. Masturbation is a regular part of normal adolescence. Most young teenagers discover that masturbation is sexually pleasing and recognize that self-stimulation is an expression of their own developing sexuality.

Although the myths surrounding masturbation have been scientifically dispelled, they still persist. A child who masturbates is *not* oversexed, promiscuous, or sexually deviant. Nor will he go blind or insane, grow pimples or warts, or become sterile. Nevertheless, many cultures still actively discourage masturbation, partly because of the general moral constraints often placed on sexual behavior.

When parents of school-age children discover their child's masturbatory play or activity, some react with embarrassment, anger, and even moral outrage; others take it in stride and recognize it as developmentally normal behavior. Ideally, this discovery provides a wonderful opportunity for teaching children about their own sexuality and about the differences between public and private activities.

Excessive or public masturbation may indicate a more serious psychological or personal problem. It could be a sign that the child is stressed, is overly preoccupied with sexual thoughts, fantasies, or urges, or is not receiving adequate attention at home. Sometimes masturbation is a means of providing himself with personal comfort when he is feeling emotionally overwhelmed. Masturbation could even be a tipoff to sexual abuse; children who are being sexually abused may become overly preoccupied with their sexuality, suggesting the need for further investigation.

What Should You Do?

"I caught my child masturbating, Doctor. What should I do?"

It is not unusual for physicians to hear this question from worried parents. However, masturbation is a part of normal human sexual experience, and children find it pleasurable. Assuming it is not excessive (not interfering with normal routines, responsibilities, or play), elimination of masturbation may not be desirable.

Nevertheless, make sure your child understands that masturbation, like many other things, is a private activity, not a public one. If you observe him touching his genitals in a public place, you might say to him: "It is not appropriate for you to be touching your penis [or vagina] here. It should be only done in the privacy of your room when no one is with you."

As you discuss masturbation with your child, do not label it as bad, dirty, evil, or sinful. This will create a sense of guilt and secrecy that may be unhealthy for his sexual development.

There are certain situations in which children should receive an evaluation by a behavioral pediatrician, child psychiatrist, or psychologist. These include:

- Frequent excessive daily masturbation, both at home and in public.

- Public masturbation that continues even after you have talked about it with your child.

- Masturbation that takes place in conjunction with other symptoms of behavioral or emotional difficulty, including social isolation, aggression, destructiveness, sadness, withdrawal, bed-wetting, or soiling (encopresis).

- Inappropriate sexual talk or other sexual activity.

PART II

NUTRITION AND PHYSICAL FITNESS

5

NUTRITIONAL NEEDS

Is your child eating a healthy diet?

Proper nutrition is one of the most important influences on your youngster's well-being. A varied, balanced diet—containing vitamins, minerals, protein, carbohydrates, and even some fat—promotes growth, energy, and overall health.

Food preferences are developed early in life, mostly during early and middle childhood. Once they are established, they are hard to break. Thus, the earlier you encourage healthful food choices for your child, the better.

From early on, your child will watch you for clues to proper food choices. She will copy many of your habits, likes, and dislikes. During the middle years, the model you provide at home will be extremely important in both guiding and reinforcing good eating habits. However, as children spend many hours a day away from home, in school and with friends, a variety of social and other factors influence what and when children eat. As they hurry to catch the school bus in the morning, they may speed through breakfast, leaving a half-full plate as they rush out the door. For lunch at school—despite the school's effort to offer healthy choices—youngsters might choose high-fat or sugar-laden foods that do not contribute to a balanced diet. They also might become much more susceptible to pressures from friends to choose soft drinks rather than milk, or a candy bar instead of fresh fruit.

Even at this young age, children in competitive sports may be misled by a Little League coach or other authority figure to adopt certain questionable eating habits, on the premise that these might improve performance. A major influence on children is television advertising, which often promotes unhealthy food selections.

MONITORING FOOD NEEDS

In general, it is the parents' job to monitor what their child eats, while the child is in the best position to decide how much to eat. Normally, healthy and active children's bodies do a good job of "asking" for just the right amount of food, although their minds may lead them astray when choosing which foods to eat.

You can easily overestimate the amount of food your child actually needs, especially during the younger years of middle childhood. Youngsters of this age do not need adult-sized servings of food. However, if you are unaware of this, you might place almost as much food on your child's plate as on your own. As a result, your child must choose between being criticized for leaving food on his plate, or for overeating and running the risk of obesity.

Weighing your children occasionally is one way for you to monitor your youngsters' nutrition. There is rarely a reason for you to count calories for your children, since most youngsters control their intake quite well. As the middle years progress, children's total energy needs will increase and thus their food intake will rise, especially as they approach puberty. Between ages seven and ten, both boys and girls consume about 1,600 to 2,400 calories per day, although caloric needs obviously vary considerably even under normal circumstances. Most girls experience a significant increase in their growth rate between ages ten and twelve and will take in about 200 calories more each day, while boys go through their growth spurt about two years later and increase their food intake by nearly 500 calories a day. During this time of rapid growth, they will probably require more total calories and nutrients than at any other period in their lives—from calcium to encourage bone growth, to protein to build body tissue.

At most ages boys require more calories than girls, primarily because of their larger body size. But appetites can vary, even from day to day, depending on factors like activity levels. A child who spends the afternoon doing homework, for example, may have fewer caloric needs than one who plays outdoors after school. Every child's caloric needs are different.

PICKY EATERS

Some children simply do not eat as much as their peers. Their appetite may not be as large, and/or they may be finicky eaters, unwilling even to taste certain types of foods.

At one time or another these characteristics seem to be a normal part of middle childhood. Appetites may fluctuate as youngsters grow. Even within the same family, brothers and sisters may vary considerably in the amounts and types of food they desire. Generally, children increase their food consumption considerably as they enter the growth spurts associated with puberty; until then, however, a child's appetite may be unpredictable.

Some children are less open to trying new foods than others. You might have more success introducing new foods as part of familiar foods that your child already enjoys. For instance, a child who dislikes hot cereal may be more receptive if you add bananas or raisins to it. While he may not enjoy cooked carrots, he still might eat them when they are part of a stew, meat loaf, or soup. Avoid special rewards or strong, coercive encouragement for trying something new ("You're going to bed early tonight unless you try the chicken!"). If you introduce foods in a confrontational way, you and your child may become caught up in a battle, and he may stubbornly resist these foods even more. Offering rewards for particular foods may give your youngster the impression that the food would otherwise be undesirable.

As frustrating as your child's picky eating habits may be, keep in mind that you, too, may have foods you like and dislike. In most cases, go along with your child's wishes, as long as he likes enough foods to achieve a balanced diet.

HEALTHY FOOD CHOICES

How can you ensure that your child is well nourished? Here are some guiding principles to keep in mind when planning and preparing meals for the family, based on recommendations from the U.S. Department of Agriculture and the U.S. Department of Health and Human Services.

Variety

Your child should consume a variety of foods from the five major food groups that make up the "Food Pyramid" on page 81. Each food group supplies important nutrients, including vitamins and minerals. These five groups and typical minimum servings are:

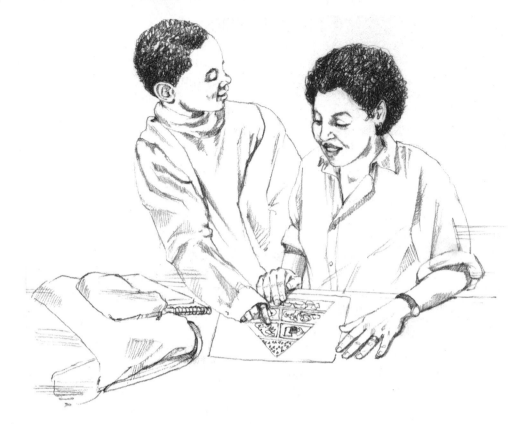

Teach your child the importance of eating a variety of foods from the five major food groups.

- Vegetables: 3–5 servings per day. A serving may consist of 1 cup of raw leafy vegetables, $^3/_4$ cup of vegetable juice, or $^1/_2$ cup of other vegetables, chopped raw or cooked.

- Fruits: 2–4 servings per day. A serving may consist of $^1/_2$ cup of sliced fruit, $^3/_4$ cup of fruit juice, or a medium-size whole fruit, like an apple, banana, or pear.

- Bread, cereal, or pasta: 6–11 servings per day. Each serving should equal 1 slice of bread, $^1/_2$ cup of rice or pasta, or 1 ounce of cereal.

- Protein foods: 2–3 servings of 2–3 ounces of cooked lean meat, poultry, or fish per day. A serving in this group may also consist of $^1/_2$ cup of cooked dry beans, one egg, or 2 tablespoons of peanut butter for each ounce of lean meat.

- Dairy products: 2–3 servings per day of 1 cup of low-fat milk or yogurt, or $1^1/_2$ ounces of natural cheese.

Eating Well with the Food Pyramid
(minimum number of recommended servings)

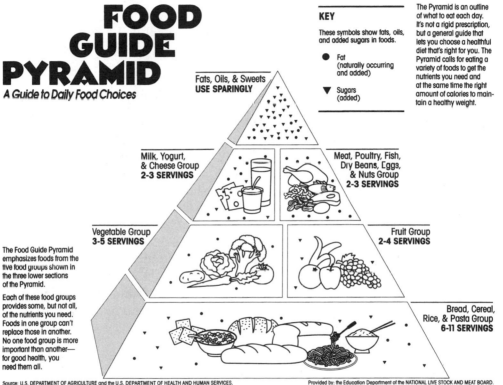

FOOD GUIDE PYRAMID
A Guide to Daily Food Choices

KEY

These symbols show fats, oils, and added sugars in foods.

● Fat (naturally occurring and added)

▼ Sugars (added)

The Pyramid is an outline of what to eat each day. It's not a rigid prescription, but a general guide that lets you choose a healthful diet that's right for you. The Pyramid calls for eating a variety of foods to get the nutrients you need and at the same time the right amount of calories to maintain a healthy weight.

Fats, Oils, & Sweets
USE SPARINGLY

Milk, Yogurt, & Cheese Group
2-3 SERVINGS

Meat, Poultry, Fish, Dry Beans, Eggs, & Nuts Group
2-3 SERVINGS

Vegetable Group
3-5 SERVINGS

Fruit Group
2-4 SERVINGS

Bread, Cereal, Rice, & Pasta Group
6-11 SERVINGS

The Food Guide Pyramid emphasizes foods from the five food groups shown in the three lower sections of the Pyramid.

Each of these food groups provides some, but not all, of the nutrients you need. Foods in one group can't replace those in another. No one food group is more important than another—for good health, you need them all.

Source: U.S. DEPARTMENT OF AGRICULTURE and the U.S. DEPARTMENT OF HEALTH AND HUMAN SERVICES.

Provided by: the Education Department of the NATIONAL LIVE STOCK AND MEAT BOARD.

Fiber

Fiber is a carbohydrate component of plant foods that is usually undigestible. It is found in foods like fruits, vegetables, whole-grain breads, cereals, brown rice, beans, seeds, and nuts. In adults, increased fiber has been linked with a reduction of chronic gastrointestinal problems, including colon cancer, irritable bowel syndrome, and diverticulitis. In children, however, fiber's only proven benefit is its ability to ease constipation—providing bulk that can promote regular frequency of bowel movements, soften the stools, and decrease the time it takes food to travel through the intestines. However, since food preferences and eating habits may be established early in life, and since high-fiber foods contain other nutrients, parents should include these foods in children's daily diets.

Protein

Your child requires protein for the proper growth and functioning of his body, including building new tissues and producing antibodies that help battle infections. Without essential amino acids (the building blocks of protein), children would be much more susceptible to serious diseases.

Protein-rich plants—such as dried beans and peas (legumes), grains, seeds, and nuts—can be used as valuable sources of protein. Other protein-rich foods include meat, fish, milk, yogurt, cheese, and eggs. These animal products contain high-quality protein and a full array of amino acids.

Bear in mind, however, that red meat and shellfish are not only rich in protein and an important source of iron but are high in fat and cholesterol as well. Thus, your child should consume them only in moderate amounts. Select lean cuts of meat and trim the fat before cooking. Likewise, remove skin from poultry, and excess fat from fish, before serving.

Fat

Humans cannot live without fats. They are a concentrated source of energy, providing essential fatty acids that are necessary for a variety of bodily processes (metabolism, blood clotting, vitamin absorption).

However, high fat intake—particularly a diet high in *saturated* fats—can cause problems. Saturated fats are usually solid at room temperatures and are found in fatty meats (such as beef, pork, ham, veal, and lamb) and many dairy products (whole milk, cheese, and ice cream). They can contribute to the buildup of atherosclerotic plaques and lead to coronary artery disease later in life. A diet rich in saturated fats also can increase blood cholesterol, particularly in people who have inherited a tendency toward high cholesterol levels.

Making Healthier Food Choices

Eat more often	Eat only occasionally
Baked potato	French fries
Low-fat frozen yogurt	Ice cream
Baked or grilled chicken	Fried chicken
Bagels or English muffins	Doughnuts and pastries
Graham crackers, fig bars, vanilla wafers	Chocolate chip cookies
Pretzels, plain popcorn	Potato chips

For that reason, after age two, children should be served foods that are lower in fat and saturated fats. Chances are that your child's favorite foods are higher in fat than is desirable. Prudent eating means relying more on low-fat, low-cholesterol foods like poultry, fish, and lean meat (broiled, baked, or roasted; not fried), soft margarine (instead of butter), low-fat dairy products, and low-saturated-fat oils from vegetables, while limiting egg consumption.

As a general guideline, fats should make up less than 30 percent of the calories in your child's diet, with no more than about one third or less of those fat calories coming from saturated fat, and the remainder from unsaturated (that is, polyunsaturated or monounsaturated) fats, which are liquid at room temperature and include vegetable oils like corn, safflower, sunflower, soybean, and olive. Some parents find the information about various types of fat confusing. In general, oils and fats derived from animal origin are saturated. The simplest place to start is merely to reduce the amount of fatty foods of all types in your family's diet.

Sugar

Keep your child's sugar consumption at moderate levels. Sugar has plenty of calories, but dietitians often call them empty calories because they have very little additional nutritional value. Even so, many children consume sugar in great quantities, usually at the expense of healthier foods—that is, when youngsters drink sodas, they are usually leaving the milk in the refrigerator; when they eat a brownie, they may be overlooking the bowl of fruit, a good source of complex carbohydrates, on the kitchen table.

Salt

Table salt, or sodium chloride, may improve the taste of certain foods. However, researchers have found a relationship between dietary salt and high blood pressure in some individuals and population groups. High blood pressure afflicts about 25 percent of adult Americans and contributes to heart attacks and strokes.

The habit of using extra salt is an acquired one. Thus, as much as possible, serve your child foods low in salt. In the kitchen, minimize the amount of salt you add to food during its preparation, using herbs, spices, or lemon juice instead. Also, take the salt shaker off the dinner table, or at least limit its use by your family.

Because of the preservative properties of salt, processed foods often contain large amounts of it. Salt-rich foods may include processed cheese, instant puddings, canned vegetables, canned soups, hot dogs, cottage cheese, salad dressings, pickles, certain breakfast cereals, and potato chips and other snacks.

DOES YOUR CHILD NEED VITAMIN SUPPLEMENTS?

Vitamins and minerals are important elements of the total nutritional requirements of your child. Because the human body itself is unable to produce adequate amounts of many vitamins, they must be obtained from the diet. The body needs these vitamins in only tiny amounts, and in a balanced diet they are usually present in sufficient quantities in the foods your youngster eats. Thus, in middle childhood, supplements are rarely needed.

For some youngsters, however, pediatricians may recommend a daily supplement. If your child has a poor appetite or erratic eating habits, or if she consumes a highly selective diet (such as a vegetarian diet containing no dairy products), a vitamin supplement should be considered. Chewable tablets are available for children who have difficulty swallowing pills.

These over-the-counter supplements are generally safe; nonetheless, they are drugs. If taken in excessive amounts (in tablets, capsules, or combined with other supplements), some supplements—particularly the fat-soluble vitamins (A, D, E, and K)—can be toxic. Scientists are finding that in some special situations and diseases, vitamin supplementation can be an important contributor to health. However, so-called megavitamin therapy or orthomolecular medicine—in which vitamins are given in extremely large doses for conditions ranging from mental retardation to hyperactivity to dyslexia—has no proven scientific validity and may pose some risks. Vitamin C, for example,

How to Reduce Dietary Fat and Cholesterol

Family eating habits determine what your child will learn to eat and enjoy. Here are some ways you and your family can limit fat and cholesterol in your diets:

- Keep fresh fruits and vegetables available.

- Serve whole-grain bread and cereals.

- Rely on low-fat milk and low-fat yogurt. Select cheeses that are lower in fat, for example.

- Include starchy foods (potatoes, pasta, rice) in your meals.

- Avoid high-fat and high-calorie toppings, including butter, margarine, sour cream, and gravy. Instead, use herbed cottage cheese, grated parmesan cheese, or low-fat yogurt as toppings.

- Serve lean meats, such as chicken, turkey, fish, lean beef cuts (lean hamburger, top loin, top round, eye of round), and lean pork cuts (tenderloin, loin, chops, ham). Cut away visible fat and remove the skin from poultry.

- Select margarine and vegetable oils (canola, corn, olive, sunflower, and soybean oils).

- Choose frozen fruit bars, angel food cake, or low-fat frozen yogurt instead of rich, creamy desserts.

- When cooking, use nonstick vegetable sprays to cut down on added fat.

- Choose fat-free cooking techniques, such as baking, broiling, poaching, grilling, or steaming when preparing meat, fish, and poultry. Do not use butter or margarine when preparing or serving vegetables.

- Serve vegetable-based and broth-based soups. Choose low-fat milk when making cream soups.

WHERE WE STAND

The American Academy of Pediatrics believes that healthy children receiving a normal, well-balanced diet do not need vitamin supplementation over and above the recommended dietary allowances. Megadoses of vitamins—for example, large amounts of vitamins A, C, or D—can produce toxic symptoms, ranging from nausea to rashes to headaches and sometimes to even more severe adverse effects. Talk with your pediatrician before giving vitamin supplements to your child.

when consumed in megadoses in hopes of undermining a cold, can sometimes cause headaches, diarrhea, nausea, and cramps. Always consult your pediatrician before giving your child supplements. And don't leave a bottle of vitamins on the table as though they were a condiment like salt or pepper; taking vitamins should be done with careful consideration.

As much as possible, try to maximize the vitamins your child receives in her regular meals. Following are some of the vitamins and minerals necessary for normally growing children, and some of the foods that contain them.

Vitamin A promotes normal growth, healthy skin, and tissue repair, and aids in night and color vision. Rich sources include yellow vegetables, dairy products, and liver.

The *B vitamins* promote red blood cell formation and assist in a variety of metabolic activities. They are found in meat (including liver), poultry, fish, soybeans, milk, eggs, whole grains, and enriched breads and cereals.

Vitamin C strengthens connective tissue, muscles, and skin, hastens the healing of wounds and bones, and increases resistance to infection. Vitamin C is found in citrus fruits, strawberries, tomatoes, potatoes, Brussels sprouts, spinach, and broccoli.

Vitamin D promotes tooth and bone formation and regulates the absorption of minerals like calcium. Sources include fortified dairy products, fish oils, fortified margarine, and egg yolks. Although vitamin proponents insist that large doses of vitamin D—far greater than the U.S. Recommended Daily Allowances—can build even stronger bones, there is no evidence to support this claim, and excessive quantities of vitamin D are potentially toxic. Sunlight also contributes to dietary sources of vitamin D, stimulating the conversion of a naturally occurring compound in the skin to an active form of the vitamin.

Especially during periods of rapid growth, *iron* is essential for the production of blood and the building of muscles. When iron levels are low, your child may demonstrate symptoms such as irritability, listlessness, depression, and

Determining Fat Percentages

The American Academy of Pediatrics recommends a diet in which fat comprises no more than 30 percent of total daily calories. Here we show how to determine the *percentage of fat calories* in one serving of a particular item. Even so, do not let the numbers confuse you; the goal should be to cut down on fat. In the example below, we have used the information found on the label of a container of low-fat strawberry yogurt:

Serving size	6 ounces
Calories	180
Fat, g	2

Every gram of fat contains 9 calories. So to calculate the percentage of fat calories in this serving of yogurt:

1. Take the total number of grams of fat in the serving (2 grams) and multiply that number by 9 calories per gram of fat (9×2 grams = 18). Thus, in this example, each 6-ounce serving contains 18 calories from fat.

2. Divide that number (18) by the total calories in a serving (18 fat calories divided by 180 calories = 0.10).

3. Finally, multiply that figure by 100, which will convert it to a percentage. In this particular example, 10 percent of the calories in the yogurt is in the form of fat.

an increased susceptibility to infection. However, a deficiency of iron is much more common in adolescence than in middle childhood. Once girls begin menstruation, they need much more iron than boys do. The best sources of iron include beef, turkey, pork, and liver. Spinach, beans, and prunes also contain modest amounts of iron. Some cereals and flour are enriched with iron.

As your child matures, **calcium** is necessary for healthy bone development. An inadequate calcium intake during childhood can not only affect present growth but might also help contribute to the development of weakened and porous bones (osteoporosis) later in life. Low-fat milk, cheese, yogurt, and sardines are excellent sources of calcium. Some vegetables, such as broccoli and spinach, also contain modest amounts of calcium. Some fruit juices are now fortified and provide a good source of calcium.

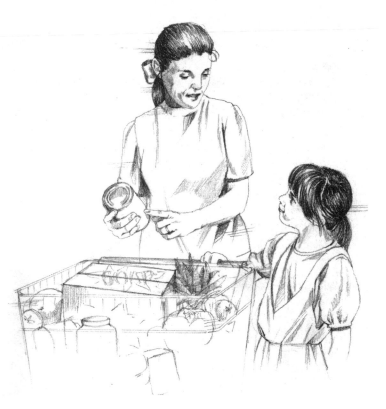

Reading food labels when shopping is part of teaching children good nutrition.

READING FOOD LABELS

By spending a few additional minutes in the supermarket to read product labels, you can help ensure a nourishing, well-balanced diet for your youngster. The specific information provided on labels can vary, but by carefully reading the amounts of fat, cholesterol, sodium, vitamins, and minerals, and the percentage of calories from fat, you will find that products on the store shelves differ greatly in their contents.

When reading this nutritional information, also pay close attention to portion sizes, which can sometimes cause confusion. For example, breakfast cereal packages often provide the nutritional content of the cereal when *combined* with half a cup of milk; thus, the serving may seem nutritious, even though the cereal itself provides little nutritional value (see adjoining table). Also, keep in mind that because these listed portion sizes are arbitrary, they may not be equivalent to the portions actually consumed by your own family. When comparing different products, make sure the portion sizes on the labels are equal, or do some quick refiguring of your own.

Let's look at the nutrition information on a box of popular corn flakes and determine their nutritional value:

Serving Size: 1 oz. (28.4 grams, about 1 cup)

	Cereal	With ¹/₂ cup vit. A & D skim milk
Energy (kcal or calories)	100	140
Protein, g	2	6
Carbohydrate, g	24	30
Fat, total, g	0	0
Cholesterol, mg	0	0
Sodium, mg	290	350
Potassium, mg	35	240

The carbohydrate listing is a combination of fiber, sugars, and complex car-bohydrates; if the manufacturer made a claim about the fiber on the cereal package, the precise amount of fiber would have to be listed.

Individuals on a low-sodium diet should compare labels to find a cereal with a reduced amount of sodium. Also, while this label provides information for a serving with half a cup of no-fat (skim) milk, fat and cholesterol levels will be greater if low-fat or whole milk is used.

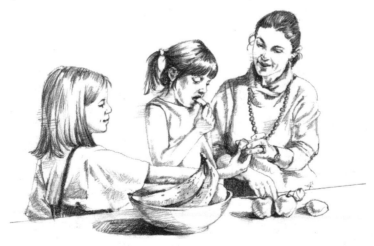

Encourage children to choose healthy snacks (especially fruits and vegetables).

CHOOSING HEALTHY SNACKS

Many children arrive home from school and head straight to the refrigerator for a snack. There is nothing wrong with moderate snacking, since youngsters have high levels of activity and may need more calories than three meals a day provide to meet their energy needs. For many children—particularly those who are quite physically active—snacks can help round out their nutritional requirements and provide as much as one fourth of their calories. In general, occasional snacks will not ruin their appetites for regular meals, as long as the snack is not eaten shortly before they sit down to lunch or dinner. Snacks are another opportunity for parents to provide healthy food choices to their children while reinforcing good eating habits—learning to get hungry, rather than eating to feel full all the time.

When snacking, children often reach for the closest food at hand. If your cupboard has cookies in it, that is probably what your child will eat. However, if there are healthier items in the refrigerator or on the kitchen table, your youngster will become accustomed to snacking on these foods. The healthiest and simplest choices are fruits and raw vegetables, which require little if any preparation. Encourage your child to make healthy snacks a habit by keeping fruit and cut vegetables (carrots, cucumbers, celery, peppers, broccoli) handy.

Children in the older range of the middle years also can learn some simple cooking techniques. As they prepare snacks for themselves, you can teach them to differentiate between healthy and less healthy choices. However, be sure they learn appropriate safety precautions for the use of a stove, oven, microwave, or other cooking appliance.

FAST FOODS

More than in previous generations, today's families eat many of their meals away from home, often in fast-food restaurants. On a given day about one fifth of the American population dines at these fast-food eateries. In most cases, they are consuming quickly prepared and uniform meals, convenient and reasonably priced, and usually consisting of hamburgers, cheeseburgers, fried/ breaded chicken and fish, and French-fried potatoes. These meals tend to be relatively high in calories, salt, total fat, and the percentage of fat calories.

While these items are often called junk food—implying that (like candy and pastries) they have no nutritional value other than calories—that is usually a misnomer, since some fast foods are as nutritious as the food you may cook at home, even though they may be high in fat and calories. For instance, a fast-food hamburger may be prepared with a salt and caloric content similar to other common lunch alternatives, such as a tuna-salad sandwich with mayonnaise or a peanut butter and jelly sandwich.

When eating with your children at a fast-food restaurant, talk with them about the benefits of making lower-fat selections. Encourage them to start their meal with a salad. Many of these restaurants now have salad bars; although this is an excellent option, minimize the use of high-calorie dressings and high-fat cheeses. Choose grilled rather than fried foods, thus avoiding items like fried hamburgers, French fries, and deep-fried chicken. If your child

Healthy Snacks for Any Mood

Your child's snacking moods may vary, but he can still consistently maintain healthy snacking habits. For instance, if his snacking mood is:

Thirsty! Cold skim or low-fat milk, mineral water with lime, chilled vegetable juice, fruit juice (apple, grape, grapefruit, orange, pineapple, raspberry).

Smooth! Yogurt, banana, papaya, mango, custard, cottage cheese, "fruit smoothie." (*"Fruit smoothie" recipe:* Blend one cup of skim milk, three ice cubes, your favorite fresh fruit, and a dash of vanilla, cinnamon, and nutmeg in a blender.)

Crunchy! Raw vegetables (asparagus, bell pepper, broccoli, cabbage, carrots, cauliflower, celery, zucchini), apples, corn on the cob, unbuttered popcorn, puffed-rice cakes, wheat crackers.

Juicy! Fresh fruit (berries, cantaloupe, grapes, grapefruit, kiwi, nectarine, orange, peach, plum, watermelon, frozen juice pops, tomato, pear).

Fun! Fruit, frozen grapes, frozen bananas.

Really hungry! Hard-boiled eggs, granola, sandwich, cereal with milk, bran muffin, peanut butter (on crackers or bread), nuts, cheese.

---

finds hamburgers irresistible, order a simple one rather than a double burger with extra dressings. A baked potato, unless it is covered with butter and sour cream, is a good choice now available at some establishments. Also, select low-fat milk or orange juice rather than high-fat milk shakes, and keep creamy sauces to a minimum.

Remember, children learn most from example. Preaching good nutrition is unlikely to be effective in guiding your child's eating habits. Practice balance, variety, and moderation in your own and your family's diet, and your children are likely to follow suit.

Cooking with Your Children

One of the best ways to familiarize your child with good food choices is to encourage her to cook with you. Let her get involved in the entire process, from planning the menus to shopping for ingredients to the actual food preparation and its serving.

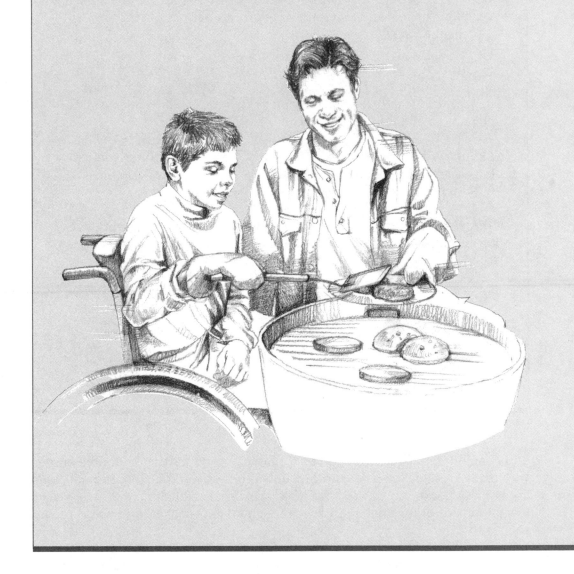

When you are planning meals with her, refer to the Food Pyramid on page 81, and try to include items from the important food groups. Explain the importance of making low-fat choices whenever possible, choosing chicken and fish rather than red meat in most cases, or choosing low-fat cheeses over higher-fat varieties. Particularly in her first few efforts at helping in the kitchen, let her select recipes that she and other family members have enjoyed in the past, so she can see what's involved in preparing them.

In assigning tasks to your child, keep in mind that they need to be age-appropriate. For instance, you wouldn't give a six-year-old a sharp knife to chop vegetables, although she can certainly wash the lettuce. Nor would you let her remove a hot, heavy casserole pot from the oven, although she can carefully open the oven door for you.

Here are some other guidelines to keep in mind:

- Make certain that you or another adult is in the kitchen at all times when your child is helping out.

- When your child pares vegetables, show her how to point sharp edges away from her to avoid accidents.

- Explain how she should weigh and measure ingredients.

- Use the rear burners when cooking on the stove. Make sure that pot handles are turned inward so children can't accidentally knock them off the stove.

- Teach your child the importance of using potholders when touching hot saucepans and other items.

- Shut off the oven and burners when you're finished cooking.

6

SPECIAL DIETS, SPECIAL NEEDS

Too many children in America are overweight, and too many people are on diets. Those may seem like contradictory statements, but they are not. Dieting as it is usually practiced is not an appropriate or successful way to deal with being overweight.

IS YOUR CHILD OVERWEIGHT?

Studies show that today's youngsters tend to be heavier than their counterparts were a generation ago, and that over 30 percent of America's school-age youngsters are now overweight. That can contribute to physical problems such as high blood pressure, limit a child's athletic abilities, and impair self-esteem. We live in a society that emphasizes thinness, and an overweight child is likely to be teased by peers. Studies show that as early as the kindergarten

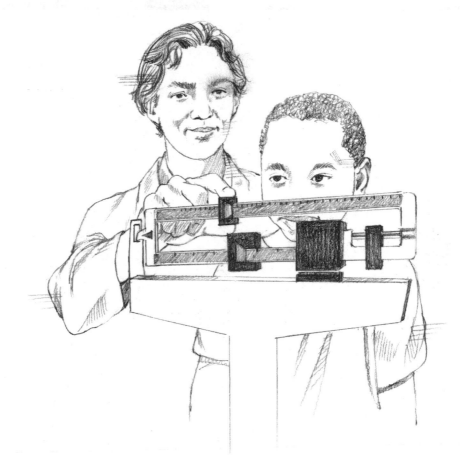

Your child's pediatrician can help you determine the appropriate weight range for your child.

years, children have an aversion to obesity and describe their overweight classmates as less likable.

What, then, is a reasonable approach to this problem? First, you need to determine if your child is overweight. Talk with your pediatrician, who will consult growth charts to determine the most appropriate target weight range for your youngster. This ideal range will depend on a number of factors, including your youngster's sex, age, height, and body build. Obesity is usually defined as more than 20 percent above ideal weight for a particular height and age. Youngsters who are greater than 40 percent overweight are generally recommended for a physician-guided weight-loss program.

Children tend to gain weight at a fairly steady rate through the middle years, with an increase in weight gain and growth during, and just prior to, puberty. Parents and their children should not become alarmed by this increase in weight and initiate dieting at this time.

Various factors can influence the likelihood of a child's becoming overweight. A family history of obesity increases your youngster's chances of weight problems later in life. A child who is physically inactive is more likely to have a weight problem. If your family's meals tend to emphasize high-calorie foods, that can cause excess weight gains. Although certain metabolic and endocrine disorders may contribute to obesity, they are the culprits in only about 5 percent of obese children.

Stress can also play a role in some overweight problems. Adults change their lifestyles in response to feelings, both when they feel good and when they feel bad. They may work harder or less intensively, engage in active exercise and social activities or become more sedentary, indulge in the use of substances such as alcohol and tobacco or abstain from them. Adults use food in similar ways—some people eat more under stress or when they are happy or excited, while others lose their appetites. Children have less control over their lives and thus have fewer options with which to respond to emotional peaks and valleys. They may be prone to changing the way they eat as their moods and behavior change— for instance, when they are bored, anxious, depressed, or even extremely pleased with things.

If your child is obese, do not ignore the problem. A lifetime of poor eating habits and obesity can increase your youngster's chances of developing serious diseases that could shorten his lifespan. Together, you and your child should set some realistic goals. In middle childhood actual weight *loss* may be an inappropriate objective for many overweight youngsters. Indeed, the goals you agree upon should not be principally about weight, but rather about healthy living—eating appropriate amounts and kinds of food, exercising, and dealing with personal and social factors that encourage poor lifestyle habits.

As part of a comprehensive program, your pediatrician may suggest the *maintenance* of current weight, keeping your child's weight at its present level while he continues to grow in height, thus causing him to slim down. However, for children who are more than 40 percent overweight for their age, sex, and height, your doctor may recommend a comprehensive plan, including dietary changes aimed at small increments of weight loss. Obese youngsters should avoid fad diets and instead consume a variety of foods relatively low in calories but high in nutritional value. Foods like vegetables, fish, and poultry fit this description. While you can limit portion sizes, do not *severely* restrict your youngster's caloric intake or you may run the risk of impeding normal growth.

Support your child by your own good eating habits. Cook low-calorie meals for the entire family. You cannot expect your youngster to successfully change his eating and exercise habits on his own, particularly if others in the household are not setting good examples. Your goal should be to help him learn and adopt healthier *lifetime* eating habits that can keep his weight permanently under control.

Also, encourage your overweight child to become more physically active.

Regular exercise can play an important role in the maintenance of a healthy weight over the long term. You can become a good role model for physical activity, even involving your child in your own exercise program, perhaps bicycling, swimming, or brisk walking as a family. It is probably better to encourage your child to exercise as part of a fitness program, not as part of a diet. Diets are short-lived, but fitness is a lifelong goal. Encourage your child to exercise, knowing that as he becomes more physically fit, his overall sense of well-being and his feelings of self-worth are likely to improve.

Finally, don't ignore the effect that obesity can have on a child's self-concept. The most successful programs concentrate not only on dietary modifications and exercise, but also on boosting a youngster's self-esteem.

WHAT ABOUT A FORMAL WEIGHT-LOSS PROGRAM?

Many community hospitals and specialized clinics offer formal weight-loss programs for children. For some obese youngsters, these programs may be worth considering. The best candidates are children who are at least 30 to 40 percent overweight and who are in basically good health, without any significant physical or psychological problems. Families of these youngsters must be willing to provide support and help their offspring implement and follow through on the eating and exercise plans that are recommended.

When you're evaluating a particular weight-loss program, keep in mind that the most effective ones tend to be those that help children adopt behavioral strategies to counteract their weight problem. Doing so in a group setting not only provides support but helps youngsters develop their social skills too. These programs also should help a child increase her physical activity.

As children enter a program, they should be assessed by a number of health professionals. A pediatrician should document that the child has sufficient excess weight to warrant her participation and to confirm that she has no significant underlying health problems. A nutritionist or registered dietitian should determine what the child's nutritional habits are and create a personalized eating plan. A psychologist or other mental health professional should evaluate the youngster to identify any existing psychological difficulties, as well as to determine whether family problems may be interfering with the child's efforts at weight control.

Once your child begins participation in a formal weight-loss program, her success will require you to make certain aspects of the program part of your family's day-to-day life—from making sensible food choices to encouraging the entire family to become more physically active together. Also, with guidance from the program's staff, encourage your child to set reasonable, short-term

Elements of a Weight-Control Program

Here are some sensible guidelines for healthy weight management:

- Have your child participate in daily vigorous physical activity, sufficient to increase his heart rate and make him sweat. He should start with at least fifteen minutes daily and increase to at least thirty minutes. He can try fast walking, jogging, bicycling, and skating. Team sports are fun, but not all are vigorous enough to be sufficient alone for weight management.

- Monitor your child's diet by writing down what he eats and drinks. Review this record each day, and find foods that he could eliminate by substituting healthier, lower-fat, lower-calorie choices. Do not rely on "diet foods" alone, but rather switch to leaner cuts of meat, poultry, fish, lower-fat cheeses, and nonfat milk. Add more vegetables and fiber to his diet, and use fruits as desserts rather than cake, pie, cookies, pudding, and ice cream. Watch the size of each serving, and avoid second helpings.

- If weight *loss* is the goal, set reasonable weight-loss targets (usually no more than one-half to one pound of lost weight per week), and monitor your child's progress. Periodically use rewards for achieving short-term goals. Do not use a long-term goal of a large amount of weight loss as the only criterion for success.

- Support your child's efforts by eliminating undesirable foods from the household. "Cleaning up" the food environment is critical. Keeping high-calorie foods in the house for special occasions or for other family members is cruel and will undermine the child's efforts. There is no acceptable reason for breaking this rule.

- As a parent, you are not the "food police," and thus you should not remind, cajole, or scold. If you yourself practice healthier habits and keep undesirable foods out of the house, you need only provide praise to your child, not negative reinforcement.

(week-by-week) goals that she has a high likelihood of achieving. Changes in eating and exercising—and the accompanying improvements in weight—should be slow and gradual.

Provide your child with rewards, too, as she meets those goals. These rewards should be given immediately upon achieving the goals rather than setting them off in the distance (such as a visit to the amusement park next month, or a trip next summer). The best rewards are not monetary or material but those that provide the child with additional, enjoyable times with the family, such as outings and sports activities.

HIGH BLOOD CHOLESTEROL LEVELS

Atherosclerosis (or "hardening of the arteries") usually becomes apparent in adulthood. The physiological processes that cause plaques to form on the walls of the arteries, clogging the arteries and thus interfering with blood flow, begin in childhood. Blood cholesterol levels may be one indicator of this ongoing disease process.

In adults, high levels of total cholesterol and of low-density lipoprotein (LDL or "bad") cholesterol are associated with a higher risk of atherosclerosis. Interestingly, *low* levels of high-density lipoprotein (HDL or "good") cholesterol are also associated with developing atherosclerosis, while having increased amounts of this HDL cholesterol is protective. Though high blood levels of LDLs promote the deposit of cholesterol and other fatty substances in the walls of the arteries, HDLs act as scavengers in the bloodstream, removing the cholesterol that could damage the arteries.

Studies are not as conclusive about the meaning of cholesterol levels in childhood. There seems to be a weak link between a youngster's elevated cholesterol and his risk of having high cholesterol as an adult.

At present, the American Academy of Pediatrics does not recommend routine cholesterol screening for all children. It does advise screening those children whose parents have a history of high cholesterol levels or early heart attacks (prior to age fifty).

What about treatment for a child with high cholesterol levels (hypercholesterolemia)? Some forms of this disease (familial hypercholesterolemia) are inherited and are caused by abnormal metabolism of fats, leading to abnormally high levels of blood fats, including cholesterol. They usually require intensive therapy during childhood, including dietary changes, exercise, and medication.

Some noninherited forms of hypercholesterolemia, however, are usually less severe, and the treatment remains controversial. Your doctor may recommend moderate dietary modification, aimed at reducing both fat and cholesterol consumption. As mentioned earlier, the American Academy of Pediatrics suggests an average of 30 percent of calories from fat (with less than one third of those from saturated fats) and a cholesterol intake of no more than 300 milligrams per day. (Dietary cholesterol is found only in foods of animal origin. Some of these foods have a very high cholesterol content: One egg has 270 milligrams of cholesterol; a 3.5-ounce serving of liver has 390 milligrams.)

Studies of adults have also shown a link between weight reduction and a decline in both total and LDL cholesterol. Increases in regular physical activity, including aerobic exercise, have been associated with increases in HDL ("good") cholesterol levels too.

FOOD ALLERGIES

Many types of food can cause allergic reactions in middle childhood. The most common of these are cow's milk and other dairy products, egg whites, poultry, seafood, wheat, nuts, soy, and chocolate.

Allergies are caused by antibodies that the body's immune system produces, which react to a component of a particular food and then release chemicals that cause allergic symptoms like a runny nose, sneezing, coughing, and itching. Children may also experience stomach pain, bloating, cramping, diarrhea, skin rashes, and swelling. Although these reactions can occur almost immediately after consuming these foods, they may be delayed for hours or sometimes even days.

Diagnosing food allergies is not easy. Identical symptoms may be caused by other disorders, and pinpointing the offending food can be difficult. Your pediatrician may refer your child to an allergist, who has several diagnostic options. The allergist might suggest an elimination diet, a procedure in which suspicious foods are removed from the diet for a period of time and symptoms are closely monitored to see if they subside. After several weeks the foods are reintroduced one by one, and allergic responses are again evaluated to determine which food, if any, is really the cause of the problem.

Your doctor might also use skin and blood tests. He or she might prick the skin on your child's back or arm, and then introduce a liquid extract of the suspicious food to see if a response—swelling and itchiness, for example—takes place. However, while the validity of this test is widely accepted in diagnosing airborne allergies, there is controversy about its reliability in detecting food allergies.

Some doctors also use the RAST test, in which a sample of your child's blood is mixed with food extracts. Then the blood is evaluated to determine whether antibodies to that food are present. The reliability of this test may vary from laboratory to laboratory.

Once an offending food has been identified, your doctor will probably recommend that it be removed from your child's diet. This means not only eliminating eggs, for example, but also all products that contain them. As a result, you may have to become more diligent reading labels in the supermarket. A child allergic to wheat gluten, for instance, may have to avoid most grains, including cookies, pies, cakes, and pasta, as well as processed cheese, salad dressings, and many other foods. The situation becomes even more challenging if your child is allergic to several food items.

Ask your doctor to suggest alternatives to the foods to which your child is allergic. Can egg substitutes be used for a youngster allergic to eggs? When a child is allergic to milk, should she eat additional protein-rich foods (legumes, chicken, fish, meat) and calcium-rich items (sardines, broccoli, spinach)? Can other products be consumed in place of cow's milk? If your child is allergic to wheat, can you cook with corn flour or rice flour instead?

VEGETARIANISM

In recent years vegetarianism has grown in popularity. School-age children become more conscious that animals must be killed in order to obtain meat, and that knowledge may prompt them to choose a vegetarian diet. Vegetarian diets tend to be high in fiber and polyunsaturated fat, and low in cholesterol and calories.

If your child is following a vegetarian diet, you need to guard against nutritional deficiencies. There are various degrees of vegetarianism, and the strictness of the diet will determine whether your youngster is vulnerable to nutritional shortcomings.

Following are the common categories of vegetarians. Although none eat meat, poultry, or fish, there are other areas in which they vary:

- *Lacto-ovo-vegetarians* consume eggs, dairy products, and plant foods.

- *Lacto-vegetarians* eat dairy products and plant foods but not eggs.

- *Vegans* eat only plant foods, no eggs or dairy products.

Children can be well nourished on all three types of vegetarian diet, but nutritional balance is very difficult to achieve if dairy products and eggs are completely eliminated. Vegetarians sometimes consume insufficient amounts of calcium and vitamin D if they remove milk products from their diet.

Also, because of the lack of meat products, vegetarians sometimes have an inadequate iron intake. They may also consume insufficient amounts of vitamin B-12, zinc, and other minerals. If their caloric intake is also extremely low, this could cause a delay in normal growth and weight gain.

Vegetarians may also lack adequate protein sources. As a result, you need to ensure that your child receives a good balance of essential amino acids. As a general guideline, his protein intake should come from more than one source, combining cereal products (wheat, rice) with legumes (dry beans, soybeans, peas), for example; when eaten together, they provide a higher quality mixture of amino acids than if either is consumed alone.

Other planning may be necessary. To ensure adequate levels of vitamin B-12, you might serve your child commercially prepared foods fortified with this vitamin. While calcium is present in some vegetables, your child may still need a calcium supplement if he does not consume milk and other dairy products. Alternative sources of vitamin D might also be advisable if there is no milk in the diet. Your pediatrician may recommend iron supplements, too, although your child can improve his absorption of the iron in vegetables by drinking citrus juice at mealtime.

A Zen macrobiotic diet usually presents many more problems than a vegetarian diet. With a macrobiotic program, important foods (animal products, vegetables, fruit) are severely restricted in stages. This diet is generally not recommended for children. Youngsters who adhere to it may experience serious nutritional deficiencies that can impair growth and lead to anemia and other severe complications.

NUTRITION AND SPORTS

Even in middle childhood some youngsters participating in competitive sports are looking for an edge that might make them run a little faster or throw a little harder. Often they will turn to nutrition for help.

However, there is no magical food or supplement that can transform an average athlete into a superstar. No matter what the age of your youngster, optimal performance depends more on a balanced diet, sufficient nutrients to meet the demands of physical activity, and adequate rest. Sports activities may require increases in:

- *Caloric (Energy) Intake.* Without adequate calories your child may feel weak and fatigued, and her athletic performance may suffer. To raise caloric consumption, your child should rely primarily upon carbohydrates (potatoes, rice, pasta, beans, bread), which are excellent sources of energy during exercise.

- *Protein Intake.* The protein needs of an athlete may be only a little higher than those of a more sedentary individual. Even so, some evidence suggests that a small increase in protein, in conjunction with exercise, may be important when trying to increase muscle mass and lean tissue. Often, simply by increasing caloric intake in a well-balanced diet, a child will obtain any additional protein she may require.

- *Fluid Intake.* Additional liquids are often overlooked, both by children engaged in sports and by their coaches. Yet during exercise, perspiring youngsters lose fluid that must be replaced to prevent dehydration and overheating. Children should drink plenty of water before exercising, and then drink again every ten to twenty minutes during exercise itself, even if they are not thirsty. This is particularly important when exercising in hot weather.

Fluid intake needs can vary widely from child to child, based on his or her body size, level of physical activity, and the weather. These requirements generally range from 1.5 to 3 quarts per day of fluid; your child should drink an extra 8 to 12 ounces of water for every half hour of strenuous physical activity.

Thanks to persuasive advertising, many children and their coaches believe that commercially prepared electrolyte or sports drinks have some advantages over water. These drinks do provide some replacement for the salts and sugars that are lost with vigorous exercise. However, they may be high in sugar, which can sometimes cause cramps, nausea, and diarrhea. Despite its simplicity, water is usually the best choice.

If your child is involved in a sport where his weight is important—perhaps wrestling or gymnastics—he might be drawn to unhealthy weight-management strategies, perhaps adopting a crash diet, taking laxatives, or consuming special supplements. Wrestlers, for example, in an attempt to "make weight," may be tempted to fast, which is potentially harmful. You might choose to consult your child's pediatrician or a registered dietitian to evaluate the adequacy of your child's diet. The doctor will probably advise against rapid reduction in body weight.

7

PHYSICAL FITNESS AND SPORTS

Our parks and playgrounds may seem as though they are filled with children, but many American youngsters are still much too sedentary. Only about one third of children participate in daily physical education at school (and with continued budgetary constraints, that figure may decline even further). At home, many youngsters watch hours of television and play video games incessantly, often at the expense of exercising outdoors.

As a result, today's youth are less fit than they should be. Studies show that the average percentage of body fat among school-age children has increased significantly during the past twenty years. For parents who want to start their children off right, this should be of great concern: Children who do not exercise today are less likely to be physically fit adults. They are creating a pattern of inactivity—often with parental complicity—that can continue for the rest of their lives.

When a group of children recently took the fitness test of the President's Council on Physical Fitness, the results were very discouraging. In the six- to twelve-year-old age category, only 64 percent of boys and 50 percent of girls could run/walk a mile in less than ten minutes. In the same age group, just 60 percent of boys and 30 percent of girls could perform more than a single chin-up. One study found that only 2 percent of children qualified for the President's Challenge award, in which they needed to perform well in sit-ups, chin-ups, a one-mile run/walk, and a shuttle run.

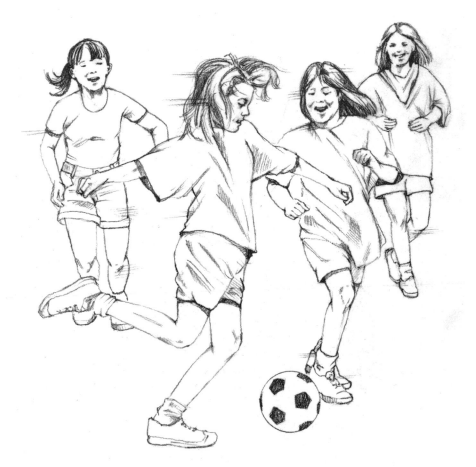

ACTIVITY AS A WAY OF LIFE

As a parent, you need to encourage healthy habits—including exercise—in your youngsters. Physical activity should become as routine a part of their lives as eating and sleeping. Reassure them that sports such as cycling (always with a helmet), swimming, basketball, jogging, walking briskly, cross-country skiing, dancing, aerobics, and soccer, played regularly, are not only fun but can promote health. Some sports, like baseball, that require only sporadic activity are beneficial in a number of ways, but they do not promote fitness. Physical activity can be healthful in the following ways:

Increase Cardiovascular Endurance. More Americans die from heart disease than any other ailment; regular physical activity can help protect against heart problems. Exercise can improve your child's fitness, make him feel better, and strengthen his cardiovascular system.

Aerobic activity can make the heart pump more efficiently, thus reducing the incidence of high blood pressure. It can also raise blood levels of HDL (high-density lipoprotein) cholesterol, the "good" form of cholesterol that removes excess fats from the bloodstream. Even though most cardiovascular diseases are thought to be illnesses of adulthood, fatty deposits have been detected in the arteries of children as young as age three, and high blood pressure exists in about 5 percent of youngsters.

At least three times a week, your middle-years child needs to exercise continuously for twenty to thirty minutes at a heart rate above his resting level. As a guideline, the effort involved in continuous *brisk* walking is adequate to maintain fitness.

Each exercise session should be preceded and followed by a gradual warm-up and cool-down period, allowing muscles, joints, and the cardiovascular system to ease into and out of vigorous activity, thus helping to guarantee a safe workout. This can be accomplished by stretching for a few minutes before and after exercise.

Improve Large Muscle Strength and Endurance. As your child's muscles become stronger, he will be able to exercise for longer periods of time, as well as protect himself from injuries—strong muscles provide better support for the joints. Modified sit-ups (knees bent, feet on the ground) can build up abdominal muscles, increase lung capacity, and protect against back injuries. For upper body strength, he can perform modified pull-ups (keeping the arms flexed while hanging from a horizontal bar) and modified push-ups (positioning the knees on the ground while extending the arms at the elbow).

Increase Flexibility. For complete physical fitness, children need to be able to twist and bend their bodies through the full range of normal motions without overexerting themselves or causing injury. When children are flexible like this, they are more agile.

Although most people lose flexibility as they age, this process can be retarded by stretching to maintain suppleness throughout life, beginning in childhood. Stretching exercises are the best way to maintain or improve flexibility, and they can be incorporated into your child's warm-up and cool-down routines.

What About Strength Training?

When most people think of strength training, their minds focus upon a high school or college football player pumping iron to get that extra edge on the line of scrimmage, or a bodybuilder lifting weights to increase muscle size. Such weight training involves lifting maximal weights and should not be part of the exercise regimen of a child in the middle years.

For the youngster in middle childhood, is there a system of strength training that is safe and effective? Some manufacturers are beginning to produce down-sized strength-training machines, but most are made for adults, not children. Although free weights (dumbbells or barbells without any external support or a machine) are another option, they present some risks for children who have not yet reached puberty; there is a much greater chance of injury in children than in adults. The American Academy of Pediatrics does not recommend the use of free weights in this age group, and strongly discourages children from power lifting of maximal weights. Encourage your child to participate in other approaches to strength building—for instance, sit-ups, push-ups, pull-ups, stationary jumps, and hill runs.

In most stretching exercises, your child should stretch to a position where he begins to feel tightness but not pain, then hold steady for twenty to thirty seconds before relaxing. He should not bounce as he stretches, since this can cause injury to the muscles or tendons.

Maintain Proper Weight. Twelve percent of children in the prepuberty years are overweight, but few of these youngsters are physically active. Exercise can effectively burn calories and fat and reduce appetite.

Ask your pediatrician to help you determine whether your youngster has a healthy percentage of body fat for his or her age and sex. (For a more complete discussion of weight problems, see Chapter 6, "Special Diets, Special Needs," and Chapter 27, "Eating Disorders.")

Reduce Stress. Unmanaged stress can cause muscle tightness, which can contribute to headaches, stomachaches, and other types of discomfort. Your child needs to learn not only to recognize stress in his body but also to diffuse it effectively. Exercise is one of the best ways to control stress. A physically active child is less likely to experience stress-related symptoms than his more sedentary peers. (For more information, see Chapter 17, "Stress and Your Child.")

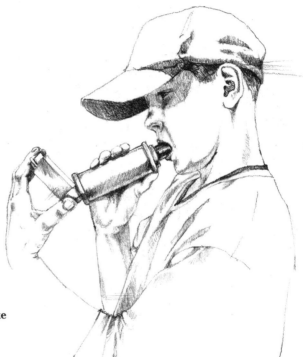

A child with a chronic disease like asthma can still participate in sports as long as he follows the instructions of his pediatrician.

IF YOUR CHILD
HAS A CHRONIC DISEASE

Exercise is a way for children to keep fit, have fun, build self-esteem, and relate to other children. Even children with a serious chronic disease can enjoy the benefits of participating in safe and appropriate physical activity.

Talk with your pediatrician about whether restrictions are necessary for your child with a chronic illness; if they are, explain the situation fully to your youngster before imposing them. Obviously, she should not be in an athletic environment where her limitations place her in danger or significantly limit her opportunity to have some success. Nearly every child can find an appropriate level of activity in which she can participate successfully and without frustration, while developing muscle strength and coordination. Every child should be encouraged to become as active as possible.

Most chronic health problems actually require few, if any, restrictions. Children with asthma, for example, can usually participate in sports, although they may have to follow carefully their doctor's guidelines for medication administration before exercising. Youngsters with well-controlled seizure disorders can enjoy nearly all sports, from baseball to basketball to soccer—although if a child has occasional seizures, it is probably sensible to avoid activities such as rope climbing, high diving, and workouts on parallel bars, where a fall could cause a serious injury; while swimming, these children should be supervised by an adult who is in the water with them.

Children with heart disease or high blood pressure can participate in most sports, although your child's cardiologist may have specific recommendations about how strenuous an activity should be. Youngsters with musculoskeletal problems like scoliosis can also lead an active life, as can most children with rheumatoid arthritis.

Some youngsters have impaired, uncorrectable vision in one eye. In these cases, talk to an ophthalmologist about protecting the good eye from injury. Special protective eyewear may be suggested. Children who participate in sports where eyes are frequently injured, such as baseball, racquetball, and handball, are also advised to use protective eyewear.

The Special Olympics program offers unique, exciting experiences for disabled children, providing opportunities for physical fitness, competition, and enjoyment. Through their participation, children can enhance their self-esteem, and parents can connect with a valuable support system.

SPORTS PROGRAMS

Childhood sports programs have grown significantly in recent years. Millions of boys and girls are now involved in Little League baseball, youth soccer, community basketball leagues, competitive swimming teams, and similar types of activities. Happily, sports programs are becoming increasingly available for girls, whose need for such activities and whose ability to participate is equal to that of boys.

If your own child joins one or more of these programs, he will have a wonderful opportunity for fun and fitness. At the same time, however, a youngster poorly matched to a sports team—or who must deal with unrealistic expectations from a parent, a coach, or even himself—can have a very negative sports experience, filled with stress and frustration.

Before your child enters a youth sports program, evaluate his objectives as

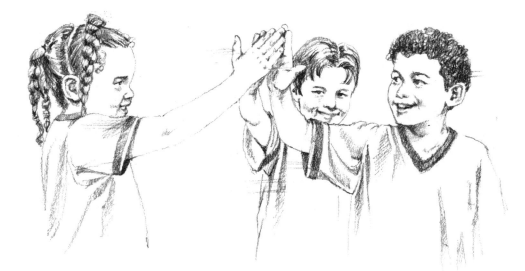

Participation in sports can boost your child's self-confidence and help develop friendships.

well as your own. Although both child and parent may fantasize about using this as a stepping-stone toward becoming a professional athlete or an Olympic champion, few participants have the talent and dedication to reach those heights. Even more modest goals are far from guaranteed: Only one in four outstanding elementary school athletes becomes a sports standout in high school. Only one in more than 6,600 high school football players will ever rise to the professional football ranks.

Nevertheless, there are other, more important reasons for your child to participate in organized sports. Sports can contribute to physical fitness and develop basic motor skills. Also, participation in the sports activity that best suits your child's capabilities can develop leadership skills, boost self-confidence, teach the importance of teamwork and sportsmanship, and help him deal with both success and failure. In addition, by participating in sports, children often find exercise enjoyable and are more likely to establish lifelong habits of healthful exercise. However, not all sports meet the requirements for promoting overall fitness. Also, there are many ways for children to be fit and become active without participating in a team sport.

Talk with your child about his interest in youth sports, and what his reasons may be for wanting (or in some cases, not wanting) to participate. His goals may be different from yours. Most children—particularly the younger ones— might say that they simply want to have fun. Others may add that they want to be active and hope to spend time and share experiences with friends. You may have all of these goals, too, along with the desire that your youngster develop an appreciation for sports and fitness.

If either you or your child places winning at or near the top of your list of goals—and if you put pressure on your child to win a tournament or kick a goal—your priorities are out of line. Winning certainly adds to the fun and excitement of sports, but it should *not* be a primary goal.

Choosing a Sports Program

Once your child has decided that he wants to become involved in a sports activity, he will have to decide which one to select. Of course, he should choose one that *he* will enjoy; even though your first love may be baseball or softball, let him choose soccer if that is what appeals to him.

Some children prefer individual sports rather than team sports. These individual activities—such as swimming, running, tennis, and cycling—can become lifetime sports, offering enjoyment and health advantages throughout adulthood. Many of these same activities (running and swimming, for example) can provide an aerobic workout too.

If your child selects a team activity, investigate the programs available in your community. There are both contact and noncontact sports (see table), and you and your child should evaluate which is more appropriate for his or her size, interests, and abilities. Many team sports (basketball, soccer) involve at least some contact, although others (T-ball, swimming, tennis) are purely noncontact activities. The nature of how some sports are played changes with a child's age. For example, soccer for younger children is played without much contact and rarely results in collisions. As a general rule, children up to the age of eight should participate only in noncontact sports; beginning at age eight, contact sports are acceptable alternatives. However, children should not participate in "collision" sports (football, hockey) earlier than age ten.

As you might expect, there is a greater chance of injury in contact and collision sports, but many children still enjoy these activities, particularly if the coach emphasizes participation, not winning. Also, take into account your youngster's physical maturity. His ability to compete with his peers—particu-

Classification of Sports by Contact

Contact/ Collision	Limited Contact	Noncontact
Basketball	Baseball	Archery
Boxing*	Bicycling	Badminton
Diving	Cheerleading	Body Building
Field hockey	Canoeing/kayaking	Bowling
Football	(white water)	Canoeing/kayaking
Flag	Fencing	(flat water)
Tackle	Field	Crew/rowing
Ice hockey	High jump	Curling
Lacrosse	Pole vault	Dancing
Martial arts	Floor hockey	Field
Rodeo	Gymnastics	Discus
Rugby	Handball	Javelin
Ski jumping	Horseback riding	Shot put
Soccer	Racquetball	Golf
Team handball	Skating	Orienteering
Water polo	Ice	Power lifting
Wrestling	Inline	Race walking
	Roller	Riflery
	Skiing	Rope jumping
	Cross-country	Running
	Downhill	Sailing
	Water	Scuba diving
	Softball	Strength training
	Squash	Swimming
	Ultimate Frisbee	Table tennis
	Volleyball	Tennis
	Windsurfing/surfing	Track
		Weight lifting

*Participation not recommended.

larly in the collision sports—depends more on body size and weight than on age. A late-maturing junior high school youngster, for instance, may have fewer skills and be much more susceptible to injury in contact or collision sports than his more mature teammates and opponents. Do not pressure your child to participate in a sport for which he may lack the proper maturity level.

What Is Your Child's Physical Maturity Level?

Throughout middle childhood, children grow at varying rates and at different times. At first glance you might think that the early maturers would have clear physical advantages over their later-maturing peers. However, both groups of children face certain difficulties.

Youngsters who mature early are more likely to experience athletic success during the elementary and junior high years. Yet, with time, their peers will catch up with them, eliminating any advantages the early maturers once had and, often, deflating their self-esteem in the process. Formerly a star athlete, the early maturer has to adjust to being just one of the gang.

If your children fall into this category, you can help ease them through the adjustment process by encouraging them to participate in athletic activities with children who are also early maturers. Their maturity level is a more important factor than age. Also, urge your youngsters to develop other interests in addition to sports—areas in which they can excel and activities they can enjoy even when their maturity status no longer gives them an advantage over their classmates.

Late-maturing children face different types of challenges. These children, smaller than most youngsters their age, tend to lag behind in their strength level and motor skills. Regardless of their size, these youngsters should be encouraged to participate in athletic activities, choosing those where maturity level and strength are not as important—perhaps tennis, gymnastics, or certain track events. Later, when they catch up with their earlier-maturing peers, they can participate in sports where size plays a more significant role.

You, your child, and your pediatrician should discuss the most appropriate activities or sports for your youngster, and whether the advantages of a contact or collision sport outweigh the potential risks.

What Else Should You Consider?

Before making a final decision on the right sport for your child, investigate the philosophy of the program under consideration. Here are some questions to ask:

- Do all team members get equal playing time? (Studies show that children would prefer to play regularly on a losing team rather than be relegated to the bench of a winning one.)

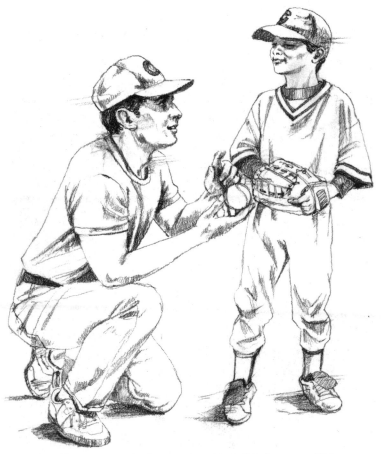

Coaches can serve as important role models for your child.

Commonly Asked Sports Questions

Should I allow my child to quit a team?
Sometimes a child's interest in a sport will fade. Or her participation may become a negative experience, perhaps because of a volatile coach, frustration in not playing as much as she would like, or a mismatch between her own physical size and that of the players against whom she competes.

In cases like this, find out the exact reasons why your child wants to quit. Listen to her and discuss her concerns. Working together, decide on the best course of action. Although it may not be wise for your child to make a habit of avoiding difficult situations, dropping out of a program may be the most sensible option in some instances.

If my child is having trouble keeping her grades up, should she still be permitted to participate in sports?
In most cases, the answer is yes. All children need physical activity as part of their day. Without this physical outlet, many have difficulty concentrating on their academic work. If practices and other sports-related demands are excessive, however, talk to the coach about your child's need to devote adequate time to studies.

There is another important factor to consider: Sometimes, children who have difficulty with schoolwork can use a boost in self-esteem, which sports often can provide. As they feel a sense of

- Does the program emphasize mastery of the sport rather than winning? Is each child encouraged to reach his or her own potential in terms of skills development?

- Are youngsters given unconditional approval, with good efforts praised and mistakes met with gentle encouragement?

- Is the teaching of good sportsmanship emphasized?

- Are the needs of the children taken into consideration? For example, are practices at a convenient time and place, and are they limited to a reasonable length of time? Will the time demands prevent the children from participating in other activities and assuming other responsibilities?

accomplishment in athletics, this renewed self-confidence can often carry over to other areas of their life, including academics.

My child is finding her sports participation too stressful. How can I alleviate her anxiety?
Sports can be stressful, but so can other childhood activities, such as school exams and band solos. However, you should try to minimize the stress in your child's athletic endeavors in the following ways:

- Emphasize that sports participation is fun; do not let a "win at all cost" attitude interfere with your child's enjoyment of the game.

- Let your youngster know that she is not being judged by her success (or lack of it) on the athletic field. When she strikes out or misses a free throw, be supportive and praise her for trying her best.

- Help your child improve her athletic skills, which will reduce her stress levels during competition; if necessary, ask for some outside instruction from a cooperative coach.

- Stay away from coaches who are abusive toward your child.

- Speak with other parents to see if there is a common problem that needs to be addressed.

- Are safety rules adhered to during practices and games? Is appropriate equipment available? Are children matched with others of the same size and strength? (This is particularly important in contact sports.)

- What expenses are involved, including the costs of equipment and travel?

- What are the expectations and demands on the parents' time?

Also, investigate the coach or coaches for whom your child will be playing. They can serve as important role models for your youngster. They should enjoy being with children and communicate well with them. They should respect each member of the team as an individual, not showing favoritism toward the best athletes on the team. They should be knowledgeable about

The ICE Treatment

As soon as an injury occurs, use the three-step "ICE" first-aid treatment to minimize swelling:

1. *I*ce: Apply an ice bag or a plastic bag of ice over the injured area. (Caution: Overuse of ice can cause skin damage; never apply ice for longer than twenty minutes, or more often than every two hours.)

2. *C*ompression: After removing any part of the child's clothing that covers the injured region, wrap a damp, cold elastic bandage around the skin. The last section of the bandage should be wrapped firmly around the ice bag. Maintain compression even after ice is removed.

3. *E*levation: Raise the injured leg or arm higher than the level of the heart, keeping it elevated as much as possible until the pain or swelling subsides.

This is the only treatment you should apply on your own until a doctor has diagnosed the injury. Do not tape or splint an injured arm or leg. Do not administer any drugs that have not been prescribed by a doctor. When helping your child leave the field of play, keep him or her from using or putting weight on the injured part.

the game they are coaching, not only in order to help children learn the sport properly but also to minimize the chance of injury. Their practices should be instructive, safe, and enjoyable, and games should emphasize participation, learning, and fun—not winning. Even when their players do not perform up to expectations, the coaches should provide support rather than react angrily.

Keep in mind that responsible parenting involves evaluating your children's athletic needs and expectations, investigating the sports that are available and which ones are most appropriate for them, estimating the quality of your youngsters' experience, and deciding whether a particular activity lends itself to a lifelong habit of exercise. Sports are one aspect of your child's life in which being an active advocate can have big payoffs.

SPORTS INJURIES

Improvements in the quality of protective equipment—such as padding and helmets—have made sports participation safer than ever before. Even so, children's bodies are still vulnerable to injury. As youngsters move through middle childhood—becoming bigger, stronger, faster, and more aggressive—the incidence of injuries rises. Studies show that each year, 2 to 3 percent of five- to seven-year-olds experience injuries that require more than a few days of rest and recuperation; that figure increases to 5 to 10 percent among nine- and ten-year-olds.

Injury prevention should be a paramount concern. Your child should be wearing a well-fitted helmet, mouthpiece, face guard, padding, eye gear, protective cup, or other equipment appropriate for the sport.

The majority of sports-related injuries involve the body's soft tissues rather than the bones. About two thirds of all injuries are strains (overstretching or overextension of the muscles) and sprains (wrenching of a joint with partial tear of the ligaments).

Many injuries are caused by overuse of or repetitive stress on the affected body part. When a child overdoes it or trains inappropriately—for example, pitching too many innings or throwing improperly—the stress placed on the joints, tendons, and muscles can cause damage.

Overuse injuries can often be prevented by advising your child to stop exercising at the first sign of discomfort. "No pain, no gain" may be a catchy phrase, but it is bad advice. "Slow but sure" makes a lot more sense.

Once an injury occurs, it needs to be properly diagnosed and treated. Even children with injuries that appear to be quite minor may benefit from being examined by a pediatrician. In addition to recommending specific types of treatment, the doctor may suggest that your child reduce the level of athletic participation for a while, allowing the injury to heal while maintaining some use of the injured body part. Improperly treated and incompletely healed sports injuries can set the stage for lifelong problems. Because youngsters in middle childhood are unable to contemplate the future seriously, parents have to be firm to ensure that medical guidelines are followed.

It is also important to identify the cause of the injury before returning to the sport. Was the playing field in bad shape? Was the safety equipment not being used? Was training or fitness not adequate? Was the coaching poor? If parents neglect these factors, injuries are likely to reoccur.

Children in contact sports are much more vulnerable to serious injury, with the knees bearing the brunt of more injuries than any other part of the body. The ankles, shoulders, and elbows are also particularly susceptible to injuries that can put youngsters on the disabled list during the healing process.

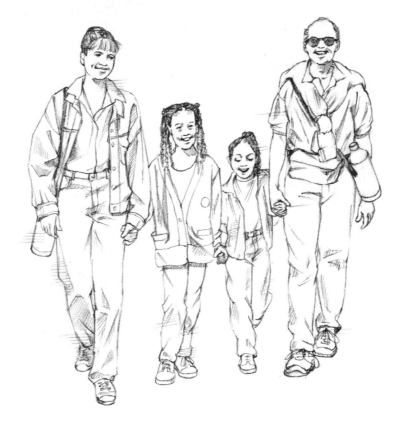

BECOME A GOOD ROLE MODEL

Perhaps the best way to get children to enjoy exercise is to make it a family affair, with parents setting a good example and encouraging the youngsters to join the fun. The entire family can participate together in many physical activities, from swimming to cycling to hiking. Not only will everyone's fitness improve, but the unity of the family can be strengthened too.

If you can get your child interested in fitness at a young age, you will improve the chances that physical activity will become a lifetime habit. Long-term health will be the ultimate result.

PART III

PERSONAL AND SOCIAL DEVELOPMENT

8

YOUR CHILD'S DEVELOPING SELF

Each year during middle childhood, the little person you're raising grows and develops, finds her place in the world, and evolves into a person in her own right. As a parent, part of your function during these years is to let your child grow and become the person she is meant to be. Guiding your youngster toward becoming more competent, self-sufficient, and self-confident means you need to accept her for herself, a growing and learning child. As you will learn in this chapter, there are some things you can change, and some things you can't.

TEMPERAMENT

Some children are "easy." They are predictable, calm, and approach most new experiences in a positive way. Other children are more difficult, not able to manage their emotional experiences and expression with ease. When a child's personality doesn't quite fit or match that of other family members, it can be a challenge for everyone. Of course no child is one way all the time, but each has his own *usual* type.

The ease with which a child adjusts to his environment is strongly influenced by his temperament—adaptability and emotional style. For the most part, temperament is an innate quality of the child, one with which he is born. It is somewhat modified (particularly in the early years of life) by his experiences and interactions with other people, with his environment, and by his health.

By the time a child has reached the school years, his temperament is well defined and quite apparent to those who know him. It is not something that is likely to change much in the future. These innate characteristics have nothing to do with your own parenting skills. Nevertheless, the behavioral adjustment of a school-age child depends a lot upon the interaction between his temperament and yours, and how others respond to him—how comfortably he fits in with his environment and with the people around him.

Characteristics of Temperament

By being aware of some of the characteristics of temperament, you can better understand your child, appreciate his uniqueness, and deal with problems of poor "fit" that may lead to misunderstandings and conflicts.

There are at least nine major characteristics that make up temperament.

Activity level: the level of physical activity, motion, restlessness, or fidgety behavior that a child demonstrates in daily activities (and which also may affect sleep).

Rhythmicity or regularity: the presence or absence of a regular pattern for basic physical functions such as appetite, sleep, and bowel habits.

Approach and withdrawal: the way a child initially responds to a new stimulus (rapid and bold or slow and hesitant), whether it be people, situations, places, foods, changes in routines, or other transitions.

Adaptability: the degree of ease or difficulty with which a child adjusts to change or a new situation, and how well the youngster can modify his reaction.

Intensity: the energy level with which a child responds to a situation, whether positive or negative.

Mood: the mood, positive or negative, or degree of pleasantness or unfriendliness in a child's words and behaviors.

Living with a "Difficult" Child

Here are some general strategies and solutions to help you live with a youngster with bothersome temperament traits:

1. First, recognize that much of your child's behavior reflects his temperament.

2. Establish a neutral or objective emotional climate in which to deal with your child. Try not to respond in an emotional and instinctive manner, which is unproductive.

3. Don't take your child's behavior personally. Temperament is innate, and your child probably is not purposely trying to be difficult or irritating. Don't blame him or yourself.

4. Try to prioritize the issues and problems surrounding your child. Some are more important and deserve greater attention. Others are not as relevant and can be either ignored or put "way down the list."

5. Focus on the issues of the moment. Do not project into the future.

6. Review your expectations of your child, your preferences, and your values. Are they realistic and appropriate? When your youngster does something right, praise him and reinforce the specific behaviors that you like.

7. Consider your own temperament and behavior, and how they might also be difficult. Think how you might need to adjust yourself a bit to encourage a better fit with your child.

8. Anticipate impending high-risk situations, and try to avoid or minimize them. Accept the possibility that this may be a difficult day or circumstance, and be prepared to make the best of it.

9. Find a way to get some relief for yourself and your child by scheduling some time apart.

10. Seek professional help, when needed, from your pediatrician or another expert in child behavior.

Attention span: the ability to concentrate or stay with a task, with or without distraction.

Distractibility: the ease with which a child can be distracted from a task by environmental (usually visual or auditory) stimuli.

Sensory threshold: the amount of stimulation required for a child to respond. Some children respond to the slightest stimulation, and others require intense amounts.

How Temperament Affects Children and Their Parents

Every child has a different pattern of the nine temperament characteristics. Many, but not all, children tend to fall into one of three broad and somewhat loosely defined categories: easy, slow to warm up or shy, or difficult or challenging. These labels are a useful shorthand, but none offers a complete picture of a child. Many parents find it more useful to think about their child in terms of the nine temperament traits, and the table on page 129 explains how the different traits may be expressed.

The *easy child* responds to the world around him in an easy manner. His mood is positive, and he is mildly to moderately intense. He adapts easily to

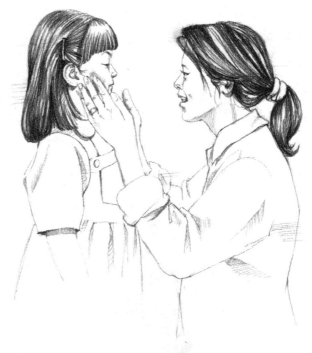

Your child's temperament determines how easily she adjusts to her environment and the people around her.

new schools and people. When encountering a frustrating situation, he usually does so with relatively little anxiety. His parents probably describe him as a "joy to be around." About 40 percent of children fall into this category.

Another temperamental profile may reveal a somewhat *slow-to-warm-up* or *shy child* who tends to have moods of mild intensity, usually, but not always negative. He adapts slowly to unfamiliar surroundings and people, is hesitant and shy when making new friends, and tends to withdraw when encountering new people and circumstances. Upon confronting a new situation, he is more likely to have problems with anxiety, physical symptoms, or separation. Over time, however, he will become more accepting of new people and situations once he becomes more familiar with them.

The *difficult* or *challenging child* tends to react to the world negatively and intensely. As an infant he may have been categorized as a fussy baby. As a young child he may have been prone to temper tantrums or was hard to please. He may still occasionally be explosive, stubborn, and intense, and he may adapt poorly to new situations. Some children with difficult temperaments may have trouble adjusting at school, and their teachers may complain of problems in the classroom or on the playground. When children have difficult temperaments, they usually have more behavioral problems and cause more strain on the mother and family.

Of the three types of temperament, parents are most concerned—and often exasperated—when they have a child with the attributes of a difficult or challenging temperament. Without doubt, a child who is negative and intense, adapts poorly, and is strong-willed can be challenging for his parents. Most mothers and fathers will feel overwhelmed, guilty, angry, or inadequate. However, once parents recognize that these characteristics are innate to the child—and, while not caused by the parents, can still be intensified or moderated by them—then mothers and fathers are more likely to change their expectations and begin efforts to help the youngster do and feel better.

It is important to distinguish a difficult temperament from other problems. For instance, recurrent or chronic illnesses, or emotional and physical stresses, can cause behavioral difficulties that are really not a problem with temperament at all. Parents also sometimes interpret a child's style of interacting as inherently bad. However, a youngster's temperament is only a problem when it conflicts with the expectations of his parents, other family members, friends, or teachers. For example, if a parent is intense and ambitious, and his or her youngster is mild-mannered and easygoing, the parent may feel disappointed, frustrated, and angry. The child, pressured to behave in ways foreign to his basic inclinations and innate personality, may resist and cause conflict within the family.

What Parents Can Do

The problem is on its way to being resolved when you recognize and accept the reality that there is a mismatch of temperaments. Once you acknowledge that your personalities are different, any tendencies to blame either the child or yourself should ease. You need to know that nothing is wrong with your child, nor are you an inadequate parent in the way you are raising him or responding to his temperament. Your challenge is to understand your own responses to him and to adjust your expectations to meet his capabilities. You need to modify your childrearing strategies to some extent to ensure a better "fit" between you and your child. At the same time, you need to help him learn to compromise, adapt, and expand his repertoire of acceptable social responses and behavior.

Once you realize that your child's behavior is, to some extent, an innate pattern and beyond his control, you can make an effort to become more patient and thus diminish the stress and strain your youngster feels. When you think of your child's temperament in objective terms rather than react to it emotionally and instinctively, you and your child will get along better. If your child has a difficult temperament as a preschooler, and if you understand and respond appropriately, he will probably modify his behavior, and may not remain as difficult during his school-age years. His intensity can become part of his enthusiasm, determination, charm, and zeal as he feels better about himself and his relationship with others. For that to happen, your own attitudes and behaviors can play a major role in how he adapts and expresses his feelings.

Also, in the weeks and months ahead, avoid labeling your child as bad or difficult. Labels stick, and not only may family members unfairly prejudge your youngster, but he may come to see himself as different, undesirable, or just not fitting in. This negative self-image can further interfere with efforts—both yours and his—to improve his way of responding to difficult situations and can lead to more serious emotional conflicts.

How Temperamental Traits Can Be Expressed

Temperamental Trait	Positive Characteristics	Difficult or Challenging Behaviors	What to Do
High Activity Level	Energetic, vigorous. Investigates his environment. Remains active even in boring circumstances.	Restless, very active. May be impulsive, reckless. Easily distracted from tasks.	Anticipate high-activity. Use safety precautions if necessary. Practice distraction techniques. Provide opportunities to burn off energy and cool down.
Low Activity Level	Is unlikely to disrupt activities in small, cramped spaces.	Slow pace in performing tasks; often labeled "lazy." Gives appearance of drowsiness.	Provide additional time to finish tasks. Make tasks realistic within the designated time frame. Avoid criticism of child's slow pace.
Irregularity (Low Regularity)	May not be upset by disruptions in daily routine activities.	Unpredictable patterns of eating, sleeping, using the toilet.	Identify child's patterns and adhere to them as much as possible. Don't force the child to eat or sleep when not ready; require child to follow routines of coming to the table or going to bed without forcing eating or sleeping.

Initial Withdrawal	Demonstrates caution in risky circumstances.	Rejection of people, food, situations. Very shy or clingy. Slow to accept change.	Introduce new things gradually, talk about them beforehand, let child proceed at own pace.
Slow Adaptability	Lower likelihood of being affected by negative influences.	Difficulty with changes and transitions. Takes a long time to adapt and adjust.	Establish daily consistent and predictable routines. Avoid unnecessary changes and prepare the child in advance. Try multiple brief exposures.
High Intensity	Child's needs get the attention of caregivers.	Expresses emotions in extremes instead of cries. Yells rather than talks. Intensity is sometimes mistaken for desire.	Learn to be tolerant. Model more appropriate responses, give general feedback, and provide alternative responses.
Negative Mood	Concern may get parents involved in issues surrounding the child.	Fussy, complains a lot, appears very serious and displays little pleasure in words and actions. Parents may overestimate importance of a child's complaint.	Understand that mood is a major part of temperament. It is not your fault. Adjust expectations or demands that intensify mood. Encourage positive responses.

Inattention and Distractability	Can soothe the child easily.	Doesn't listen. Has difficulty concentrating and studying. Gets pulled off task easily, and needs reminders.	Keep tasks, instructions, and explanations short and simple. Remove distractions and competing stimuli. Practice good communication skills: Get his attention, address by name, use eye contact, repeat, clarify, and review. Provide frequent breaks and require the child to return to the task at hand when reminded. When necessary, redirect your child without anger or shame. Provide praise for completing the task.
Low Sensitivity Threshold	High awareness of changes in surroundings and of nuances in the feelings and thoughts of others.	Overreacts even to normal stimuli (light, noise, smells, textures, pain, social-emotional events).	Reduce level of stimulation. Anticipate problems and prepare child. Respect child's preferences when possible.

SELF-ESTEEM

Self-esteem plays a central role in a child's motivation and achievements in school, athletics, and social relationships, as well as in her resiliency (the ability to bounce back). It influences her chances of becoming involved in drug or alcohol abuse and sexual activity, and her vulnerability to unhealthy or negative peer pressure.

Children develop a self-concept and self-esteem very early in life. Almost from the start, some have learned generally positive feelings about themselves, and have acquired a sense of importance and self-worth. They can acknowledge and appreciate their individual talents, achievements, and physical appearance. They can also accept their shortcomings and mistakes and realize that occasional failure is a natural part of life and learning.

Other children, however, feel quite different about themselves. They have been taught a sense of inadequacy and inferiority and have come to believe they are incapable of achieving or creating changes in their lives. They may be withdrawn and cautious, not willing to expose themselves to public scrutiny or to the risk of failure.

What Is Self-Esteem?

By definition, self-esteem is the way in which an individual perceives herself— in other words, her own thoughts and feelings about herself and her ability to achieve in ways that are important to her. This self-esteem is shaped not only by a child's own perceptions and expectations, but also by the perceptions and expectations of significant people in her life—how she is thought of and treated by parents, teachers, and friends. The closer her perceived self (how she sees herself) comes to her ideal self (how she would like to be), the higher her self-esteem.

A child's self-esteem grows from an interaction between her biological, inborn traits (such as temperament, intelligence, physical characteristics) and environmental influences (such as her parents' parenting style and economic status, and her relationships with other adults and peers). As early as the first few months of life, a child begins to develop a sense of "I," a concept of the self, and feelings of mastery over certain aspects of her environment. For instance, an infant soon learns that a cry or a smile brings an immediate and, hopefully, positive response from a parent, which reinforces her sense of trust, security, control, and self-importance. As she moves through the toddler and preschool stages, her self-concept will continue to evolve, influenced in large part by her parents' verbal and nonverbal responses to her: their praise and criticism, smiles, other facial expressions, and hugs. Other major influences include her level of independence and her sense of achievement.

By the middle years of childhood, a youngster needs a positive sense of self to do well in the world outside the family—that is, achieving in school and interacting successfully with her peers. Her self-concept at this age will be a major influence on her accomplishments, social interactions, and emotional status throughout childhood and adult life.

A child's self-esteem can fluctuate from day to day, or from situation to situation, although over the course of many years, it tends to remain relatively constant. In general, a child will usually seek out those activities and interactions that make her feel successful, and that can act as a buffer against stress and help her maintain a positive sense of well-being when she's not doing well. A youngster with high self-esteem will perceive herself as a capable individual who can set realistic goals and achieve them. A child with poor self-esteem will tend to settle for more modest accomplishments in the classroom and later in life. She may feel shame, depression, or inadequacy over what she perceives as a lack of appropriate or satisfying achievement, and the inability to earn recognition and respect from others. At the same time, her low self-esteem will make her more likely to conform to her peer group and to seek their favor, adopting their behavior and values in order to gain acceptance, a sense of belonging and self-worth. The behavior and values she conforms to may or may not be positive or healthy.

Some children have special stresses and challenges that make it more difficult for them to develop strong self-esteem. Perhaps they have a physical handicap, a chronic illness, a learning disability, or an attention problem. Or they might face discrimination because of their ethnic origin or religion. Environmental and social stresses like poverty, a neglectful parent, alcoholism, or intense sibling rivalry can further erode a child's self-esteem. Even so, these youngsters *can* develop positive self-esteem, but the need to succeed and earn the acceptance and appreciation of parents and others will be even more important than for a child without additional challenges.

Furthermore, some children appear to be very resilient and have a more positive outlook than their peers. These are children who have met and overcome hardships, setbacks, and challenges, and who tend to elicit positive responses (affection, admiration, respect) from adults. As a consequence, they are eager to explore new situations and seem able to adapt to change with greater ease. If the "fit" between parent and child temperaments is good and if parents set expectations that children can meet, their self-esteem is likely to be even further enhanced. Even in the face of great hardships, these children emerge with their self-esteem still intact and healthy. They appear to be almost invulnerable.

You know your own child better than anyone and should be able to pick up the signs—through behavior and words—if your youngster has a low self-esteem problem. Sometimes, however, you might be too close to her, or you might have difficulty seeing the world through her eyes. In cases like this, teachers, coaches, relatives, and friends might be able to help. Also, use the information in the box on page 137 as a guide.

Components of High Self-Esteem

Spend some time thinking about how your child deals with success and failure. Many children with low self-esteem may attribute their successes in life to luck, fate, or other influences beyond their control, thus eroding their confidence and reducing their chances of being successful in the future. When these same youngsters make a mistake or experience failure, they again may look beyond themselves for a cause ("I had a bad day" or "The teacher doesn't like me"). This makes it harder for them to create new and more successful strategies or to seek help or advice.

And what about a child with high self-esteem? She probably sees her successes largely as a result of her own efforts and abilities. She feels a sense of self-control and becomes motivated to do better when she experiences failure. She'll accept her mistakes, while realizing that she needs to make changes and work harder, and she will avoid blaming others.

For healthy self-esteem, children need to develop or acquire some or all of the following characteristics:

- *A sense of security.* Your child must feel secure about herself and her future. ("What will become of me?")

- *A sense of belonging.* Your youngster needs to feel accepted and loved by others, beginning with her family and then extending to groups such as friends, schoolmates, sports teams, a church or temple, and even a neighborhood or community. Without this acceptance or group identity, she may feel rejected, lonely, and adrift without a "home," "family," or "group."

- *A sense of purpose.* Your child should have goals that give her purpose and direction and an avenue for channeling her energy toward achievement and self-expression. If she lacks a sense of purpose, she may feel bored, aimless, even resentful at being pushed in certain directions by you or others.

- *A sense of personal competence and pride.* Your child should feel confident in her ability to meet the challenges in her life. This sense of personal power evolves from having successful life experiences in solving problems independently, being creative, and getting results for her efforts. Setting appropriate expectations, not too low and not too high, is critical to developing competence and confidence. If you are overprotecting her, and if she is too dependent on you, or if expectations are so high she never succeeds, she may feel powerless and incapable of controlling the circumstances in her life.

- *A sense of trust.* Your child needs to feel trust in you and in herself. Toward this goal, you should keep promises, be supportive, and give your child opportunities to be trustworthy. This means believing your child, and treating her as an honest person.

- *A sense of responsibility.* Give your child a chance to show what she is capable of doing. Allow her to take on tasks without being checked on all the time. This shows trust on your part, a sort of "letting go" with a sense of faith.

- *A sense of contribution.* Your child will develop a sense of importance and commitment if you give her opportunities to participate and contribute in a meaningful way to an activity. Let her know that she really counts.

- *A sense of making real choices and decisions.* Your child will feel empowered and in control of events when she is able to make or influence decisions that she considers important. These choices and decisions need to be appropriate for her age and abilities, and for the family's values.

- *A sense of self-discipline and self-control.* As your child is striving to achieve and gain more independence, she needs and wants to feel that she can make it on her own. Once you give her expectations, guidelines, and opportunities in which to test herself, she can reflect, reason, problem-solve, and consider the consequences of the actions she may choose. This kind of self-awareness is critical for her future growth.

- *A sense of encouragement, support, and reward.* Not only does your child need to achieve, but she also needs positive feedback and recognition—a real message that she is doing well, pleasing others, and "making it." Encourage and praise her, not only for achieving a set goal but also for her efforts, and for even small increments of change and improvement. ("I like the way you waited for your turn," "Good try; you're working harder," "Good girl!") Give her feedback as soon as possible to reinforce her self-esteem and to help her connect your comments to the activity involved.

- *A sense of accepting mistakes and failure.* Your child needs to feel comfortable, not defeated, when she makes mistakes or fails. Explain that these hurdles or setbacks are a normal part of living and learning, and that she can learn or benefit from them. Let your supportive, constructive feedback and your recognition of her effort overpower any sense of failure, guilt, or shame she might be feeling, giving her renewed motivation and hope. Again, make your feedback specific ("If you throw the ball like this, it might help") and not negative and personal ("You are so clumsy," "You'll never make it").

- *A sense of family self-esteem.* Your child's self-esteem initially develops within the family and thus is influenced greatly by the feelings and perceptions that a family has of itself. Some of the preceding comments apply to the family in building its self-esteem. Also, bear in mind that family pride is essential to self-esteem and can be nourished and maintained in many ways, including participation or involvement in community activities, tracing a family's heritage and ancestors, or caring for extended family members. Families fare better when members focus on each other's strengths, avoid excessive criticism, and stick up for one another outside the family setting. Family members believe in and trust each other, respect their individual differences, and show their affection for each other. They make time for being together, whether to share holidays, special events, or just to have fun.

For your child, one experience can establish a way of responding to subsequent events and can either boost or damage her self-esteem. For instance, if a child performs poorly in school, that can cause frustration and damage her self-confidence. In an attempt to prevent further pain and failure, she may work less hard and avoid doing her schoolwork, causing even poorer performance and even more difficulties with her self-esteem. If unaddressed, this may become a repeating cycle and make her feel, think, and act like a nonachiever, living up to this new self-image.

This cycle also can work in positive ways. If a child performs well and her success is acknowledged, her belief in her own abilities will grow, and she may feel motivated to work harder and achieve even more as she responds to the intrinsic pleasure and external rewards of success. As that occurs, her accomplishments will increase, instilling in her even stronger feelings of control over her life. Pushed along by her own desire to improve, she will keep trying and succeeding, and her self-confidence will grow even more. She soon feels, thinks, and acts in a way that fits her self-image.

Keep in mind that throughout childhood, your youngster and her attitudes toward herself will be molded by your own expectations and responses. If she brings home a report card filled with B's and you praise her effort and accomplishments, she will probably feel good about herself and what she has achieved. However, if you react with disappointment—"Why didn't you get A's in arithmetic and spelling?"—her self-esteem will suffer, even though the report card in both situations is the same. Be sensitive to the power of your own reactions and words.

Signs of Low Self-Esteem

To help you determine if your child has low self-esteem, watch for the following signals. They could be everyday responses to how your child relates to the world around him, or they might occur only occasionally in specific situations. When they become a repeated pattern of behavior, you need to become sensitive to the existence of a problem.

- Your child avoids a task or challenge without even trying. This often signals a fear of failure or a sense of helplessness.
- He quits soon after beginning a game or a task, giving up at the first sign of frustration.
- He cheats or lies when he believes he's going to lose a game or do poorly.
- He shows signs of regression, acting babylike or very silly. These types of behavior invite teasing and name-calling from other youngsters, thus adding insult to injury.
- He becomes controlling, bossy, or inflexible as ways of hiding feelings of inadequacy, frustration, or powerlessness.
- He makes excuses ("The teacher is dumb") or downplays the importance of events ("I don't really like that game anyway"), using this kind of rationalizing to place blame on others or external forces.
- His grades in school have declined, or he has lost interest in usual activities.
- He withdraws socially, losing or having less contact with friends.
- He experiences changing moods, exhibiting sadness, crying, angry outbursts, frustration, or quietness.
- He makes self-critical comments, such as "I never do anything right," "Nobody likes me," "I'm ugly," "It's my fault," or "Everyone is smarter than I am."
- He has difficulty accepting either praise or criticism.
- He becomes overly concerned or sensitive about other people's opinions of him.
- He seems to be strongly affected by negative peer influence, adopting attitudes and behaviors like a disdain for school, cutting classes, acting disrespectfully, shoplifting, or experimenting with tobacco, alcohol, or drugs.
- He is either overly helpful or never helpful at home.

If Your Child Needs Help

The most important component of self-esteem comes from the success of doing and achieving. Children need close supervison and opportunities to meet the expectations of the adults around them. Since middle childhood is a period of great industry, children's competency and self-confidence grow through their success in mastering challenges and activities. The lifelong rewards of early success and competency are self-confidence and self-esteem.

If you and/or your pediatrician or other professional have concluded that your child could use help with her self-esteem, start with some positive steps of your own. You can become the most influential person in getting your child's self-concept back on track.

First, review the various components of self-esteem described in this chapter, which will help you identify and better understand your child's particular needs and then develop some strategies and solutions. If your youngster's problems are not too serious, and you have a good relationship with her, you often can intercede on her behalf in various circumstances. Do not protect her from difficult situations, but rather help her confront them in a manner that will yield more success than in the past. Assist her in dealing with the problems at hand (for example, troubles with reading or science at school). Help her identify changes she wants to make or skills she wants to improve upon, and then assist her in setting up challenging but realistic goals and a timetable for achieving them.

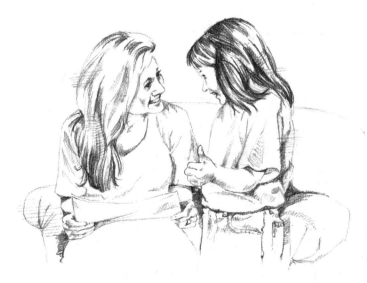

A child's self-esteem can be strengthened by encouragement and support from her family.

To meet these goals, develop a plan of action with her. For instance, if the goal is to improve reading, she should commit herself to spend extra time with her books, starting with an extra fifteen minutes per day and increasing that gradually. Teachers, family members, and perhaps a tutor should be available to provide the youngster with support. At the same time, however, avoid the temptation to run the show, superimposing your own directives over the entire process; instead, give your child as much control and responsibility as possible. This will build competence, confidence, and trust and demonstrate your respect for her.

At the same time, find other areas of strength in your child and build upon them. For example, make sure she has opportunities to do things she is good at doing. Single out something from which she derives pride and pleasure, nurture it, help her develop it, and let her appreciate her achievement. These experiences will show her, more than words, that she is capable of accomplishment.

Also, try to expand your child's interests and talents. If she is bored, she will tend to become bogged down in her apathy and self-pity. By contrast, new experiences will probably increase her motivation.

In the weeks ahead, assess your child's feelings about herself from time to time. If there still seems to be a problem with her self-confidence or self-esteem, repeat some of the interventions mentioned above if they still appear appropriate but simply need to be tried again or in a slightly different manner. Or consider alternative strategies if she is not making progress, all the while reaffirming your faith in her ability to succeed. Consider modifying goals and expectations if they have been too difficult to meet. When she ultimately reaches a goal, give her praise, and if it seems appropriate, offer her a reward (perhaps money, a gift, or special privileges). Reassure her of your faith and confidence in her ability to attain what she sets out to accomplish. As her efforts continue to pay off, she will feel encouraged and motivated by her successes, and her sense of personal competence will grow.

Here are some additional suggestions:

- Spend time with your child. Find activities you can do together that will make her feel successful—and that are fun, too, without winners and losers. Attend her soccer games and music recitals. Show her that you are interested in her and what she accomplishes. By giving time and energy to your child, you will convey a powerful message of love and acceptance.

- Treat your child as an important person. Encourage her to express herself, listen without judging, accept her feelings, and treat her with respect.

- Whenever possible, allow your child to make decisions and assume more responsibility in her life. Show your trust in her.

- Build close family relationships, and make your child feel that she is contributing to the family unit.

- Do not expose your youngster to, or confide in her about, adult topics or family/marital tensions that will cause her stress. Try to minimize her anxieties related to family crises and changes, providing her with as much continuity and stability as possible.

- Encourage your child to provide service to others—perhaps through Scouting or a similar type of program—in order to increase her sense of community, her feeling of belonging and being appreciated, and her sense of importance and personal worth.

- Teach your child to praise herself. She should feel pride in her accomplishments.

- Tell your youngster how much you love her, and what a good and lovable child she is—without any conditions or strings attached. Although parents' actions and efforts convey love indirectly, children also need to hear the words "I love you."

Boosting your child's self-concept will not happen overnight. It may take months or years, and it is an ongoing process. If your child is not responding to your attempts at helping her, however, and worrisome or serious problems persist, talk to your pediatrician about the need for professional assistance.

No matter what your child's self-esteem may be, your goal should continue to be to help her feel as good as possible about herself. Remain sensitive to what she is feeling, recognize and acknowledge her efforts and gains, and remain flexible and supportive in the way you approach her difficulties. Accept your child as the person she is, and help her feel good about herself and the person she is becoming. Keep in mind that the single most important factor in maintaining a child's self-esteem is the presence of an adult who demonstrates respect and acceptance and who provides support that conveys the message "I believe in you."

GENDER IDENTITY AND GENDER CONFUSION

Does your daughter refuse to wear dresses and like throwing a football with the boys in the neighborhood? Does your son have an interest in girls' clothes or cosmetics?

When middle-years children exhibit these kinds of behavior, their parents often are concerned, and many questions arise: Is my youngster's behavior abnormal? Should I be trying to change him or her? Does he or she need professional help?

Youngsters actually begin developing strong gender identities long before middle childhood. A child's awareness of being a boy or a girl starts in the first year of life. It often begins by eight to ten months of age, when youngsters typically discover their genitals. Then, between one and two years old, children become conscious of physical differences between boys and girls; before their third birthday they are easily able to label themselves as either a boy or a girl as they acquire a strong concept of self. By age four, children's gender identity is stable, and they know they will always be a boy or a girl.

During this same time of life, children learn gender role behavior—that is, doing things "that boys do" or "that girls do." Before the age of three they can differentiate sex-stereotyped toys (trucks, dolls) that are identified with boys or girls. By three years of age they have also become more aware of boy and girl activities, interests, and occupations; many begin to play with youngsters of their own sex in activities identified with that sex. For example, you probably saw your daughter gravitating toward dolls, playing house, and baking. By contrast, your son may have played more aggressive and active games and might have been attracted to toy soldiers and toy trucks. These gender role behaviors, including the toys children play with and activities in which they engage, are influenced by how youngsters are raised and what expectations are made of them.

In middle childhood, gender identification continues to become more firmly established, not only in children's interest in playing more exclusively with youngsters of their own sex, but also in their interest in acting like, looking like, and having things like their same-sex peers. During this time of life you will see your child express his or her gender identity through gender-specific role behavior, some of which began during the preschool years:

1. Through his or her toys, play activities, household tasks, and family roles. Most often, boys will choose to play "boy games" with masculine attributes, while girls will select "girl activities" with feminine characteristics.

2. Through social behavior that reflects varying degrees of aggression, dominance, dependency, and gentleness.

3. Through the manner and style of behavioral and physical gestures and other nonverbal actions that are identified as masculine or feminine.

4. Through social relationships, including the gender of the friends your child chooses and the people he or she decides to imitate. During the elementary-school years, children continue to be most involved with children of their own sex: boys playing mostly with other boys, and girls playing mostly with girls. Boys often voice a strong dislike of girls, and vice versa, during the early school years, perhaps as a means of strengthening their own gender identification.

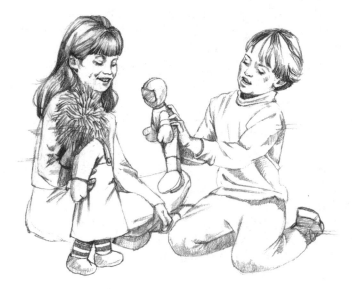

The gender-role behavior of children seems to be strongly influenced by their identification with the males and females in their lives. All children pick up characteristics from the men and women around them, incorporating these traits into their own personalities and value systems. They are also influenced by TV and sports heroes and adults in all other activities in their lives. Over time, the combined effect of these many influences may determine many of their masculine and feminine qualities. Perhaps more than any other factor, the subtleties of every child's relationship with his or her father and mother—and the attitudes of the parents toward each other and toward the child—will influence his or her gender-related behaviors.

Sexual Stereotypes

Stereotypes of masculine and feminine behaviors and characteristics permeate our culture. And when a child's aptitudes and interests deviate from these accepted norms, he is often subjected to discrimination and ridicule.

As a parent, it is natural for you to have concern about whether your youngster is accepted socially. You will probably find yourself trying to teach him social behaviors that will allow him to function well in this culture, even if they sometimes seem to run counter to his own interests and talents. However, you need to weigh your well-meant efforts at promoting conformity against your child's need to feel comfortable with and good about himself. Even if he

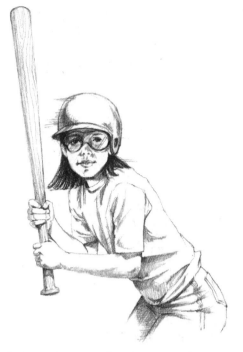

doesn't fit the accepted stereotypes—that is, even if your son doesn't excel in sports or even have an interest in them, for example—there will still be many other opportunities and areas in which he can excel. Each child has his own strengths, and at times, they may not conform to society's or your own expectations. Yet they can still be a source of his current and future success and self-satisfaction.

Ironically, social stereotypes evolve over time. In recent decades, there has been a tidal wave of change in gender roles and behaviors. Today, women are expected to be more assertive and "feminist" than their mothers and grandmothers were. Men are allowed and perhaps even expected to express their "softer," more compassionate, and more "feminine" side.

Thus, rather than force your own child into the mold of current or traditional gender behavior, help him fulfill his own unique potential. Don't become excessively concerned with whether his interests and strengths coincide with the socially defined gender roles of the moment. Let him evolve in his own way.

When Gender Identities Become Confused

Occasionally, children seem to display gender-role confusion. More than just lacking an interest in sports, for instance, some boys actually tend to identify with females. Likewise, some girls identify more with masculine traits. Conflicted about their gender, they may deny their sexuality. Rather than learn to accept themselves, they may come to dislike that part of themselves that is a boy or a girl.

At the extreme, a boy may seem more effeminate and have one or more of the following characteristics:

- He wants to be a girl.

- He desires to grow up to be a woman.

- He has a marked interest in female activities, including playing with dolls or playing the roles of girls or women.

- He has an intense interest in cosmetics, jewelry, or girls' clothes and enjoys dressing up in girls' apparel.

- His favorite friends are girls.

- On rare occasions, he may cross-dress and actually consider himself to be a girl.

Effeminate boys are sometimes ridiculed, teased as being "gay," and shunned by their peer group. This rejection may intensify as the boys get older. As a result, they may become anxious, insecure, or depressed and struggle with their self-esteem and social relationships.

On the other hand, girls who identify with boys are thought of as "tomboys." They usually encounter less social ridicule and peer difficulties than effeminate boys do. For many girls, some tomboyishness seems to be a very natural course toward healthy adolescent gender identity. Yet there are rare girls who exhibit one or more of the following traits:

- They express a wish to be a boy.

- Their preferred peer group is male.

- When playing make-believe games, they prefer male roles over female ones.

These traits suggest a conflict or confusion about gender and relationship with peers of the same sex. The possible causes of these variations are speculative and controversial. Research demonstrates a role for both biological factors and social learning in gender-identity confusion.

Family and parenting influences also might contribute to gender confusion. Family studies indicate that effeminate boys often have unusually close relationships with their mothers and especially distant relationships with their fathers. Research suggests that the mothers of some effeminate boys actually encourage and support "female" activities in their sons.

Parents of these children often ask whether gender confusion will influence their youngster's sexual preference and orientation later in life—that is, whether their child will become a homosexual. Long-term studies suggest that some (but certainly not all) effeminate boys and tomboyish girls do become bisexual or homosexual in late adolescence and adulthood.

What Should You Do?

If your middle-years child seems to have distortions and confusions in gender identity, discuss boy and girl, male and female behavior directly with him or her. For instance, talk with your child about the specific gestures or behavior that may provoke reactions from others, and identify together some that might be more appropriate. Through a sensitive dialogue, you might be able to help your child better understand his or her behavior and why it gets the responses it does from peers. Providing a lot of support for your child can bolster his or her self-esteem and counteract the social and peer pressures he or she might be facing.

In addition to your own efforts, talk with your pediatrician, who may suggest that you consult a child psychiatrist or child psychologist to help overcome the youngster's confusion and conflict. Consultation with a mental-health professional may be necessary when there are questions of gender identity, especially when any of the following are present:

- The child refuses to accept his or her biological sex.

- The child plays exclusively with youngsters of the opposite sex.

- The child is socially isolated at school and/or is teased or ridiculed by peers.

Early professional intervention can be helpful to the child and family by helping work through the confusion that may exist about a child's gender identity. However, there is little evidence that mental-health services can influence gender identity in the middle years.

Our society continues to move toward breaking down many of the sexual stereotypes that direct and limit our behavior, and creating an environment of greater sexual equity and balance. The need or desire for professional help should be guided to some extent by the discomfort of your family, and to a greater extent by the social discomfort of your child.

Sexual Orientation

A child's sexual orientation is a related area that may be of concern for some parents. A youngster's interests and behavior during middle childhood may cause mothers and fathers to worry that their offspring might be homosexual. They may inappropriately discipline the child or seek professional help to ensure that he becomes heterosexual.

However, this is a time when acceptance and support for your child should be paramount. An individual's physical and emotional attraction to a member of the same or the opposite sex appears to be a biological phenomenon. Some recent research has shown that the brains of homosexual men—specifically, the amount of tissue in parts of their hypothalamus—differ from those of heterosexual men. Only rarely, if ever, is sexual orientation caused by personal experiences and environment.

Your own child's sexual orientation is actually established quite firmly by the middle years. But since there is little opportunity to test and act out this orientation, it may not be evident to the family until adolescence or even later. Meanwhile, keep in mind that many children try out different ways of relating to their peers, and these can be confused with heterosexual or homosexual orientation.

The greatest difficulty for children and adolescents who are homosexual is the social pressure they feel to behave heterosexually, and the discrimination they may experience because of their sexual orientation. This may isolate them from their peers and even their family, and their self-esteem and self-confidence can suffer terribly in the process. A large proportion of teenage suicide attempts is linked to issues of gender confusion and to perceived rejection of an adolescent with a homosexual orientation.

Sexual orientation cannot be changed. A child's heterosexuality or homosexuality is deeply ingrained as part of them. As a parent, your most important role is to offer understanding, respect, and support to your child. A nonjudgmental approach will gain your child's trust and put you in a better position to help him or her through these difficult times. You need to be supportive and helpful, no matter what your youngster's sexual orientation may be.

9

DEVELOPING SOCIAL SKILLS

Good social skills are necessary for success, security, and adjustment in life, whether in the home, the classroom, the playground, or the community. When a child is able to interact well with others, she will develop and maintain resiliency when encountering stress and will be better able to compensate for shortcomings or failures in other parts of life. On the other hand, inadequate or inappropriate social skills—and the peer rejection that they may cause—can contribute to social, behavioral, emotional, and academic problems.

What are social skills? They are the verbal and nonverbal behaviors that occur during everyday social interactions. Some are innate; most are learned. Usually, children learn their social skills at home, with friends in the community, at school, or in places of worship. However, as these institutions change, the development of these skills is being affected. The American family structure, for instance, is in transition. More than ever before, mothers are working, and

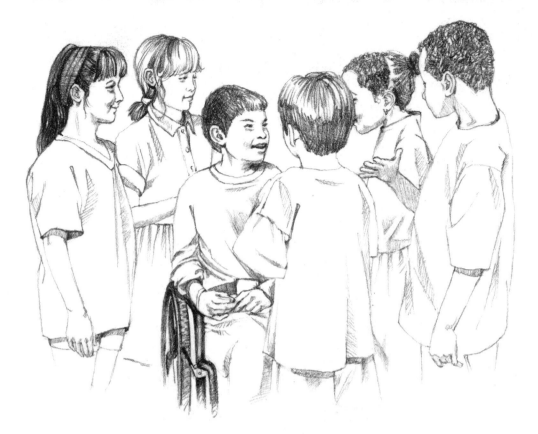

many children live in households with a single parent or as part of a stepfamily. No matter how the family is structured, it is not immune to marital, financial, or health-related stresses, which can interfere with a family's time together. Yet families are the primary place in which children learn social skills.

America's schools are also changing. The diversity of students is increasing, and schools are being called upon to respond to an ever-widening range of individual abilities and needs. School personnel, who are having to cope with budget changes, redistribution of funds, and increasing class size, have new and increasing responsibilities, including the need to attend to the complex emotional and social needs of children. As schools stretch limited resources to address the academic needs of their students, the development of social skills may not get all the attention it deserves.

Furthermore, children increasingly spend more time outside the family in a variety of peer-group organizations such as day care and preschool and after-school programs. As a result, time spent with other children is on the rise, increasing both the opportunity to learn and the need for good social skills.

Does Your Child Have Problems with Social Skills?

If you suspect that your child has difficulties with social interactions, the following questions might help pinpoint the problem.

Does your child have difficulty

- Entering and joining a group?
- Keeping a friend?
- Dealing with teasing and provocation?
- Effectively managing major conflicts?
- Successfully participating in group activities?
- Responding to failure or disappointment?
- Responding to success?
- Meeting the expectations of peers, parents, and teachers?
- Considering other people's feelings?

To help you understand how your child relates to others, talk to her teachers, coaches, and even friends (in a confidential, discreet manner). What are her strengths? What are her difficulties? Do the difficulties appear to be isolated incidents, related to a specific difficult situation or stress? Or are they long-term problems, repeated patterns that are leaving her unpopular and unhappy? If they tend to fall into the latter category, you'll need to take some action. Try to pinpoint the components of social interactions that create the most problems for your child—for instance, does she have trouble reaching out and "breaking the ice," even with just simple statements such as "How are you today?" Does she have difficulty keeping a conversation (or a game) going, settling disagreements without physical or verbal violence, and ending an activity pleasantly and appropriately? Answer the questions in the box above to get a better sense of where problems may lie.

IF YOUR CHILD HAS A PROBLEM

As a first step, find a quiet place to raise your concerns with your child. Ask some general, open-ended questions that might allow him to raise social issues that concern him. As sensitively as possible describe to him what you have heard and observed, and help him to discuss how he feels about it. With his help, identify the specific difficulties he is experiencing. Be sure to focus on specific behavior in a calm, supportive way so as not to make him feel worthless or hopeless. Even if his poor social skills irritate you or other family members, it is important not to make him feel ashamed and even more insecure. Avoid statements like "You'll never have a friend," "No wonder no one likes you," or "You're acting like a jerk."

Quite often, in order to maintain their self-esteem or avoid pain and embarrassment, children will deny that a problem exists in their lives, no matter how obvious. Even when a problem is acknowledged, they may have difficulty accepting responsibility for it and for its resolution. But the first, necessary step toward making the situation better is for both of you to acknowledge that a difficulty really exists, although it may take several attempts on your part.

Once the problem is identified and acknowledged, then there are actions you can take to help your child overcome his difficulties. Social skills can be learned. Be sure he really understands what the problems are, explaining them (without blame) in words that make sense to him. Avoid predictions of doom and gloom, and instead maintain an optimistic and hopeful outlook.

Here are some other suggestions:

- Teach him to think in terms of actions and consequences. If he alters his behavior in a particular way—for example, if he is willing to share his toys and games with the neighborhood children—help him see the positive consequences of that action, including a greater likelihood that he will be accepted and liked by his peers.

- Help him identify alternative behavior to replace the actions that are causing the difficulty. For example, if he tries to resolve conflicts by hitting other children, discuss more productive, socially acceptable ways of approaching the same situation, such as taking turns, walking away, or knowing when to back off before things heat up.

- Relate your child's particular problem—and its solution—to circumstances he is likely to face in the future. Help him anticipate situations that may arise, and discuss or even practice how he will respond to them. Remind him that everything will not necessarily always proceed according to plan, however, and that he will need to be flexible and adapt to unexpected turns of events.

- Remind him that social skills are not developed overnight, but are learned through practice, observation, discussion, and more practice until they become automatic and natural. He may find that practice works best when done in a role-playing situation, where a parent, sibling, or trusted friend plays the role of the child in order to demonstrate an alternative or appropriate behavior. Then the "players" switch roles so the child can practice and rehearse.

- Encourage your child to bring a playmate or classmate to your home, where you can observe their interactions and teach them some appropriate social behavior. Teaching children that "to have a friend you must be a friend" can be very powerful when opportunities are made to practice at home. If your child agrees that you can watch him play in order to help him make friends, you will have a powerful teaching opportunity.

- Assign your child a friend to be a "tutor" or "coach." Or have him observe peers with good social skills and talk with you or a teacher about what he sees.

- Help your child develop a skill or interest that will allow him to fit in with peers. This should be done in a way that suits your child and does not force him to change in ways that make him feel uncomfortable.

- Highlight your youngster's strengths and talents that make you proud of him, and that might be used to help overcome his social difficulties. Remind him that most of his peers probably have areas that they need to work on too.

SHOULD YOU SEEK PROFESSIONAL HELP?

Sometimes other problems are causing or contributing to your child's poor development of social skills. These might include family discord and stress, medical problems, emotional difficulties (depression, anxiety), or your youngster's speech and language difficulties or attention deficits. If you suspect that problems like these are making things worse, seek out advice from your pediatrician or other professional.

To deal with your child's specific difficulties with social skills, consider involving her in formal social skills training programs, which are available through behavioral psychologists or behavioral pediatricians. They are frequently offered in small group settings, so that children with similar problems can support one another as well as learn successful strategies for dealing with their own areas of concern. In general, those who fare best in these groups tend to be insightful and open to new ideas, have a good intellectual understanding of their situation, and are willing to discuss or role-play their problem with other youngsters who are learning to cope with similar difficulties.

Whether your child works with a therapist in a group or an individual setting, the professional should regularly assess your youngster's progress as she continues to meet new and more challenging situations.

Peer acceptance is one of the most gratifying experiences for children. By contrast, peer rejection or ridicule can take an enormous toll on a child's self-esteem and sense of security. As you help your child, remember to remain sensitive and supportive at every step. Set expectations at a realistic level; offer lots of praise, encouragement, and rewards for efforts and even small improvements. Your child's greatest reward for these efforts will be the gift of friendship.

FRIENDS

Children need friends. Through friendships, youngsters broaden their horizons beyond the family unit, begin to experience the outside world, form a self-image, and develop a social support system.

During the preschool years, play provides positive social encounters and increasing amounts of cooperative activity, which are the foundations of friendship. Aggressive behavior increases between ages two and four but then declines. Rules and social roles become increasingly important, and sex differences in social activities become more obvious. The stability of friendships also increases as children approach school age, and girls seem to develop more intense relationships with a few other children than do boys, who scatter their affection across a larger number of youngsters.

Between the ages of five and twelve, making friends is one of the most important missions of middle childhood—a social skill that will endure throughout their lives. Developmentally, school-age children are ready to form more complex relationships. They become increasingly able to communicate both their feelings and their ideas, and they can better understand concepts of time—past, present, and future. At this age they are no longer so bound to the family or so concerned mostly about themselves but begin relying on peers for companionship, spending more time with friends than they did during the preschool years. Day by day they share with one another the pleasures and frustrations of childhood.

Friends play many roles in a child's life, serving as companions, confidants, and allies, sharing advice and feelings, and providing stability and support in difficult times. Friends also supply feedback that allows children to measure, judge, and make adjustments within themselves, while answering the nagging and important question "How am I doing?" In some natural sequences, chil-

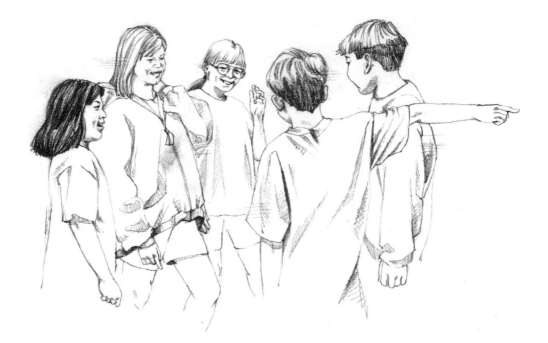

Making friends is one of the most important missions of middle childhood—a social skill that will endure throughout their lives.

dren move through stages in which their friendships first emphasize common activities and similarities in outlook, then are characterized by shared values and rules; finally, as puberty approaches, they focus on understanding others, self-disclosure, shared interests, and stronger emotional bonds.

Even so, youngsters differ in the rate at which they develop social skills. Also, some desire and need friends more than others. While certain children may be quite content spending most of their time by themselves, with family members, or with just a single best friend, others may be much more gregarious, forming and maintaining many friendships. The average school-age youngster has about five close friends. However, a child's preferences and needs may change from year to year and even from month to month. In most cases there is no reason for concern when a child decides to limit the number of his friends, unless he also seems depressed or is being rejected by his schoolmates.

Children also form friendships with siblings, especially in large or close families, or when families are isolated from other children and families. These sibling friendships may replace outside friends and the need for them.

Late in the middle years, peer influence is very evident. Friendships often evolve into highly exclusive cliques in which children strongly influence one another. At most schools there are a variety of cliques, each with its own hierarchy of members. Youngsters' attraction to particular friends may be based on anything from personality to extracurricular interests, from athletic ability to appearance. In these preadolescent years, youngsters in tightly knit inner circles may feel quite secure with one another, creating their own group identity by looking and talking alike, perhaps creating a secret handshake, and feeling much more "with it" than those on the outside looking in. These youngsters often feel a strong pressure to dress and talk in a particular way, listen to certain music, and wear their hair in a specific style. This peer pressure begins to compete (and sometimes clash) with the influence of parents and their values.

Pre-adolescents also tend to be quite judgmental, labeling others and at the same time becoming increasingly concerned about what their friends think of them. If a peer is even just a little different, they may conclude, "He's terrible; I just hate him."

In the early elementary school years, friends are almost always of the same sex. During the latter years of middle childhood, however, girls and boys begin to spend a little more time together. Girls may gossip with their girl-friends—and boys with their boyfriends—about whom they like and who is cute; even so, at this age there is no real dating, even though kids may talk of "going together." Sometime during adolescence they will finally begin to pair off in a more serious way.

Choosing Friends

A number of factors play a role in determining whom a child befriends. Some research shows that the friends a youngster chooses tend to share mutual traits with him and/or possess characteristics that he would like to have. Thus, as a child's preferences and goals change—which they inevitably do as he grows—he will make new friends to satisfy his evolving needs and desires and fit his own self-image.

Children also select friends with similar temperaments and patterns of play. Shy youngsters tend to be attracted to others like themselves; loud and boisterous children usually choose boisterous friends. Youngsters interested in the same activities and hobbies are drawn together as well.

Particularly in your youngster's early years, you as a parent often will arrange opportunities for him to spend time with playmates of your choosing. With the passage of time, however, he will begin making more choices of friends on his own, and you need to know with whom he is spending time, actively monitoring (if not supervising) that play.

A number of factors can come into play as your youngster selects his friends. If he feels good about himself, and if he has been loved and respected within the family, he is more likely to make good choices of friends. If you and your spouse relate to each other well, and if your child has caring and supportive relationships with his brothers and sisters, he will have seen and experienced positive examples of how people can relate, and he will carry these impressions over into his own friendships, including the friends he chooses. On the other hand, if those family experiences have not been supportive and confidence-boosting, he is likely to seek out peers who have similar types of troubles.

Take some time to help your child understand why he chooses the friends he does. This is an opportunity to discuss his own values, feelings, and behaviors.

A healthy friendship is one in which both children are on an equal footing. Neither child should dominate the other or make all the decisions on what activities to pursue. They should share and make an effort to please each other. They should also be capable of problem-solving on their own: If one boy wants to play with a particular toy that belongs to his buddy, they will probably work out a time schedule so that each can have a turn. Or they might devise alternative activities that they can do together.

Language skills are essential for building and solidifying a good friendship. During middle childhood, friends learn to communicate clearly with one another, sharing secrets, stories, feelings, and jokes. Children with language or speech problems often have difficulty making friends, frequently using inappropriate words and missing out on subtle messages and cues—verbal as well as nonverbal—from their peers.

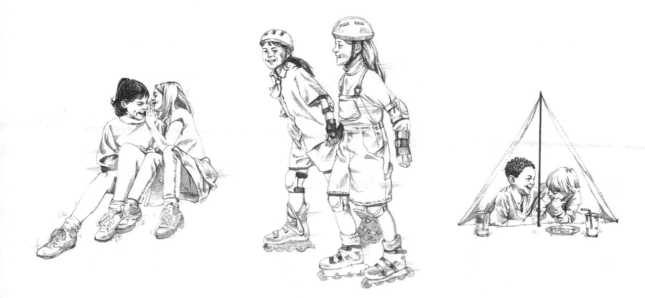

A "Best" Friend

In middle childhood some youngsters concentrate their social activity on a single best friend. In these relationships children usually match themselves with someone with whom they feel completely compatible, someone who is capable of meeting their needs for companionship, approval, and security.

These can be wonderful friendships, the kind that seem as though they will last a lifetime—sometimes they actually do. Even though parents often worry that exclusive friendships can be confining and stifling, and that their child has too much invested in this single relationship, most experts disagree. Sharing experiences, thoughts, and feelings with one special pal can often be more satisfying than spending time with a large group, as long as these two friends are having a positive influence on each other and are not excluding themselves from a broad range of experiences.

Dealing with Negative Peer Influence

What should you do if your child wants to play with the neighborhood troublemaker? What if he starts hanging out with a youngster who lies, destroys property, or bullies other children? What if he begins expressing values or attitudes you do not like? What if he adopts behaviors that are worrisome?

Dealing with negative peer influence is a challenge, but there are solutions. Some parents may demand that their own youngster stop spending time with this "bad influence," but this may not be the best strategy. Typically, children adamantly defend such a friend, and they may trivialize or rationalize his faults or shortcomings. They may ignore their parents, finding a way of seeing this playmate anyway. And if they do abide by their parents' wishes, other problems may ensue, since the children's own judgment and ability to make wise decisions independently are affected.

In most cases a better strategy is to reinforce positive friendships with other children whose behavior and values meet with your approval. Encourage your youngster to invite these children over to your house to play. Arrange activities that are somewhat structured, mutually enjoyable, and time-limited, such as bowling, bicycling, or watching a sporting event. Also, arrange summer events (camp, special weekend trips) that bring the children together.

At the same time, do not hesitate to express your displeasure over the less desirable playmates. Speak calmly and rationally when you explain why you would prefer that your child not spend time with them, focusing on specific behavior rather than generalizing or criticizing their character. Let him know the consequences if he ends up adopting the unacceptable behavior that you have seen in these other children, while still not absolutely forbidding him to play with them. This approach will teach your youngster to think more logi-

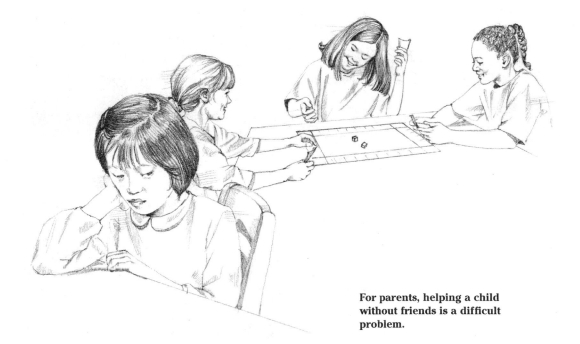

For parents, helping a child without friends is a difficult problem.

cally and assume responsibility for his actions, and show that you trust his growing capacity to make the right decisions.

CHILDREN WITHOUT FRIENDS

At one time or another, most children enjoy spending time alone. Perhaps after a long day at school or a busy weekend, they prefer just to relax by themselves, reading a book or playing a video game.

As normal as this type of behavior is, there may be cause for concern when a child has *no* friends, and especially when she feels lonely or socially inadequate. She may not get invited to parties, often sits alone during school lunch, is not picked to be part of a team, and receives few, if any, telephone calls.

Most children want to be liked, yet some are slow in learning how to make friends. Others may long for companionship but might be excluded from one group or another, perhaps picked on because of the way they dress, poor personal hygiene, obesity, or even a speech impediment. Youngsters are often rejected by peers if they exhibit disruptive or aggressive behavior. Still other children may hover on the fringes of one clique or another but never really get noticed. These neglected children spend most of their time alone.

In some cases, children do not have opportunities to make friends, which requires time and energy. They are too programmed in highly structured activities, live far away from school, live in areas without children's facilities or activities, or are bound tightly to their families.

A child without friends is, for parents, a difficult and painful dilemma. The problem is not uncommon; as many as 10 percent of school-age children say they have no best friend. These children may feel lonely and socially isolated and, as a result, have emotional and adjustment difficulties or fail to master the social skills so necessary for success with peers or adults.

To help your child resolve these social dilemmas, you will need skill and sensitivity. If your child senses that you are agonizing over—or are too intrusive toward—the problems in her social life, she may become overly anxious or defensive, perhaps even feeling that she has let you down by her inability to make friends. In response to your attempts at intervention, she may withdraw or deny that any problem exists. If she says, "Everything is just fine, Mom," she still may be aching for some friendships.

Understanding Your Child's Problems

As a parent, try to discover why your child is not happy with or is rejected by peers. From your adult perspective, your child's world may seem quite simple, but actually it is complex and demanding. For instance, on a playground your child may have to accomplish many tasks: entering a group, maintaining conversations, coordinating play, dealing with teasing and other forms of provocation, and resolving conflicts with others. Those are a lot of issues to handle, and if she is not adept at them, she may have difficulty making or keeping friends.

There are a variety of child-centered reasons why she may not have friends, including being rejected, neglected, or simply being a shy child. Rejected youngsters are overtly disliked by their peers and are constantly made to feel unwelcome. They often tend to be aggressive or disruptive and very sensitive to teasing. They may be bullies and rule-violators, or they may be so unsure of themselves that they invite the rejection of others. They might also be rejected because of their impulsive and disruptive behavior. Some of them may have attention deficits or hyperactivity.

Neglected children, on the other hand, are not overtly rejected and teased but are often just ignored, forgotten, not invited to parties, and are the last ones picked for a team. These youngsters may be perceived as loners but might be passive and detest their isolation. Others may actually prefer to be alone. This latter group might be respected and admired by others but simply feel more comfortable in solitary pursuits or in spending time with parents, siblings, other adults, or even pets. They may also lack the social skills and self-confidence necessary for them to enter social arenas, often because of limited social experiences. Or they may be more shy, quiet, and reserved than most of their peers.

Shyness

Although childhood shyness is commonplace, it concerns many parents, especially those who place great value on sociability. Some children become shy because of harsh life experiences, but most are born that way. For some middle-years children, social situations and interactions can be terrifying. When they come in contact with new children, they rarely feel at ease. Typically, they are unwilling or unable to make the first move, preferring to abandon a potential friendship rather than reach out to the unfamiliar. A few of these timid children may be emotionally distressed, but they are in the minority. In fact, some children are just naturally withdrawn and slow to warm up in new situations.

In some cases, shyness can be disabling. Extremely shy children often do not adapt as well as most of their peers in the classroom and on the playground. The longer this pattern exists, the more difficult it is for children to change. Shyness can increasingly lead to purposeful avoidance of social settings and withdrawal, and ultimately create an inability to function effectively as a social adult. If your child's shyness becomes debilitating, it may be caused by an anxiety disorder or a temperament pattern; then an evaluation by a child mental-health professional would be helpful.

Most shy children, however, do well in relationships and in social settings once they are past an initial period of adjustment. Children who have difficulty establishing and maintaining relationships even after the ice-breaking period merit more concern and attention. Eventually, many (and perhaps most) children who are shy learn to conquer their tendency. They function in ways that are not obviously timid or reticent, although inside they may still feel shy. Parents can gently guide or direct their children into social situations in which they can learn to successfully interact.

The Influence of Parenting Styles

Parents have their own temperaments, social skills, and parenting style that can influence a child's social abilities and her acceptance by peers. If you are highly critical, disapproving, rejecting, or aggressive, your child will tend to mimic your style and behave in a hostile and aggressive manner with her peers. By contrast, if you are generous, accepting, and patient, your child probably will adopt these same characteristics and do much better in making friends.

Some experts have categorized parenting into three styles:

Authoritarian parents tend to overcontrol their children, instituting a set of absolute rules and standards. As they emphasize a high degree of control, they may deemphasize warmth and trust. They also tend to assert their power by restricting privileges and even withdrawing love or approval. This parenting style may cause the child to feel rejected and isolated. She may develop only adequate social skills and will tend to remain dependent on her mother and father.

Permissive parents are at the other end of the spectrum. They demonstrate considerable warmth and affection, are generally very accepting, exercise a low level of control over their children, and make few demands upon them. Their children tend to become moderately independent and achieve modest degrees of social success.

Authoritative parents fall between these two extremes. While exercising considerable control, they also exhibit warmth and affection and seem to have appropriate expectations for their children. As their youngsters move through the middle years of childhood, the parents recognize the growing maturity of their offspring, encourage appropriate levels of responsibility, and use reason and negotiation in resolving differences. Their children tend to be independent and socially successful.

The way you relate to your child also can be influenced by the child herself. If your child is temperamentally difficult, for instance, you may react by becoming more anxious, aggressive, negative, and controlling, and less nurturing and less likely to respond positively. As a result, your child may grow up insecure and lacking appropriate social skills, and she may experience difficult interactions with peers.

Social Influences

Although children sometimes feel they are the sole cause of their lack of friends, that is not the case. Friendship is a two-way, dynamic process that depends on how children perceive one another. In middle childhood, youngsters tend to see one another in absolute terms, often lacking appreciation for more subtle individual differences or unique characteristics—a situation that sets the groundwork for rejection or neglect.

Often, an unpopular child develops a self-image or a reputation among her peers that is difficult to alter. Even if the youngster makes improvements in her social style, labels and peer perceptions are hard to change. Children may decide to cling to their biases, and thus even when the unpopular youngster has finally moved into a group, she may not be fully accepted or welcomed. So although technically she may no longer be an outsider, she still may experience feelings of loneliness, isolation, and diminished self-esteem.

While some unpopular children can change their behavior, others cannot and continue to behave in a way that interferes with their ability to make friends. Some youngsters simply have difficulty acquiring the new social skills they need. Others actually are not even aware that they are having trouble with relationships. Still others have come to expect rejection as part of their lives, and these expectations become self-fulfilling prophecies keeping them from behaving in ways that would promote friendships. Sometimes several of these influences are at work at the same time, reinforcing one another.

When families live in rural, isolated areas far from school, there may be few opportunities for children to socialize after school or on weekends. Some communities do not have activity programs in which youngsters can participate together. A family's financial stress, or frequent changes of jobs and homes, can add to the difficulty of making friends.

What Parents Can Do

When your child seems to be lacking friends and is hurting because of it, you need to get involved as soon as possible. As a first step in helping your child overcome her loneliness and isolation, you and your youngster need to acknowledge that a problem exists. In a sensitive, supportive manner, talk about this situation together. Although denial, sadness, embarrassment, or rationalization are normal responses, you and your child need to get beyond them.

Maintain Open Communication at Home. Encourage your youngster to talk openly about her concerns and difficulties regarding friendships. She is much more aware of her social scene than you are, so be a good listener. At the same time, this is an extremely sensitive subject, and problems may be difficult for your youngster to acknowledge. Her own insights and understanding of the group dynamics may be limited.

Avoid downplaying the social problems that your child is having with her peers. When your youngster is in pain, if you offer only simple reassurance, you may communicate that you neither understand nor care. For example, if peers are calling her a wimp or a nerd, do not advise her just to ignore them. That is like asking an adult not to be concerned when she loses her job. Be accepting, nonjudgmental, and very sympathetic.

Find Balance Between Empathy and Responsibility. In many cases your child may be able to solve her social problems without your direct intervention. If she is being excluded from the basketball games at the playground on Saturday afternoons, for instance, nothing could be worse for her stature among her peers than for you to show up and insist that she be allowed to play. ("Look who needs her mommy to stick up for her!") Also, if you constantly rescue her, she will become overly dependent on you, or resent your well-intentioned efforts, rather than find solutions on her own.

Ask Some Key Questions. Parents can ask some direct questions of their child, but there is a fine line between being interested and being intrusive and interrogating. Cautiously try to get a sense of how your child views the situation she finds herself in. Pose questions like:

- Are you pretty popular?

- Who is popular? Why are they popular? Is it because other kids like them, or is it because they want to be like them?

- Are there any children you can really talk to and trust?

- Do the children you know call each other names? What kinds of names do they use? Do you ever get called names?

- Is there a particular group you would like to be part of, or someone you would like to be friends with?

- Do you worry about what other children think of you?

Observe Your Child. If appropriate—and without embarrassing your youngster—observe your child when she is with some of her peers, perhaps at a pizza parlor restaurant, an athletic event, or a movie. See how she comes across, what her mood is like, and what actions may create conflict or isolation.

Later, talk with your child about what has occurred and together see if there are other ways she might have interacted with her friends. Focus on specific, concrete behavior, and use real-life examples. For instance: "At the pizza parlor I noticed that you took a few sips out of Emily's soft drink. How do you think she felt about that? What might you have done differently? Did you feel you were being yourself with your friends, or were you trying to act differently because they were there?"

In order to help your child when she is having difficulty making friends, you must understand the specific problems she faces. Besides observing her interactions in various situations, you might tactfully gather information from siblings and peers. Find out about the peer groups and cliques with which your youngster has to deal. Also, learn as much as you can about what takes place at particularly vulnerable sites, away from adult supervision, like bus stops, lunchrooms, and bathrooms. You might even videotape your child's social interactions—at a birthday party, for instance—so you can study them more closely.

Peer Relationship Skills

Successful peer interactions require a variety of skills and special ways of interacting. Parents should look for these skills in their children and help develop and model them.

Coping with failure and frustration

Coping with success

Coping with change and transitions

Coping with rejection and teasing

Managing anger

Using humor

Forgiving

Apologizing

Refusing to accept a dare

Thinking up fun things to do

Expressing affection

Avoiding dangerous situations

Defending himself

Comforting someone

Sharing

Making requests

Self-disclosure

Giving a compliment

Expressing appreciation

Coping with loss

Sticking up for a friend

Doing favors

Asking for help

Helping others

Keeping secrets

Get Information from School. Ask your child's teacher or the playground supervisor at school how she interacts with other youngsters. Inquire about her social interactions, not only in the classroom but also in those vulnerable ar-

Why Some Children Don't Have Friends

Children may have social problems for a wide variety of reasons, some of which are outside their control—and yours. Following are some of the factors that might be contributing to your child's difficulty in making or keeping friends.

Child-Related Influences

Temperament (difficult, shy)

Attention problems/hyperactivity

Learning disabilities

Social skill problems

Communication skill difficulties

Delayed physical, emotional, or intellectual development

Physical handicap

Chronic illness, frequent hospitalizations, school absenteeism

Poor gross motor skills, limiting participation in group activities

Emotional difficulties (depression, anxiety, low self-esteem)

Poor personal hygiene

Unattractive physical appearance

Child chooses or prefers to be alone

Child derives social satisfaction and friendship mainly from family members

Cultural values do not fit those of peers

Parent-Related Influences

Parenting style (too authoritarian, too permissive) adversely affects child's social development

---

eas. The bus driver may provide some useful information about interactions in the bus.

The teacher may have impressions of whether your youngster comes on too strong, or whether she is withdrawn. You may find that she has some eccentric habits that make her the butt of jokes or bullying among her peers. The teacher may have some suggestions on what your child can do to make friends or identify other children with like interests. Also, a group of young-

Parent keeps child too busy with programmed activities, chores, or jobs that limit time, energy, or opportunities for developing friendships

Parent is overly critical or negative of child's choice of friends

Parent has poor social skills; child does not have a good role model

Parent has depression or mental illness

Parent has substance abuse problem

Parenting style includes domestic chaos or violence

Parents experience marital stress, tension, abuse

Parent overprotects child or imposes excessive limits on activities

Parent has difficulty adjusting to child's individuality or special needs

Social-Environmental Influences

Family lives in rural, isolated area

Family residence is far from school

Neighborhood has few other children

Family goes away all summer

Family experiences financial stress and frequent moves

Family has cultural or language differences

Community has few opportunities or programs for children to gather and socialize

Danger of violence in usual play areas prevents children from interacting

Child's peer group perceives differences in dress, values, and behavior

sters with similar needs might benefit from a few sessions with a qualified professional.

Initiate a Plan. With this information in hand, you might be able to focus on specific problems and guide your child in appropriate directions, perhaps developing a strategy for entering into a group activity and practicing how to start and maintain conversations and deal effectively with minor and major conflicts.

Spend a few minutes talking with her about the perspective of other children—what they might think of her and what they consider important. By encouraging her to talk with you about her struggles with friendships, you will have the opportunity to guide and teach her how to get along. And if you maintain and nurture other areas of gratification and success, you can help your child become resilient and persistent in her attempts to gain success in the social domain.

Direct Your Child. A child in this position needs help and guidance to find social events or initiate activities. Guide her into situations where she is likely to meet other youngsters and develop friendships. Encourage her to invite someone in her class to spend the night at your home, or to accompany your family on an outing to the beach.

To increase your child's likelihood of success, suggest that she spend time with peers whose temperaments and interests are similar to her own. More active girls, for instance, tend to have greater camaraderie with equally active playmates. Try to assist your youngster's entry into the group by encouraging her to build one or two special friendships. Pick the friend your child seems closest to, and one who seems to have a similar temperament, and provide them with opportunities to spend time together, first in relatively brief, structured activities, and then in progressively less structured ones. Short visits and structured activities are usually the easiest first steps.

As a starting point, invite your child's friend to go bowling or to a sporting event, a movie, or a play—something where the two of them won't have to engage in much conversation *face to face* but can do something together *side by side.* Let them warm up gradually with an activity that has a definite end, rather than an open-ended day at the beach or "spending the afternoon." Usually if the activity itself is pleasurable and time limits are brief, the odds of success increase dramatically. Unstructured activities can follow if the initial encounters are successful and might be at a selected place—a park or a playground—or simply be at home without designated things to do. Your own discreet monitoring may be necessary to prevent any potential problems.

As these friendships develop, get to know your child's playmates better. Encourage your youngster to invite them over to your house to play. Also, make contact with the parents of her friends. Keep the lines of communication open between families.

Identify Your Child's Strengths or Interests. Encourage your child to use her strengths to make friends. If she has a good sense of humor, for example, she might be able to take advantage of it in a class play or other situation where she is likely to be appreciated by peers. If she likes animals, she might meet others with the same interest, go to the zoo with them, watch nature/wildlife videos together, or do a group project.

Carefully Select Social Activities. Encourage your child to avoid situations that are likely to lead to embarrassment. For instance, if your youngster is poorly coordinated, organized sports may be a poor choice. Instead, help her take advantage of her strengths, selecting activities where she can excel. Or involve her in individual noncompetitive sports activities.

Ask your child if she would like to sign up for a Scouting program or other group activity, an excellent way to meet and share experiences with a group of children the same age. Look into the group composition and activities of the Scout troop beforehand, making sure that your child fits in with the other youngsters. Be cautious of activities that are so competitive that conventional friendships are not emphasized.

For shy children, a summer camp can also bring them out of their shell. Camp can be particularly useful if it keeps youngsters involved without appearing to force them to interact.

Finding the right camp is critical. For a child who is very shy, or who has never been away from home before and may experience homesickness, a day camp may be best for the first camping experience. A child who is physically inept might not do well in a typical camp; there are alternative camps that specialize in computers, writing, and nature study.

When a child is having social difficulties, describe them beforehand to the adult leaders (camp counselors, church leaders) of the programs in which she participates. Ask these adults to give your youngster a little more attention if problems arise, and to provide you with ongoing feedback.

Tutor a Skill. If your child has some skill but not enough to satisfy her own need to succeed or to be admitted into the circle of children with better skills, individual lessons may be helpful. Depending on the skill, a relative, local coach, teacher, or older student may help your child develop her skills to the point where they may build her self-esteem and enhance her popularity. These skills might include sports, music, or writing. Or again, a specialized camp or weekend workshop may be the ideal niche.

Seek Professional Help. When your child has serious difficulties making friends, and when your own initial efforts at helping her are unsuccessful, seek the help of your pediatrician, a child psychologist, or another professional with expertise in behavioral problems. These professionals might suggest programs to help your youngster develop her social skills. Child counseling or family therapy can often help point a youngster in the right direction toward developing positive friendships. Parent training might be part of these therapeutic efforts, helping you to recognize, reinforce, and reward your child's positive behavioral changes.

Other problems (like attention deficits, learning disabilities, or emotional problems) might be contributing to social difficulties. Children with these problems can benefit from professional help.

Remember that your child's ability to make and maintain friends is closely intertwined with her success and self-esteem. If she is hurt and frustrated by her loneliness and isolation, you must help her acquire the confidence and social skills she needs in order to get along with her peers and enjoy the benefits and pleasures of friendships.

10

RAISING A SON,
RAISING A DAUGHTER

W hat are the unique challenges parents face in raising sons versus daughters? Even in these "gender-neutral" times, you've probably noticed significant differences between your sons and daughters (besides the obvious physical ones). Your own boys and girls may have varying interests. Their skills and aptitudes may differ. So might their styles of play, and the way they relate to friends.

In fact, boys and girls *are* different. Researchers, however, disagree on whether these differences are attributable to nature or nurture. Are they the result of genetics? Or is social conditioning primarily responsible? In this ongoing debate, there are no definitive answers. Some investigators believe differences between the sexes can be traced back to the womb, where the developing brains of boys and girls are exposed to varying hormones. But other investigators insist that these variations are primarily environmental in nature. After all, they say, boys and girls are often treated differently by the adults in their lives, including parents and teachers who often praise them for "gender appropriate" behavior and activities. At the same time, as children move through the middle years, they turn increasingly to their culture—peers and the media—as a guide to how they're supposed to look and behave.

Certain gender differences, while present in the first years of life, become even more evident in school-age children. In this chapter, we'll take a look at the differences between boys and girls ages five to twelve. Keep in mind, of course, that the descriptions that follow are generalizations. Although *most* boys and girls have these gender-specific characteristics and patterns of behavior, all boys are not alike, nor are all girls.

SONS

That cute baby boy whom you cuddled in your arms shortly after his birth has changed dramatically since then. Now, during his school-age years, here are some of the characteristics you may see in him.

Play

All children engage in pretend play. However, the themes of this play tend to differ between the sexes. Boys may assume the role of a heroic character (perhaps one that they've seen on television), and engage in fantasy activities that involve righteous combat or danger. They may want to wear a Superman cape, put on a Batman costume, play with swords, or wrestle with playmates. They might pretend to be cowboys, soldiers, or policemen. Boys in the middle years are also drawn to toys that move; that's why they like to play with trucks and balls.

In general, boys need opportunities to express themselves physically. They are more prone to engage in roughhousing than girls. In nearly every culture that has been studied, boys are more aggressive than girls on the playground.

One study found that boys spend much of their playtime participating in games, the majority of which are competitive; in fact, during play, fourth- and fifth-grade boys engage in competitive games about fifty percent of the time, compared to one percent for girls. Boys are also very focused on the rules of the games they're playing, and often argue with playmates over them ("You broke the rules!"). Boys are typically allowed and sometimes encouraged to be assertive, outspoken and loud, and their excesses are dismissed with the explanation, "Boys will be boys." However, you should guide your son toward channeling his aggressiveness in constructive ways, including burning off energy in physical play rather than confrontation. Roughhousing and fighting, although common among boys in this age group, tend to decline during the later years of middle childhood.

Remember that although these gender-specific patterns are commonplace, individual differences can be strong and often supersede group identities.

Friends and Social Relationships

There are both similarities and differences in the way boys and girls form and nurture their friendships. In the middle years, same-sex playmates are more the rule than the exception for boys as well as girls (just as it was during the preschool years). Even in school settings where children have a wide choice of friends, they are about ten times as likely to play with youngsters of the same sex. On the playground, boys and girls tend to play apart. In school cafeterias, there appear to be unofficial "boys' tables" and "girls' tables."

Boys need a peer group in which they can be part of a group, where they can relax and yet feel powerful. They tend to choose friends who have interests similar to their own, perhaps a shared love of soccer or collecting baseball cards, while girls may look for friends with compatible personalities. Boys are likely to play outdoors with friends, and they tend to "run in a pack" of boys. Compared with girls, boys are less likely to have a "best friend." (Also see "Friends," pages 152–157.)

Academics

Even in elementary school, teachers treat boys and girls differently. Academic expectations tend to be higher for boys; both teachers and often their own parents expect them to do better in school. Boys are called upon more frequently in class. They also get more of everything from the teacher—time, praise, and criticism.

Boys do better than girls with visual tasks, which is one reason why boys are attracted to video games. But boys are also more likely to have learning disabilities and problems with language. Even so, academic failure by boys is often attributed to external influences, while success is attributed to their abilities. (Also see "Academic/Teacher Problems," pages 493–494.)

Emotional Development and Self-Esteem

Boys in the middle years tend to lag behind girls in many areas of emotional development. Because they may have been encouraged to "be tough," many boys have difficulty articulating their feelings, and thus they are inclined to express themselves physically. By the age of nine, in fact, many boys have learned to repress their feelings—except for anger. For example, research has found that in the first year or two after their parents divorce, boys tend to become more aggressive, a phenomenon not commonly seen among girls in divorced families. However, when pressed, an obviously troubled boy may say something like, "I don't know how I feel." And they honestly don't know! Boys of this age are adventurous and rambunctious, and generally not inclined toward introspection and talking about their feelings.

Although boys and girls in the middle years have very similar rates of mental health problems, boys are more likely to receive mental health services. That's generally because their symptoms—including aggressive and hyperactive behavior—are more often visible to their parents and other adults.

Boys need as much or more emotional support and guidance as girls. They need to have emotional opportunities to foster their awareness of feelings and their ability to express their needs. One of your tasks as a parent is to make sure that your son is prepared to meet the challenges of childhood and adulthood with a more well-rounded perspective than, "I can only react by being tough . . . by suppressing my feelings." Let him know that it's often appropriate to say things like, "This scares me," that he doesn't have to hide these kinds of feelings.

In raising a son, show him respect, have a sense of humor, and make an effort to stay close and connected. Frequently, it takes an older male—a father, an uncle, or another role model—to support a boy's emotional maturation, and help him grow into a socially responsible, sensitive adult. (Also see "Self-Esteem," pages 132–140.)

Sports and Physical Activity

Both boys and girls require plenty of opportunities for physical activity. More children of both sexes are participating in organized sports than ever before. These activities are an opportunity for them to master physical skills. But perhaps more important, sports are ways in which sons and daughters can develop self-esteem and discipline, and learn social skills like teamwork and sportsmanship.

Competitive physical activities offer middle-years youngsters opportunities to develop their personalities and self-confidence. Boys, especially, are inclined to judge themselves by whether they're equal or superior to their peers on the Little League or youth soccer fields. Competition is also a way for boys and girls to learn to deal effectively with pressure and stress. Encourage your child to stay physically fit, which can enhance self-esteem and a sense of well-being.

In general, boys are more interested in sports than girls are, even as spectators. They are more likely to watch games on television, wear T-shirts with the names of their favorite teams emblazoned on them, and collect trading cards featuring baseball or other sports stars. (Also see "Sports Programs," pages 110–120.)

DAUGHTERS

Play

During play, your daughter is less likely to pretend to be the heroic figure commonly seen among boys; instead, the play of girls often revolves around school or domestic themes (they may rock their "baby" to sleep or apply a Band-Aid to their doll).

During play, your daughter is less inclined than her brother to physically fight with playmates. Instead, she'll settle differences by talking them out. If there are disagreements about the rules, girls are more likely than boys to suggest a compromise, saying "Let's make the rules different," or "Let's play a different game." They are less likely to yell at one another, feeling it's more important to maintain the relationship than to prevail during a disagreement. Their games are more inclined to involve turn-taking than those of boys.

Keep in mind that children learn from their play, so guide your daughters (and your sons) into a broad array of experiences. They should be given toys and directed into activities that go beyond the stereotypes of their sex. Thus, while it's fine to give your daughter a doll, also present her with traditional boys' toys, as well as with materials that she can play creatively with, giving her opportunities to make something with clay, cloth, or feathers.

Friends and Social Relationships

There seem to be fundamental gender differences between the way girls and boys perceive themselves and relate to the world around them. Compared with boys, girls are far more likely to have their personal identities tied to their friendships, which are primarily with other girls. Their sense of self is organized around being able to make and maintain these relationships. Much more than boys, girls appreciate and seem to need connections to other people. Because of this tendency, girls generally judge themselves as successful when they are caring and responsible. Girls also tend to talk about and assess their friendships much more than boys do.

In our culture, girls are raised to relate in so-called face-to-face intimacy, and thus are inclined to have conversationally based interactions with their girlfriends. These conversations are intended to create and maintain relationships. Yes, boys talk to one another, but their interactions tend to be "side-by-side intimacy," organized around an activity (playing with a tractor or a video game) or similar interest.

More than boys, girls are likely to have a "best friend" or two, although those special friends may change frequently. They will share their secrets with and write confidential notes to their best friend. Girls often hold hands, give hugs to each other, and arrange social occasions just to be together, not because a particular activity is planned.

Your eleven- or twelve-year-old daughter may discuss her relationships at the dinner table, while boys are less likely to talk in this way. Girls are also more inclined to become emotionally distressed when a friendship breaks up or when they move away from their best friend.

The natural tendency toward gender-segregated friendships in the middle years has an unfortunate consequence. It limits the opportunities for girls and boys to get to know and appreciate one another before the sexual attraction of puberty places them together. Ideally, girls need boys as friends (and vice versa) if they are to have good relationships as teenagers and good marriages as adults. You should encourage and provide opportunities for your school-age daughter to play with boys. However, you are likely to meet with some resistance. Girls of this age simply prefer to play with girls, and boys with boys.

As girls move through their middle years and approach adolescence, they tend to be reluctant to take risks in relationships for fear of displeasing others. They may refrain from asserting themselves and taking credit for their accomplishments. They may avoid criticizing or disagreeing with others, or to make their likes, wants, and needs known. They may have trouble saying no to someone with whom they have an important relationship. When girls have conflicts, they often avoid direct confrontation, and rather retaliate by attempting to damage the other girl's friendships or social status.

Academics

School-age girls have some advantages over the boys in the classroom. In general, girls seem able to pay attention longer than boys. Verbal skills also tend to mature earlier in girls.

Traditionally, girls perform better in English and as well or better than boys in mathematics through about the fifth and sixth grades. But on the brink of adolescence, and during the teenage years, the top-performing girls often begin doing less well in math than they once did. By the time your middle-years daughter reaches high school, the top performing math students in her class will disproportionately be boys.

What's the reason for this? Teachers often have lower expectations for girls in math, and may have biases in favor of boys. Research shows that teachers are more likely to call on boys during math instruction.

The gap between girls and boys may be narrowing, however, because many school districts are making efforts to encourage and support girls in mathematics. In some schools, administrators have instituted girls-only math and science classes, believing that girls will feel more confident and less intimidated in this learning environment (some research shows that poor achievement in math is preceded by a loss of confidence in the subject).

Of course, girls *can* do well in math and science, and their own beliefs and self-confidence in this area are influenced strongly by parents (low expectations can be a self-fulfilling prophecy). Let your daughter know that your hopes for her in school are just as high as they are for her brothers, and that careers in math and science are just as appropriate for her as for boys.

Emotional Development and Self-Esteem

Girls mature emotionally earlier than boys. In the middle years, they find it easy to express their emotions verbally, and their self-esteem tends to be strong and resilient. They may be full of themselves—confident, adventurous, secure, and certain of their ability to do valuable things in the world. From their youthful point of view, anything is possible.

However, as girls approach and enter adolescence, their self-esteem can become more fragile. In about one third of girls, a decline in self-esteem becomes pronounced and long-lasting. Sadness, anxiety, and eating disorders are more prevalent in girls on the brink of becoming teenagers. Between the ages of eleven and thirteen, some girls lose much of their emotional strength and spirit. They may develop a crisis in confidence and become depressed. Their optimism dampens, and they become less likely to take chances. By adolescence, girls are much more likely than boys to say that they are "not good enough" to attain all of their dreams.

By the time girls enter high school, less than one third of them report being happy with the way they are. When it comes to body image, negative feelings can begin much earlier. As young as the age of seven, many girls start becoming self-critical of their bodies, and up to fifty percent of nine-year-old girls have already tried dieting. Some may find themselves on the fast track to eating disorders, which are often associated with depression and even thoughts of suicide.

Particularly as girls enter adolescence, they become more reluctant to assert themselves and take credit for their accomplishments. They may refrain from criticizing or disagreeing with others, or making their likes, wants, and needs known. They may set less challenging and lofty goals, and may see their futures with more uncertainty.

Of course, this need not be the case. As a parent, you should help your middle-years child hold on to her strong sense of confidence and self-worth. Recognize and reinforce your youngster's positive traits. Applaud her efforts and achievements at every opportunity. And to counter some of the messages that girls get from the media that her appearance is crucial, help your daughter value the things she *does* rather than how she looks.

Since adolescence threatens to diminish individuality, parents should help children discover their unique talents and interests. Support your child in the belief that it is okay to be different—that difference is special and valued. Talk with your youngster about things she likes about herself, and about things you particularly like as well.

Also, talk with your daughter about her dreams and her anxieties, and what may be getting in the way of feeling good about herself. Encourage her to believe that she can become anything she chooses. Help her find opportunities to experience success, and reward her when she is assertive and shows pride in her accomplishments.

Sports and Physical Activity

Most parents recognize that it's just as important for girls to be physically active and fit as boys. Fortunately, today's school-age girls have more chances to participate in organized sports—from softball to soccer to gymnastics—than their mothers and grandmothers ever did.

As with boys, girls can learn many lessons about life through their athletic participation, including teamwork, perseverance, risk-taking, and strategic thinking. Even so, girls are more likely to encounter limitations associated with their athletic participation. Parents often worry more about girls' getting hurt, and some parents still think that competitiveness (not to mention getting dirty) is neither feminine nor "ladylike." Too often, expectations are communicated that boys are inherently better equipped than girls to compete in sports.

Emphasize the positive in your daughter's physical activity, whether she's running track or dancing ballet. Encourage her to develop her athletic skills in accordance with her interests and capabilities. Sports are a valuable environment in which she can prove her competence and enjoy success.

Helping Your Daughter or Son Excel

The transition into puberty and adolescence can be difficult. You can promote your child's successful development throughout the middle years by:

1. Talking about those things your youngster values and about which he or she feels passionate.

2. Discussing the qualities your child likes about himself or herself.

3. Teaching your child to appreciate and respect his or her gender as well as the opposite sex.

4. Encouraging your child to take credit for his or her achievements.

5. Recognizing your youngster's strengths and skills, as well as limitations.

6. Pushing your child to be socially assertive, and asking for things that he or she needs or wants.

7. Encouraging your child to express feelings and beliefs.

8. Helping your youngster set limits with friends and say no to them when appropriate.

9. Providing opportunities and encouragement to develop talents and interests.

10. Encouraging your child to take leadership roles.

11. Teaching your youngster honor, respect, and integrity.

12. Being a good role model as a parent.

DOES GENDER-NEUTRAL CHILDREARING WORK?

Some families try hard to treat all their children similarly, regardless of sex. But this type of childrearing can deny inherent differences among youngsters. Also, even when gender-neutral childrearing is attempted, it is very difficult to accomplish. Friends and relatives often treat boys and girls differently, even when parents do not. Television shows, magazines, books, and toys surround children with images of what boys and girls, and men and women, are supposed to be, and experiences not only shape a child's sense of who he or she is, but also what he or she believes can be accomplished in life.

Gender-neutral childrearing has the advantage of helping parents and youngsters identify universally desirable human traits and values they would like to adopt and promote. It also might enhance relationships between boys and girls (and men and women). However, keep in mind that boys and girls are sometimes inclined toward different interests and behaviors. If you ignore biological differences, you can deny children the opportunities to build on their innate strengths.

At the same time, encourage both your sons and daughters to participate in the full range of human experience. That means girls need to know that it is all right to be angry, to get dirty, and to be physically intense. Boys need to know it is okay to care deeply about friendships and not to finish first every time. Help your child discover and develop his or her unique talents and interests.

11

DEALING WITH PREJUDICE

S adly, nearly four decades after the civil rights movement of the 1960s, our children are growing up in a society in which prejudice and bigotry are still commonplace. Although laws have been implemented and many attitudes have changed, bigotry based on racial, ethnic, and religious grounds remains too much a part of the daily lives of children and families.

Our children are growing up in a time when the racial and ethnic composition of our country is rapidly changing. In some areas of the nation, groups of people previously characterized as racial or ethnic minorities make up the majority of the population.

Children are also being exposed to different cultures through the media. They are learning and forming opinions about people and events all over the country and the world. As a result, there is more of a need and opportunity to help children learn to understand and value diversity.

Children's encounters with prejudice are not confined to ethnic and racial stereotypes and bias. Every day, children are exposed to the way some individuals are valued more or less because of their gender or age. Young children may or may not be aware of the preferential treatment boys tend to receive from their teachers over girls. But they are very much aware that their feelings, opinions, and beliefs receive less consideration because of their youth. As children approach adolescence, they also become increasingly aware of the more subtle prejudices and intolerances tied to differences in social class and religion.

Children can suffer from a climate of prejudice. Prejudice creates social and emotional tension and can lead to fear and anxiety and occasionally hostility and violence. Prejudice and discrimination can undermine the self-esteem and self-confidence of those being ridiculed and make them feel terrible, unaccepted, and unworthy. When that happens, their school performance often suffers, they may become depressed and socially withdrawn, and childhood can become a much less happy time.

It is critical that you help your child deal with diversity in a positive way. Prejudice is learned at a very young age from parents, other children, and people and institutions outside of the family. By about four years of age, children are aware of differences among people, primarily in characteristics like appearance, language, and names, but later they are aware of religious and cultural distinctions as well. To some extent, children begin to define and identify themselves through their understanding of these personal differences. This is normal.

As youngsters try to make sense of these individual distinctions, they may hear and accept simplified stereotypes about others. When that happens, they not only develop distorted views of the youngsters and adults they encounter in daily life, but they may start to deny and overlook the common, universal human elements and traits that would bring people together. As a result, intolerance may develop where there should be friendship.

TAKING ACTION

As a parent, don't ignore the prejudice to which your child may be exposed in the media or in his own experience. Keep in mind that you serve as the most powerful influence and role model for your youngster, and more than anyone else, you can mold his attitudes and his behavior toward others. Here are some guidelines to follow:

1. Your actions toward the people in your life will lay the foundation for how your child relates to his peers and others. Examine your attitudes and the way you feel about people with traits and characteristics different from your own. Consider the different roles, relationships, and responsibilities within your own household, and what forms of age or

gender discrimination may occur there. If you want your child to be free of prejudice, you need to demonstrate that attitude in your words and deeds.

2. Nothing is more powerful in dispelling myths and stereotypes than person-to-person contact. Bring diversity into your own life. Make your friends and co-workers of different races and religions regular participants in your family's activities. Let your child experience that there are more similarities than differences among people. It is valuable to expose him to cultures and holidays different from his own: For example, with the cooperation of friends and neighbors, gentile children can attend a Bat Mitzvah or Passover seder, while Jewish youngsters can go to a church service or baptism. But your child should understand that these are only limited aspects of the differences and diversity that surround them.

3. Children initially focus on differences in physical appearance. In language appropriate for your child's age, explain why people have different skin and eye color, hair type, and other features. Discuss how differences in appearance are inherited from mothers and fathers. Talk about the diversity of your own child's ethnic heritage. At the same time, point out the similarities among all people, such as the need to be loved, the need for self-respect, and feelings of happiness and sadness, anger and pain, which everyone has at some time.

4. Discuss your family's history of immigration to this country, or more recent moves to new neighborhoods and the adjustments that this required for the family. Talk to your children about their unique qualities, and the characteristics, feelings, and dreams you and they share with people all over the world.

5. Discuss the issue of prejudice with your youngster. Since many schools have curricula that promote discussions of diversity and prejudice, you may have the opportunity to reinforce this at home. Make it clear that diversity should be valued and that discrimination in any form is unacceptable. He should understand that teasing, insulting, rejecting, or diminishing another person based on race, religion, background, origin, economic status, gender, or appearance will not be tolerated. Explain that there is no need for your child to build himself up by putting others down. (This may reflect a basic insecurity or unhappiness within himself.) Mistreating others can give your child a false sense of security that will produce anxiety when he is with others who are "different," particularly since they will invariably be able to do some things better than he can.

6. If you sense that your youngster has negative attitudes toward others, or you witness or hear about any intolerant or discriminatory behavior on his part, do not ignore them. Address these prejudices by discussing

why your child feels the way he does. Let rational thinking diffuse the emotional intensity of prejudice.

At the same time, encourage positive values toward diversity and harmonious and cooperative ways of living. Love and respect your child, so he can come to value and respect others.

7. Help your youngster understand the erroneous basis of stereotypes and hatred. Call attention to negative stereotypes when they appear in the media, including television (programs and commercials), newspapers, and magazines. Some common ways in which prejudice appears in the media and even in schools include:

- Presenting other people in stereotypical roles: male doctors, black athletes, overly emotional women.

- Showing racial or ethnic minorities in only one role, such as Native Americans in traditional clothing, or people of color as poor.

- Equating different cultures with single aspects of that culture, such as food, dress, or special observances.

- Always presenting minority individuals as the "different" person within a group, rather than as one of many within their own community.

8. When choosing experiences for your child—including camps, schools, child care, and extracurricular events—seek out diversity in racial and ethnic backgrounds among the other children participating.

9. Use the library, bookshop, and video-rental store to obtain material about other people and their cultures that depict them in a positive, sensitive, humanistic light.

10. Actively work to reduce prejudice in your life and community. Establish a household in which all members are valued and respected. Participate in your child's school to assure that diversity is valued and reinforced. Join political and civic organizations and attend multicultural events, both to change the world in which your child lives and to demonstrate your commitment to addressing the prejudices that exist.

11. If your child personally experiences prejudice, he will probably feel hurt and angry. Yet because of social circumstances or his own stage of development, he may feel unable to express these emotions. You need to encourage him to vent his feelings, and you must acknowledge their validity, before trying to discuss them with reason. A child whose personhood has been attacked through prejudice needs to be supported and have his self-esteem bolstered by his family and friends. Then you can discuss the roots of prejudice with him, and how the two of you believe he should respond.

How Schools Can Diffuse Prejudice

Schools should be a place where your child learns more than academic skills. They should also promote understanding and cooperation among people, not prejudice.

Here are some questions to ask schoolteachers and administrators about your child's educational environment:

- Do learning and problem-solving tasks emphasize cooperation and team play, while minimizing excessive competition? Children should not be placed in situations where differences in gender, race, ethnicity, economic status, and academic ability are stressed, or are even allowed to be expressed in a negative, divisive way. Rather, whether the academic skill being taught is math or spelling, or the activity is drama or sports, part of each child's grade should be dependent on the achievement of the entire group. Team spirit can conquer feelings of difference and separateness that children experience among themselves.

- Does the school have a curriculum that covers the different races, religions, and cultures of present-day America? Is your youngster continuously exposed to the achievements and contributions of all Americans and cultures?

- Does the school take advantage of ethnic holidays—Chinese New Year, Cinco de Mayo, Kwanzaa, etc.—for children to actively learn customs and traditions with which they may not be familiar?

- Do teachers have open discussions in class about discrimination and negative feelings toward others? If an incident involving prejudice has occurred at school or in the community, is it used as a springboard to discuss these issues in a sensitive, nonpunitive, nonstigmatizing way that emphasizes the common human qualities of people?

PART IV

BEHAVIOR AND DISCIPLINE

12

YOU AND YOUR
CHILD'S BEHAVIOR

There are few areas that raise more concern among parents than their child's behavior. While their pediatrician may be able to prescribe an antibiotic to cure a sore throat or an ear infection, solutions for childhood behavior problems are not nearly as clear-cut, nor is there a consensus on the best approach to discipline.

While the terms *behavior* and *discipline* often carry negative connotations, they are considered neutral terms in this book. By definition, behavior is simply verbal and nonverbal communication. It is the conduct, actions, and words that children employ—a signal with which they express their thoughts, feelings, needs, and impulses. It is judged as to whether it meets social, cultural, developmental, and age-appropriate standards. Behavior can be positive or negative, impulsive or planned, predictable or unpredictable, consistent or inconsistent, and it can elicit a wide range of positive or negative responses from others.

Through her behavior, your child may be trying to communicate messages like: "That's too difficult for me. . . . I'm afraid of failure. . . . I'm afraid of disappointing you. . . . I'm bored. . . . I'm tired. . . . I'm afraid of being rejected. . . . I want you to play with me. . . . I need you. . . . I want to please you. . . . I love you. . . . I want you to pay attention to me."

Attention, of course, is one of the most important things that children desire and seek from their parents. The attention they most want is the message that they are loved, valued, accepted, and respected. Children will go to great extremes for the feeling that unconditional love is there for them.

Children will do whatever it takes to get recognition and to have their needs met. They quickly learn which kinds of behavior get their parents to respond to them and meet their needs, and if positive behavior doesn't work, they will turn to the negative. Even if their misbehavior gets them a negative reaction (such as being scolded), any recognition is better than none, in the eyes of children.

Behavior, then, does not occur in isolation. It is a form of communication, a way to express needs and feelings, and is influenced by a child's desires, temperament, and ability to adapt, as well as by her mother's and father's parenting style, family situation, and various stresses and transitions—from a minor illness to starting a new school year.

During the school-age years, children are developing rapidly, and in many ways they are trying to understand the world around them, face new demands, deal with success and failure, and communicate with their siblings, parents, and increasingly with their peers. In many cases these changes can lead to problems. Just as the middle years offer endless opportunities for children to learn and to meet new challenges, so, too, they provide an equal number of chances for them to make mistakes, to achieve and succeed, and to question or challenge parental values, rules, and attitudes. Proper parental discipline is a way to teach children what behavior is appropriate in which circumstance, or how to interact in a socially acceptable manner.

Here, *discipline* does not imply punishment or scolding. It means "to educate." Proper discipline teaches children to live in a safe, civilized, and harmonious manner with themselves and others. There are some essential elements to disciplining well, including correctly understanding the child's needs and abilities (going beyond the concrete, actual behavior), communicating effectively, and using positive and negative reinforcement appropriately. (See Chapter 14, "Changing Your Child's Behavior.")

THE MYTH OF THE PERFECT PARENT

Many people believe in the myth of the perfect parents—the ideal mother and father who raise happy, well-adjusted, problem-free children. In truth, there is no such person as a perfect parent—or a perfect child.

Problem behavior is common among school-age children and takes up a significant portion of a parent's time. At any one time, on average, school-age children have about five or six traits or behaviors that their parents find difficult. These might include not complying with simple requests, avoiding chores, spending too much time watching TV or playing videos, engaging in sibling rivalry, or having difficulty completing homework. Other common problems for parents are dealing with a temperamentally difficult child, or coping with a child who either wants too much independence or hasn't achieved enough autonomy. Parents also sometimes encounter the dilemma of a child who prefers friends or activities not approved of by his mother or father.

As a parent, you need to recognize that it is normal to feel worried, confused, angry, guilty, overwhelmed, and inadequate because of your child's behavior. That is part of being a parent. It is futile and self-defeating to try to be perfect or to raise perfect children.

Think back to how you behaved, or misbehaved, as a child, about how your parents dealt with your behavior, and how you felt about their disciplinary techniques. They were not perfect, but neither was anyone else. Do not try to overcompensate for their shortcomings by trying to be perfect yourself, and by getting caught up in statements like "I'm not going to make the same mistakes my parents made."

All parents and all children make mistakes in their attempts to communicate and deal with one another and in trying to solve problems. Parents need to trust themselves and their instincts. Mothers and fathers tend to have good intuition and knowledge of their own children. They often know more than they think they do, and they should not be afraid of making mistakes. Children are resilient and forgiving and usually learn and grow through their mistakes. Parents tend to be just as resilient and forgiving.

However, parents who "live for their children" are putting themselves in a very vulnerable position, setting themselves up for possible disappointment, frustration, and resentment. They are also being unfair to their family. Parents should not expect to receive all their personal fulfillment from their children or from the parenting role. Parents need other activities to fulfill their self-images, and other sources of love and nurturing. They need time to be adults and time for themselves—and a break from children and parenting responsibilities.

As a parent, you need to develop your own philosophy—one with which you feel comfortable—within a flexible and adaptable framework. Take into account your own expectations, parenting style, and temperament, and how they fit with each of your children and your spouse, and their own unique preferences and temperaments. Your approach and philosophy will vary from youngster to youngster, mainly because of their own particular attributes. (See "Why They Are Similar and Different," page 360.)

Along the way, remember that professional help is available if problems ever become too intense, exceed your own coping capabilities, or cause secondary difficulties such as a decline in school performance, increased family stress, or serious emotional problems.

You should take comfort in the fact that in the vast majority of cases, children do turn out well. But along the way, keep your sense of humor, trust your instincts, and seek help and advice early rather than late. While parenting is a great challenge, it can also be one of the most rewarding and enjoyable experiences of your life.

DEVELOPMENT AND BEHAVIOR

To help you better understand and deal with some of the difficult—yet often normal—behavior of childhood, you should appreciate the general developmental trends in school-age youngsters. All children desire recognition, success, acceptance, approval, and unconditional love. Younger children seek them from their parents in particular. While older children (ages ten and up) continue to have these same needs from Mom and Dad, they also increasingly desire recognition and acceptance from their peers and other adults.

At the same time, school-age children have a growing need for privacy, autonomy, and separation from their parents. To some degree they will gradually move away from the family—physically, socially, and emotionally. This is a normal part of growing up, and it is a principal goal of raising children so that eventually they succeed in the world outside the family. Nonetheless, for many parents this changing relationship can be painful, confusing, and the source of tension and behavioral conflicts.

As they grow up, children also experience a variety of challenges and transitions. Some are predictable and part of the life of every child; some are less usual. Children face transitions such as entering school, taking new subjects, changing classrooms and teachers, making new friends, trying new activities, and moving to new homes or cities. They might also include certain losses, like losing a favorite possession, a pet, or a friend. The illness or death of a family member or loss of a parent through divorce is especially traumatic. These times can be painful for school-age children, and parents need to provide support and attention.

Three Types of Behavior

Some parents find it helpful to consider three general kinds of behavior:

1. Some kinds of behavior are wanted and approved. They might include doing homework, being polite, and doing chores. These actions receive compliments freely and easily.

2. Other behavior is not sanctioned but is tolerated under certain conditions, such as during times of illness (of a parent or a child) or stress (a move, for instance, or the birth of a new sibling). These kinds of behavior might include not doing chores, regressive behavior (such as baby talk), or being excessively self-centered.

3. Still other kinds of behavior cannot and should not be tolerated or reinforced. They include actions that are harmful to the physical, emotional, or social well-being of the child, the family members, and others. They may interfere with the child's intellectual development. They may be forbidden by law, ethics, religion, or social mores. They might include very aggressive or destructive behavior, overt racism or prejudice, stealing, truancy, smoking or substance abuse, school failure, or an intense sibling rivalry.

DEVELOPMENTAL VARIATIONS: HOW THEY AFFECT BEHAVIOR

You should be aware of two less typical patterns of behavior that your youngster might exhibit, which reflect variations in development to some extent, or an inability to cope with challenges. First, very well-behaved children, too well-behaved, may be overly anxious to please, very needy of attention, love, and approval, or fearful of rejection. Sometimes these children are attempting to care for, defend, or protect a parent by being very well-behaved. They may be overly cautious, very shy, overprotected, and feel insecure and incompetent. They also may have few friends and interests that are appropriate for their age.

Another worrisome pattern is characterized by *self-defeating* behavior, such as the child who deliberately does poorly in school, breaks rules, or continually places herself in no-win situations. These kinds of behavior may stem from the youngster's need to assert her own power, to gain control of her life (or parts of it), or to reject parental authority, pressure, or expectations. They also may arise from a fear of failure or rejection, or from a need to rationalize failure or to avoid the uncertainty of taking on a new task. Quite commonly, these children have low self-esteem and lack self-confidence. (See the section on "Self-Esteem," page 132.)

This latter group of children finds it emotionally safer and more comfortable to accept the certainty of failure rather than risk the uncertainty and anxiety of attempting success. They also often blame themselves when things go wrong or when they feel rejected or unloved. They tend to think in absolute and fatalistic ways, feeling that "now is forever"—that is, if their life circumstances are unpleasant now, they will be so forever.

These children also may have difficulty seeing the world from the perspective or viewpoint of others. For instance, a parent may be having her own difficulties and is thus unable to give much love or positive feedback at a particular time. Children take this change very personally and may respond by feeling rejected, or they may inappropriately blame themselves for their parent's disregard.

Children such as these do not merely have discrete behavior problems. Rather, they have developed unsuccessful patterns of responding to and interacting with the world around them. Simple interventions by their parents are likely to be of limited value. If these descriptions seem to fit your child, you should consider seeking help from a mental-health professional or a behavioral pediatrician.

Children also often resort to negative behavior such as regressing or being very disobedient in order to communicate feelings that they otherwise cannot express, or in response to the belief that their feelings are not being acknowledged by their parents. Behavioral difficulties might also be an outgrowth of a language problem, often when a child cannot readily understand spoken language or cannot easily put feelings into words. Or they may be part of a family where verbal communication and expressing feelings through words are not encouraged. Unfortunately, some children may fear they will be punished or receive disapproval for expressing their feelings; eventually, these repressed feelings may emerge, indeed erupt, through their behavior.

EVALUATING BEHAVIORAL PROBLEMS

Parents often have difficulty telling the difference between variations in normal behavior and true behavioral problems. In reality, the difference between normal and abnormal behavior is not always clear; usually it is a matter of degree or expectation. A fine line often divides normal from abnormal behavior, in part because what is "normal" depends upon the child's level of development, which can vary greatly among children of the same age. Development can be uneven, too, with a child's social development lagging behind his intellectual growth, or vice versa. In addition, "normal" behavior is in part determined by the context in which it occurs—that is, by the particular situation and time, as well as by the child's own particular family values and expectations, and cultural and social background.

Understanding your child's unique developmental progress is necessary in order to interpret, accept, or adapt his behavior (as well as your own). Remember, children have great individual variations of temperament, development, and behavior.

Your own parental responses are guided by whether you see the behavior as a problem. Frequently, parents overinterpret or overreact to a minor, normal, short-term change in behavior. At the other extreme, they may ignore or downplay a serious problem. They also may seek quick, simple answers to what are, in fact, complex problems. All of these responses may create difficulties or prolong the time for a resolution.

Behavior that parents tolerate, disregard, or consider reasonable differs from one family to the next. Some of these differences come from the parents' own upbringing; they may have had very strict or very permissive parents themselves, and their expectations of their children follow accordingly. Other behavior is considered a problem when parents feel that people are judging them for their child's behavior; this leads to an inconsistent response from the parents, who may tolerate behavior at home that they are embarrassed by in public.

The parents' own temperament, usual mood, and daily pressures will also influence how they interpret the child's behavior. Easygoing parents may accept a wider range of behavior as normal and be slower to label something a problem, while parents who are by nature more stern move more quickly to discipline their children. Depressed parents, or parents having marital or financial difficulties, are less likely to tolerate much latitude in their offspring's behavior. Parents usually differ from one another in their own backgrounds and personal preferences, resulting in differing parenting styles that will influence a child's behavior and development.

When children's behavior is complex and challenging, some parents find reasons not to respond. For instance, parents often rationalize ("It's not my fault"), despair ("Why me?"), wish it would go away ("Kids outgrow these

Your Child's Development and Behavior: Points to Keep in Mind

1. Even among children of the same age, there is a range of what is normal in the way they develop socially, emotionally, intellectually, and physically.

2. A child's maturity level may be different for the various qualities he is developing, including social skills, athletic abilities, and learning capabilities. He might be strong in math but weak in writing (or vice versa), or good at basketball but not at golf.

3. The variations described above may be permanent, forming a child's own unique profile; or they could be evolving and thus be subject to change.

4. The way a child develops can influence his behavior, and vice versa.

5. The particular parenting style of a mother and father, as well as the child's environment, will affect the youngster's behavior and development.

problems anyway"), deny ("There's really no problem"), hesitate to take action ("It may hurt his feelings"), avoid ("I didn't want to face his anger"), or fear rejection ("He won't love me").

If you are worried about your child's behavior or development, or if you are uncertain as to how one affects the other, consult your pediatrician as early as possible, even if just to be reassured that your child's behavior and development are within a normal range.

13

COMMUNICATING WITH YOUR CHILD

S uccess as a parent, as a teacher, or in other roles with children depends a lot on being able to communicate well.

Communication is more than simply sharing information. When parents and children communicate, they are understanding one another and learning about the others' thoughts and feelings. Thus, while many people tend to think of communication primarily as talking, the most important part of it, and perhaps the most difficult to learn, is listening.

The initial communication between parent and child occurs in infancy. A baby's smile, seen by the mother or father, is an invitation to talk and smile back. At this stage, successful parents are good observers. Soon, parent-child sharing of messages moves beyond nonverbal communication to sounds and spoken words. Children and parents not only exchange information, but their communication quickly becomes a way of sharing emotions and giving support. Families that communicate well share a full range of experiences—

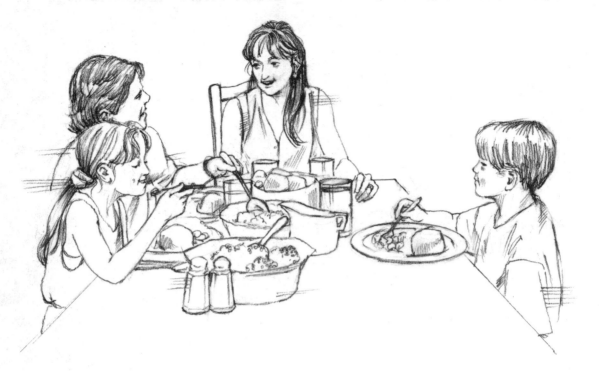

Success as a parent depends a lot on your ability to communicate well with your children.

the happy and good parts of life and also sad times, problems, and their solutions.

To be effective communicators, you and your child must practice and develop skills together. Successful communication not only allows any topic or feeling to be shared, but it uses nonverbal as well as verbal ways of expressing oneself.

As with other aspects of parenting, you probably communicate with your own child in much the same way that your parents did with you. When it comes to communication, your parents were your models—and in many families, parents were not necessarily good models.

Listen to yourself. Although it is not something you are conscious of, you probably sound a lot like your parents did when they talked to you. Try to remember what was positive and negative about their ways of communicating, and see if you can find echoes of that in your own style. You may need to train yourself to break old habits of poor listening and damaging criticism. As you do, you will not only communicate better with your youngster, but you will also be providing a model of more positive behavior, so that she will become a better communicator.

COMMUNICATION BEYOND THE FAMILY

The communication skills your child learns will affect the way he interacts not only with you but with the world at large. These skills will help your youngster to negotiate, solve problems, and learn from others. Communication can also be used to praise, punish, express feelings, and provide insights and understanding.

The *way* you communicate is part and parcel of *what* you communicate. Done well, communication is how you convey love, acceptance, respect, and approval to your child. Providing praise, for example, is not just saying words. It requires that you understand how your child thinks about himself and his behavior, and knowing when and in what way you can share with him your pride, so that he is best able to hear you and accept what you are trying to say. Successful communication is a two-person process, not merely one person saying something to another. If you consistently communicate well with your child, he will know that you think well of him. Not only will this nurture your relationship with him, but it can help him grow, develop, and live up to his capabilities as a person. (See the section on "Self-Esteem" on page 132.)

Unfortunately, too many parents do a poor job of expressing this acceptance. They may think: *If I tell my son that in my eyes he is just fine the way he is, he won't be motivated to work harder and do better in life.* But in fact, children do better once they feel relieved of the pressure of having to win their parents' approval. Rather than constantly judging and criticizing your child, let him know that you accept and love him. In turn, he will begin to like himself more, and his self-esteem will grow.

Make an effort to communicate this acceptance through both words and actions. Yes, you can demonstrate your feelings in nonverbal ways through your body language, including your facial expressions, hugs, and gestures. But you also need to *say* it.

Too often, parents choose ineffective, nonaccepting ways to communicate verbally with their children. They might give commands ("You're going to do it as I say or else!"), lecture ("When I was a boy, I had twice as many chores as you"), or preach ("You must never behave that way again"). Or they might criticize ("You are doing everything wrong today"), ridicule ("You looked silly when you struck out"), or belittle ("Someone your age should know better").

Be positive and accepting in the way you talk with your child. Offer praise often and be as specific as you can ("You did a wonderful job solving that difficult problem in your math homework tonight"). Let him know how much you appreciate him as he is, without his having to struggle to resemble your own preconceived notions of how you want him to be ("I was so proud just watching you run in the track meet today").

You can also demonstrate acceptance by *not* involving yourself in some of your child's activities. For example, if you just let him paint without giving him advice on what colors to mix together, this will convey the message that he is doing just fine on his own. In much the same way, you can listen quietly to your child at times, without interjecting your own thoughts and comments that might contradict or correct him.

THE COMPONENTS OF COMMUNICATION

Here are the elements of good communication to keep in mind as you relate to your middle-years child.

Listening Skills

An essential part of the communication exchange with your child is receiving messages from her. They can be verbal messages (questions, requests) or non-verbal ones (actions or nonactions). Listening is a learned skill, and with effort you can become better at it. In the process you will be setting a good example for your children, and they will become better listeners too.

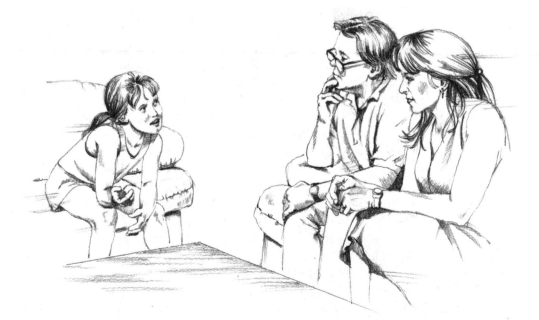

Active listening demonstrates that you think what your child has to say is important.

Active listening is the central component of communication. When you become an active listener, you are telling your child that the channels of communication are open. You are recognizing that your child has a need and/or a desire to share her feelings and thoughts, and that you are receptive.

There are several skills and techniques involved in active listening that will decrease the likelihood that you will be judgmental or critical, or will lecture or belittle. These skills allow you to help your child get in touch with what she is really feeling and thinking, analyze it, and put it in perspective so that problems do not seem bigger than they really are. It will also build a bond between you and your youngster, and make her more receptive to what is on *your* mind.

To become an active listener:

- Set aside time to listen. Block out distractions as much as possible. In order to hear and understand what your child has to say, you have to want to do so, and want to help your child with any concerns she has at the moment. Some parents and children find they can communicate best just before bedtime or when they share an evening snack.

- Put aside your own thoughts and viewpoints, and place yourself in a frame of mind to receive information from your youngster. Give her your complete attention, and try to put yourself in her place so you can better understand what she is experiencing. Make her feel that you value her thoughts and consider them important, and that you are sensitive to her point of view.

- Listen to, summarize, and repeat back to your child the message you are hearing. This is called reflective listening. When appropriate, gently state what you think she may be trying to say. Do not just parrot what you hear, but go beneath the surface to what your youngster may be thinking and feeling. Remember, the spoken words may not be the true or complete message.

  The underlying messages may include the feelings, fears, and concerns of your youngster. Assign these feelings a name or label ("It sounds to me as if you are scared . . . sad . . . angry . . . happy").

- Maintain eye contact while your child talks. Show your interest by nodding your head and occasionally interjecting "door-openers" or noncommittal responses like "Yes . . . I see . . . Oh . . . How about that." Encourage her to keep talking. Although these may seem like passive responses, they are an important part of communication.

- Accept and show respect for what your child is expressing, even if it does not coincide with your own ideas and expectations. You can do this by paying attention to what your youngster is communicating, while not criticizing, judging, or interrupting.

- Create opportunities for your child to solve the problems she may be facing. Encourage and guide her. Ask her to bounce ideas off you, which might eventually suggest solutions to problems.

When parents are active listeners, other people may describe them as having good intuition and as being "tuned in" to their children. The process of active listening will help your child understand her feelings and be less afraid of the negative ones. It will build bridges and create warmth between you and your child. It will also help her solve her own problems and gain more control over her behavior and emotions. And if your child sees you as an active listener, this will make her more willing to listen to you and to others.

You can monitor how actively you are listening by watching for cues that you are not listening well. If you find yourself feeling bored by the conversation, distracted, looking around or away, or feeling rushed, or if you feel that you are wasting time, you are not listening actively.

Even when you think you and your child are doing a good job of listening and communicating, it is a good idea to test that impression occasionally. You can ask her to repeat as best she can what you have been trying to say—either the words or the feelings. Similarly, you should try to summarize and restate what it is that you heard her say.

Talking Techniques

As you talk to your child, you should try to make it a positive dialogue, rather than impose judgment or place blame. That usually means choosing "I" messages rather than "you" messages, especially when attempting to change or encourage certain behavior.

"I" messages are statements like "I sure have trouble finding things on my desk when it hasn't been straightened up by the last person who used it." "I need more quiet when I am trying to read." "Since I am so tired, I sure would like some help cleaning up the dinner dishes."

These "I" statements communicate the effect of a child's behavior or actions upon the parent. But they are less threatening to a child than "you" messages, even though they still convey an honest feeling or message. They also communicate just how a child's behavior affects her parents and encourage her to take responsibility for straightening up Dad's desk or helping clean up the kitchen. They communicate trust—showing the parents' willingness to express their own feelings and their belief that their child will respond in a positive, responsible way.

By contrast, "you" messages are statements like "You should never do that." "You make me so angry." "Why don't you pay attention?" These messages are more child-focused and are more likely to create a struggle between you and

Causes of Poor Communication

If you are having difficulty communicating with your child, see if the problem might lie in one of these areas.

- Do one or both of you do a poor job of interpreting the messages of the other?

- Is there a poor fit between the communication styles or temperaments of parent and child?

- Do you have communication shortcomings that turn your child off? For instance, middle-years children sometimes complain that their parents talk over their heads, nag, become judgmental, do not make an effort to understand their youngster's point of view, or interrupt them constantly. If these sound like familiar complaints, you may have to work on your own listening and talking skills.

- Does your child have attention-span problems that may make it difficult for her to concentrate long enough to receive a message? Is she too impulsive, and does she talk before she thinks? If you have these problems, there is a chance your child may have them too.

- Does your youngster have a memory deficit, perhaps related to her attention problems, in which messages are received so superficially that they do not get placed into her memory? Or do memory problems prevent her from knowing what to say or finding the right phrase, or make her just a bit late with a response? Keep in mind that worry and sadness can interfere with attention and memory.

- Does your child have language or speech disabilities that make it hard for her to understand what you are saying, or to express her own ideas and thoughts in words? Or does she stutter or have another speech problem that makes it difficult for her to communicate verbally?

- Do you or your child have other worries, stresses, or preoccupations that may be interfering with your communication?

- Are you choosing the right time and place to communicate?

- Does the pace or intensity of the conversation overwhelm your child's ability to listen and respond?

your youngster, put a child on the defensive, encourage personal counterarguments, and discourage effective communication.

Even worse are the "put-down" messages that judge or criticize a youngster. They might involve name-calling, ridiculing, or embarrassing the child. These messages can have a serious negative impact on the youngster and on her self-esteem. If you communicate the message that your child is bad, stupid, inconsiderate, a disappointment, or a failure, that is how she is likely to perceive herself, not only during her childhood but for many years thereafter.

With "I" statements, however, children do get the message in a more positive light. They often say things like "I didn't realize that the noise I was making was bothering you." Or "I'm glad you told me you were so tired. I'll help you with an extra chore or two." Children often readily assume more responsible roles if they are made aware of the situation and the feelings and needs of others, and are not "put down" in the process.

Of course, even with "I" messages you are not guaranteed success. Children may disregard the message, particularly when you first begin to make use of "I" statements. If this happens, repeat your "I" message, maybe saying it in a different way and with greater intensity. Be willing to say something like "This is how I feel, and I do not appreciate having my feelings ignored."

If you have consistently shown yourself to be receptive to and respectful of your child's feelings and thoughts, she will probably be more responsive to your own "I" statements. Give it some time. Middle-years children usually catch on relatively quickly.

Also, as you communicate with your youngster, be sensitive to your tone of voice. It should be consistent with your message. Do not let your emotions confuse the message you are trying to convey.

Be as consistent as possible with all your children. You should have the same communication approach and style with every child, although the unique aspects of each relationship and each child's temperament may require some modifications. Do not appear to play favorites or be more accepting of one youngster than another.

COMMUNICATION DO'S AND DON'TS

Here are some points to keep in mind as you communicate with your child.

- Listen actively.

- Make and keep eye contact.

- Look for the underlying messages in what your child is saying. What is the emotional tone or climate?

- Show respect for his ideas and feelings. Stay away from sarcasm, hurtful teasing, blaming, belittling, and fault-finding.

- Use "I" messages and avoid "you" messages and put-downs.

- Be honest.

- Be sensitive to the times and places that are good for talking. If your youngster comes home from school tired, give him some time to rest or have a snack before you communicate what may be on your mind. If you come home tired, take a rest yourself. Choose a quiet, private area in which to talk.

- Praise or reward your child from time to time when he shows good listening habits. He may be motivated to listen more carefully and follow through on what you are saying if his efforts are recognized.

If you and your youngster have ongoing problems with communication, ask your pediatrician for some guidance. He or she may suggest having your child evaluated for problems that may be interfering, such as language and attention deficits, or family issues. Your pediatrician might also be able to refer you and your child to a family counselor who can work out the difficulties that can improve your communication skills.

CHANGING YOUR
CHILD'S BEHAVIOR

C hildren are rarely irrational; their behavior almost always has a purpose or at least a reason. However, when children misbehave, parents often do not recognize what it is their child is trying to accomplish. They also may not understand or agree with their child's reasoning, particularly when the child is under stress. Sometimes in anger or frustration a parent will yell at their child, "What were you thinking?" Rarely do parents expect a reasoned answer to that question, yet the answer can often be revealing and enlightening. Changing a child's behavior requires understanding why it occurs, and that takes time, effort, and good communication.

It is often helpful to remember what circumstances existed just before your child's unacceptable behavior occurred. Where were you and your child? What were each of you doing? Who else was present? What was said, by whom and in what tone of voice? What would have been an acceptable response or action by your child? Talking about these questions with your child can be a way to begin understanding better how your child views things. With that new knowledge, it may be easier to help your child behave in ways that you appreciate.

Often a child has one specific behavior pattern that parents find especially troubling and difficult to handle. Sometimes a parent's initial interventions may not have been successful, and occasionally they may even have made things worse.

What can parents do? Consider, for example, a child who regularly bullies a younger sibling. This child needs to be told calmly that bullying is not permitted but that disagreements and arguing are normal and acceptable. Explain and even demonstrate appropriate, alternative behavior (arguing, sharing, taking turns). She then needs to understand that if she is again aggressive toward

Setting Expectations

Does your child fully understand what you expect of her? Here are some guidelines to keep in mind when setting and communicating expectations:

- Expectations need to be stated clearly and explicitly and must be achievable and reasonable.

- There needs to be an agreement between what parents expect and what the child expects.

- Parents and child should set short-term goals that can be achieved steadily in a step-by-step manner. These goals should ensure success that will satisfy both parents and child.

- Acknowledge the child's genuine efforts, even when she doesn't fully meet expectations. Small increments of change are important and more realistic.

- Be willing to reconsider and adjust when the child is consistently unable to meet parental expectations.

- Parents should set up realistic, short-term time schedules for implementing specific behavioral goals. For example: "By the end of two weeks, Linda will be picking up her clothes four days a week" (as opposed to never picking up clothes).

- The family meeting provides an excellent forum for a discussion of appropriate expectations, methods of achieving goals, and rewards and punishments. To minimize misunderstandings, someone should write down the major points of agreement. (See "How to Have a Family Meeting" on page 336.)

her brother or sister, she will be given a warning and then will lose a privilege (TV viewing for a day; not having a friend over to visit). If the behavior recurs, carry out the consequence or punishment that has been promised.

Punishment and consequences need to be appropriate to the behavior and the child's age and abilities and of course should not be excessive. Punishments (as well as rewards) need to occur soon after the behavior in order to reduce the problem in the future. Thus, a child's punishment should be to lose a privilege that day or the next, not the next month. Effective disciplining and rewarding require that the parents be in agreement or at least not interfere with or undermine each other's priorities or efforts.

For some behavior, parents can implement a behavior modification program. This approach involves modifying both the child's and the parent's behavior. It works by discouraging negative behavior, encouraging and supporting positive behavior, and setting appropriate expectations for meeting goals and time guidelines. Even if you plan to carry out a behavior modification program on your own, you might find it helpful to consult a pediatrician or another behavioral expert for advice and support.

THE ABC SYSTEM

Here is a behavior modification program—the ABC system—that many parents find helpful. It requires effort and patience to implement but is simple to set up and very effective.

A: *Antecedent events* or activities that usually precede (and sometimes contribute to) the behavior, and the situation or the context in which the behavior occurs (for example, at the dinner table).

B: *Behavior that is problematic.* Parents will need to specify clearly the behavior that needs changing (for instance, fighting with a sibling) and note its frequency, duration, and intensity. This is information by which later success can be measured.

C: *Consequences of the child's behavior,* specifically the responses (emotional and behavioral) that the problem behavior elicits from the parents and others.

Here is how the program is implemented:

Step 1: Describe A, B, and C, and write down this information. The more specific, the better.

Step 2: Initiate a program that will eliminate, reduce, or modify conditions in A.

Positive Reinforcement Through Rewards

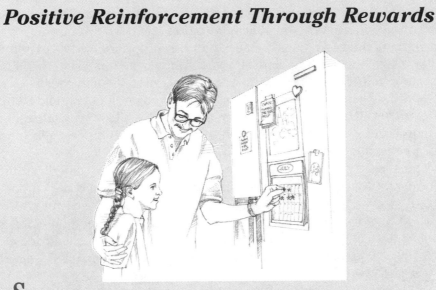

Some children need more than recognition and praise. Rewards can be effective in middle childhood, especially once you have clearly defined the specific, positive behavior goals you expect. Here are some effective strategies:

- Make or devise a chart that specifies the desired behavior, as well as the time of day or the situation in which it should be demonstrated. The calendar should cover an entire week or, for some behavior, a longer period. It should allow the activity or goal to be rated each day. Decide how many points an incidence of positive behavior will earn. In a summary col-

Step 3: Clearly state agreed-upon changes and expectations for B, including a time frame.

Step 4: Change C. This contains three components: First, the negative behavior is ignored and not reinforced or in any way rewarded by the parents' responses; ideally it gradually becomes less frequent or severe because the parents ignore it. Second, the parents reinforce *any positive change* in behavior by calling attention to it and by providing rewards that were agreed upon in advance with the child. Third, the parents carry out punishment or consequences as agreed upon and as appropriate.

Step 5: Record any changes in behavior (frequency, duration, intensity), comparing them to the original measures in B to see how successful the program is.

umn, total up the points. (Tokens, such as paper stars pasted on the calendar, tend to work better for early school-age children; points and contract systems work better for older children.) Small rewards may be given for a predetermined amount of points at the end of each day or week, with larger rewards reserved for a longer period of time or a greater number of points. Keep this behavior chart in a conspicuous place so it can serve as a source of positive reinforcement and pride.

- Make a list of the rewards your child will receive for a particular number of points. Rewards should be meaningful to your child, and she should participate actively in their selection. Be very clear about how many points or days or weeks of changed behavior it takes to earn a reward.

- It is important to keep close daily track of your child's progress. Keep her enthusiasm level high by reinforcing behavior as frequently as possible.

- Keep in mind that the chart should be used as a measure of success. Avoid penalties and demerits that are humiliating, or that discourage your child from even trying. Use other forms of mild punishment, such as timeouts. (See page 213.)

Gradually, this program can be phased out as children internalize their behavior. At that time, children usually lose interest or forget to ask for their points.

Step 6: Review the situation, progress, and overall satisfaction with all family members. Usually it takes two to three weeks to produce a change. The family's expectations and commitment should be clearly understood and stated.

Repeat the process—Steps 1 to 6—as needed and with necessary modifications.

OTHER APPROACHES

No single approach is going to work for all children or all problems. Here are behavior modification techniques that can be used with simple, specific problems that do not require the more complex, systematic ABC approach.

Extinction, or "Active Ignoring"

This approach entails briefly removing all attention from the child. It is particularly effective with children who are whining, sulking, or pestering. As part of this technique, parents provide appropriate alternative behavior for the child to use; when he adopts this new behavior, he receives parental attention again.

Positive Reinforcement

Catch the child exhibiting good behavior, and recognize and reward it quickly and as often as possible. The rewards can include demonstrations of affection, words of praise, eye contact, points, material objects, or special meals or activities. Give the youngster specific feedback about specific behavior: for example, "I like the way you shared your toys with your friend."

Giving rewards based on your child's behavior is more difficult than you might first imagine. Monitoring his behavior can consume a great deal of your time and energy. Also, material rewards can lead to your child's expectation that if he makes any behavioral change you request, he should receive a reward. There is also the danger that the good behavior will stop when the reward stops. However, without positive reinforcement, other efforts to change behavior, such as punishments, are unlikely to work. Use this technique only when you and your child think the problem is worth the effort. (See the box on pages 208–9, "Positive Reinforcement Through Rewards.")

Demonstrating Good Behavior

Parents' actions are more powerful than their words. Parents should demonstrate the desired behavior. Help out with a task. Also, do what you say, say what you mean, and mean what you say. Keep actions and words as consistent and positive as possible. When you slip up and don't match your behavior to your own expectations, show your child how you are able to learn from your mistakes.

SPECIAL TIME

Special Time is a regular, guaranteed, unconditional, and uninterrupted time that a parent spends with a child—a time when they interact without the parent's being judgmental or directive. Children of all ages want parents to pay attention to them and to feel loved and capable. Special Time is one way to fill these needs. It is a "time in," an opportunity for parents and children to spend time together.

Special Time should:

- Be given to each child every day regardless of behavior or mood.

- Be called "Special Time" or another favorite name so the child knows she is getting it.

- Be an activity of the child's choice (within reason). Older children may want to carry out an activity over several sessions.

- Engage the parent and child in an interactive activity, although occasionally a passive activity such as TV viewing is okay and even preferable.

- Be a time that is convenient for both parent and child; the time of day can vary.

- Be a consistent, fixed, short, and predetermined amount of time (to avoid boredom and fatigue) depending on age and interest (10–30 minutes). The time can be measured by using a timer.

- Not be saved up and used to extend the time on the next day. Parents should avoid promising Special Time but not fulfilling that promise.

- Be without interruption of any kind, except true emergencies. This time should be special and recognizable for the child.

- Should be adjusted. If the child is aggressive or disruptive during Special Time, she should receive a timeout or another consequence with the timer still running. If both parent and child want and agree to cancel or shorten Special Time, they should do so.

WHAT ABOUT CONTRACTS?

A contract between a parent and child can be an effective means for changing behavior, particularly for a child who is age ten or older, an age when children want to negotiate, feel more empowered and independent, and show more initiative and responsibility.

First, identify a problem that is of mutual concern, even if it is only a potential or anticipated problem. Sometimes contracts are most effective *before* a particular conflict or problem arises. For instance, if your child wants a pet, draw up a contract of responsibilities before the pet has been obtained.

Do not impose the contract on your child. He should be a participant in developing it. Children have definite and firm thoughts, opinions, and feelings and are capable of quite sophisticated negotiations if given the opportunity.

First the child and then the parents should state their needs, desires, and responsibilities. Then both child and parents should state what they feel are appropriate rewards, punishments, or consequences of the child's behavior. Next, parents and child should negotiate an agreement, probably a compromise or middle ground on which they can all agree. Then the contract should be written. It should clearly describe what the child and parents intend to do—for example, what activities are permissible, and what actions will be taken if the contract is breached or is successfully completed.

Post the contract in a prominent place so that it can serve as a reminder, as a stimulus for positive reinforcement, and as a marker for achievement and progress. If your child feels embarrassed by having it displayed, put it in a private place. It should be reviewed (and modified as necessary) on a regular basis for a specified length of time, usually until goals are reached.

WHAT ABOUT PUNISHMENT?

Your child needs you to be her parent, not her friend. Hopefully, you do not feel the need for your youngster to like you every minute; parents who have this need are destined to be ineffective, frustrated, and disappointed. Just by saying no, you will clarify who is in charge, set the boundaries, create the values, and show the parental guidance children want and need. Children need to be loved and to love, and therefore it is necessary to focus on and punish only the specific activity, not blame or criticize the child herself, which may make her feel ashamed, inept, and undeserving of love.

Punishment can be an important element in any approach aimed at changing a child's behavior. There are various types of punishment, and the one chosen must fit the need or the deed. While children have a need for parental control, that control should vary for different ages or stages of development. The form of discipline that you use with a six-year-old may not work or be appropriate when that child is ten.

Children may feel guilty about inappropriate behavior or failing to do the right thing, and a mild, appropriate punishment often relieves them of that guilt. Like everyone else, children have the right to make mistakes and learn from their experiences.

Here are some common forms of punishment:

Natural Consequences

As a result of the child's own actions, certain consequences or reactions naturally happen, unless someone intervenes. For example, not taking care of a toy may result in that toy's becoming unusable. Teasing playmates may cause the child to lose her friends, get hit, or get teased herself.

Logical Consequences

In certain situations a natural consequence may be too dangerous. For instance, bike riding in the street may result in an accident or injury. So instead, the parent provides a punishment or consequence that appears logical and demonstrates a reasonable relationship between the behavior and the consequence. For example, if the child rides her bicycle in a busy street, that may result in losing the use of the bike for a week.

Behavior Penalty

A mild punishment may be given in response to behavior for which there is no ready natural or logical consequence. The penalty should be something meaningful to the child. For instance, when a youngster does not care for her pet, she may lose television privileges. These behavior penalties should be calmly discussed before they are instituted. Rules and expectations should be clear, preferably laid out in advance, and not presented as a surprise, a threat, or punishment.

Timeout

This is an effective way of dealing with a child's impulsive, aggressive, or hostile behavior, which often includes hitting, having tantrums, throwing toys, name-calling, whining, interrupting, humiliating, or directly disobeying a request to stop a particular action. It is not useful for a child whose only recognizable problem behavior is excessive sulking, crying, or whining. For these children, it is important to discover the root or purpose of these behaviors. Occasional excesses of this sort may be emotional expressions of frustration or disappointment which are normal and should be allowed. For a youngster with an attention deficit, lesser expectations and smaller consequences are needed.

A timeout removes the attention children are getting for their behavior and thus does not reinforce the behavior. It also allows parent and child alike to

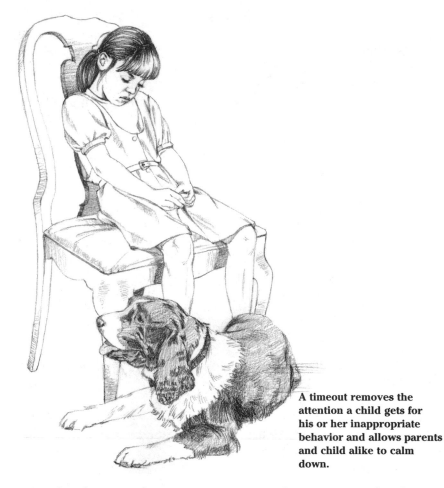

A timeout removes the attention a child gets for his or her inappropriate behavior and allows parents and child alike to calm down.

calm down, lessening the chances of angry encounters and power struggles. It permits parents to focus on the rational, specific behavior and allows interactions to return quickly to normal.

Here are some other points about timeouts to keep in mind:

- Discuss the use of timeouts—and the specific problem behavior that prompts them—with the child. Changes in behavior may need to be measured so both of you will know if timeouts are succeeding.

- Employ timeouts immediately after the specific behavior occurs. Use the rule of "ten plus the child's age"—that is, send the child to a timeout within ten seconds of the bad behavior, with no more than ten words being said (calmly). Timeouts should last about one minute per year of life, up to age eleven or twelve.

- Send the child to a preselected place that is safe, boring, and away from the busy areas of the house. Do not use a location the child finds entertaining or frightening. Do not drag or pull the child there. For each minute of protesting going to timeout, you can add a consequence.

- Use a portable timer that she can see or hear ring at the conclusion of the timeout. Let the youngster take responsibility for staying and leaving.

- Talk to your child *after* the timeout, when you are both calm, and explain the particular behavior that prompted the timeout. If the youngster is still angry or pouting, give her more time to calm down. Do not act angry or apologize, and do not ask her to apologize.

- Timeouts may require some practice before they become an effective means of modifying behavior.

- Seek professional advice for the child who refuses timeouts, leaves the room before they are over, damages the room, or continues the same behavior repeatedly despite the timeouts.

When Timeout Fails

When timeouts fail, consider the following:

- Are you using timeout correctly and consistently?

- Review the steps you took to begin the timeout. The two most common errors parents make in timeouts are (1) talking too much, and (2) getting upset and angry.

- Are your expectations realistic for your child and for the specific situation?

- Are there changes you can make in the environment that would reduce conflict? For example, must your child do homework right before dinner, when she is hungry? Is your child tired or already irritable, and in need of some quiet time before she is ready to take on a task?

- Would your spouse or another adult be more effective in doing timeout with your child or working through a disagreement with her in a particular situation?

- Are there new stresses or changes in your lives that are affecting you or your child?

Scolding and Disapproval

Use this approach sparingly, and only when the parents are in charge of their own emotions. When it is applied, it should be soon after the undesirable behavior and focusing on the particular behavior.

Scolding should never be done in a nagging, humiliating, cynical, or sarcastic manner, which can result in a child feeling shame and resentment. The problem of the actual behavior may become "lost" in this turbulent emotional climate. Parental anger is normal but should not be excessive or out of proportion to what the child did to provoke it.

Physical Punishment

Parents often ask, "Should I spank my child?" Many parents occasionally lose their patience or, in anger or fear, may spank their youngster. For instance, if a child runs out into the street, a parent may sweep the child up and, in a moment of anxiety for the child's well-being, spank her to emphasize the parent's sense of urgency or worry. Actually, it is the parent's expression of disapproval that is an effective deterrent in this situation, not the spanking.

Spanking may relieve a parent's frustration for the moment and extinguish the undesirable behavior for a brief time. But it is the least effective way to discipline. It is harmful emotionally to both parent and child. Not only can it result in physical harm, but it teaches children that violence is an acceptable way to discipline or express anger. While stopping the behavior temporarily, it does not teach alternative behavior. It also interferes with the development of trust, a sense of security, and effective communication. (Spanking often becomes *the* method of communication.) It also may cause emotional pain and resentment.

WHERE WE STAND

The American Academy of Pediatrics strongly opposes striking a child. If the spanking is spontaneous, parents should later explain calmly why they did it, the specific behavior that provoked it, and how angry they felt. They might apologize to their child for their loss of control, because that usually helps the youngster understand and accept the spanking.

THE NONCOMPLIANT CHILD

Younger children (ages five to eight) often flatly refuse to comply with a reasonable request. They may say "No!" or they may simply ignore their parents' requests.

Before imposing any punishment upon this child, make sure you have given him a specific, clearly stated, reasonable request, such as "Jason, please pick up your toys and put them on the shelf before dinner." (Statements like "Clean up your room" or "Straighten things up" are too vague and general.) If the child is preoccupied, distracted, or seems confused by the order, call him by name, make eye contact at his level, and state the command in as simple a form as possible, using a calm, rational voice. Use of the "I" message may be most effective, such as "Jason, I would be very pleased to see these toys put on the shelf before dinner." (See Chapter 13, "Communicating with Your Child.")

Wait ten seconds and maintain steady but not too intimidating eye contact with the child. If he begins to obey your command, praise him right away for this specific behavior. If he does not obey, tell him you will give him another ten seconds and then he will need a timeout. In this case it is appropriate to use timeout as a threat or warning. If the child exceeds the ten-second limit, impose the timeout right away.

Once the timeout is over, return him to the task and repeat the command in a clear, calm, task-specific manner. If he refuses again, repeat the timeout, adding an extra minute or two. This may need to be repeated several more times. If timeouts seem not to be working, you will need to reconsider how they are being used (see "When Timeout Fails," page 215).

BEHAVIOR PROBLEMS OUTSIDE THE HOME

A child's misbehavior often occurs at the home of friends or relatives, in the car, or in public places such as shopping malls and restaurants. These situations are very difficult to handle. In instances like these, anticipating the problem and taking some preventive action is best.

Decide upon the type of age-appropriate and achievable behavior you want your child to exhibit in these outside-the-home situations, and then discuss it with your youngster in terms of what you both expect. If your child is having greater difficulty in some specific situations away from home, you might modify your expectations accordingly. Do not put your child in situations that you know she cannot handle.

You may find that the most helpful approach is to use immediate rewards and praise when good behavior is exhibited. Be willing to utilize timeouts, delayed timeouts, or behavior penalties in public situations. (Delayed timeouts

Suggestions for Changing Behavior

1. Be selective about disciplining, and keep things in perspective. Behavior that causes physical or emotional harm to a child or others merits a lot of parental effort. Minor irritating behavior should receive little attention.

2. Avoid these common mistakes:

   • Parents may inadvertently punish good behavior or at least fail to reinforce good effort. For example, if their child improves her grades, raising them all to C's, they may ask, "Why didn't you get B's?"

   • They may reward or reinforce bad behavior. This often occurs when a child continually whines and pleads and then finally gets her way.

   • They may fail to reward good behavior. For instance, a child might wash the dishes and fail to be praised for accomplishing this task.

   • They may fail to stop a child's bad behavior, or they may rationalize it. Perhaps one sibling is hurting another; the parent may respond, "Well, she deserved it," or "She needs to learn to fight back."

3. Reward and punish specific behavior. Focus on the behavior, and do not criticize the child as a person ("You are such a bad child").

are those that are implemented once you return home.) The use of logical consequences is also often helpful.

Try bringing along a child's favorite toys and books, and plan to give her some positive attention on a trip or on a visit to relatives.

In general, scolding and nagging will not work. It is embarrassing to everyone, tends to reinforce negative behavior, and could spoil a family outing for everyone.

Once you find the behavior modification techniques and punishments that work, apply them at home before using them outside the house so your child is familiar with them.

4. Use punishments sparingly, and only when you are in control of your emotions. Physical punishment is harmful and not productive.

5. Children frequently experience physical and emotional stress, which can result in behavioral problems. Be sensitive to this issue, and try to eliminate the sources of stress.

6. Some children exhibit behavioral problems because they have not been taught or have not experienced appropriate alternative behavior. Teach them other, more acceptable ways to behave and respond ("If I shouldn't do this, then what should I do instead?").

7. Look beyond the concrete behavior the child is exhibiting, and understand what she might be trying to tell you. Recognize that sometimes a child's worrisome behavior is a signal that she or the family is in pain. She may be the designated family "messenger," and her behavior may be a cry for help for the entire family.

8. Recognize the state of your own emotions and your coping ability when confronting your child's behavior. That state may range from feeling competent and secure to feeling depressed and helpless. This recognition and self-awareness will help you decide if you need help or not.

9. Seek professional help when you think it is necessary. The earlier the intervention, the better the outcome. This professional input can also often provide reassurance that you are doing the right thing.

Some parents have difficulty implementing timeouts away from home, and in cases like this you and your child may have to take a timeout together. In a restaurant a timeout may require that you and your child sit in the car for a while. In a mall she might sit on a bench while you stand beside her; in a park or at the zoo, use a bench or a rock as a place for a timeout. If you are driving, stop the car at the side of the road and sit quietly until she settles down. You might use a delayed timeout when you arrive at a hotel, a restaurant, or a rest stop.

In the weeks ahead, evaluate and discuss positive changes in the frequency, duration, and intensity of any continued undesirable behavior, and point these out to the child with praise.

DEALING WITH YOUR OWN FEELINGS

Your child's difficult behavior can no doubt make you feel angry, resentful, unappreciated, inadequate, or guilty. From your experience you know that these negative emotions can interfere with effective parenting and good parent-child communication. You should not deny your feelings, and you need to learn to share them effectively and appropriately with another adult—a spouse, friend, relative, or professional.

Here are some suggestions for dealing with your own anger:

- Accept the fact that children do make parents angry, resentful, and guilty.

- Recognize that parents are entitled to these feelings without feeling even more guilty, angry, inadequate, or full of shame.

- Express your feelings without attacking or condemning your child: for instance, "I am angry when I fix a good meal and nobody comes to the table."

Successful childrearing is easier if parents also understand how and why they react to their child's behavior as they do. Often parents respond to their children in much the same way they were treated by their own parents. Even when parents intend to raise their children differently, ingrained patterns persist, and become especially evident during times of stress in the family. Sometimes particular memories are so powerful that they influence how you interpret something your child has done. Perhaps your child's behavior reminds you of a childhood playmate or a relative about whom you have strong feelings. It is natural, but incorrect, to generalize from a single behavior and react as though your child will behave in other ways or suffer the consequences that you observed in your past. Understanding your own temperament and experiences can be a great advantage in raising your child.

15

MANAGING
COMMON BEHAVIOR
PROBLEMS

DISOBEDIENCE

From time to time most children defy the wishes of their parents. This is a part of growing up and testing adult guidelines and expectations. It is one way for children to learn about and discover their own selves, express their individuality, and achieve a sense of autonomy. As they stretch their independent wings and engage in minor conflicts with their parents, they discover the boundaries of their parents' rules and of their own self-control.

Sometimes, however, these conflicts are more than occasional disturbances and become a pattern for how parents and children interact. Disobedience can have a variety of causes. At times, it is due to unreasonable parental expectations. Or it might be related to a child's difficult or intense temperament, or to school problems, family stress, or conflicts between his parents.

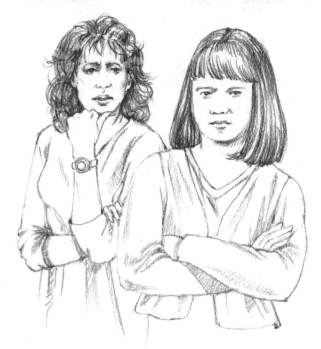

All children defy the wishes of their parents from time to time—it is a part of growing up.

In some instances these children have demonstrated a persistent pattern of disobedience throughout their development, beginning in their early years. They may resist authority by talking back to and disobeying their parents. They may stubbornly tell their parents no when asked to do something. In many cases this behavior occurs only at home; at other times it is a pattern with all authority figures (teachers, babysitters, grandparents) in all settings. This latter situation, of course, is of greater concern.

Other youngsters who are generally cooperative and agreeable may suddenly become disrespectful and disobedient during middle childhood. This is usually a sign that they are experiencing a lot of inner turmoil or that a significant new stress is occurring around them, such as abuse or school failure. Their hostility is directed toward the nearest target, those closest to them, and is a way of coping with and expressing the stress they feel.

Some children may have a lengthy history of being out of control and noncooperative. This is a serious problem. When children have been disobedient for long periods—routinely talking back to and having outbursts aimed at their parents and others—there is often conflict and disorganization within the family as a whole. This might include harsh punishment and family relationship problems, including physical aggressiveness between family members. The children may reject their parents' authority, feeling that their mother and father disapprove not only of their behavior but of them as people. Thus, these youngsters learn to be unhappy with themselves, and their self-esteem can suffer greatly. Gradually, if the family relationships continue to deteriorate, the children become even more angry, sad, hostile, and aggressive.

Many disobedient children do not adequately communicate the reasons for their sadness or discomfort, or their parents are unable to understand what they are trying to express. This breakdown in communication sometimes occurs if the child is not receiving enough parental attention, perhaps because his parents are preoccupied with their own lives, careers, and problems. (See Chapter 13, "Communicating with Your Child.")

For some children, aggressive and disobedient behavior is a response to violence they see within the family. To youngsters raised in abusive environments, aggressive behavior may seem like a reasonable way to deal with anger or frustration or seem like the way to solve problems between people. Many families with disobedient children resort to physical abuse as one of their techniques for disciplining. But physical punishment leads to more aggressive behavior by the children, and a vicious cycle is established. Children raised in this type of setting are at much greater risk for lifelong problems with interpersonal relationships and authority. (See Chapter 30, "Child Abuse.")

As a parent, you need to keep in mind that middle childhood is a vulnerable period of life. Young school-age children are quite egocentric, thinking that all events that happen around them have something to do with themselves. For example, in families where there is marital conflict, youngsters may misinterpret this problem, concluding that they themselves have been bad and have upset their parents. In the process their self-esteem may suffer, and they may be more prone to reacting inappropriately to the events around them.

What Parents Can Do

When you have a chronically disobedient child, examine the possible sources of his inner turmoil and rebelliousness. If this has been a persistent pattern that has continued into middle childhood, closely evaluate your own family situation: How much respect do your family members show for one another? Do they respect one another's privacy, ideas, and personal values? How does the family work out its conflicts? Are disagreements resolved through rational discussion, or do people regularly argue or resort to violence? What is your usual style of relating to your child, and what forms does discipline usually take? How much spanking and yelling is there? Do you and your child have very different personalities and ways of getting along in the world that cause friction between you? Is your child having trouble succeeding at school or developing friendships? Is the family undergoing some especially stressful times?

If your child has only recently started to demonstrate disrespect and disobedience, tell him that you have noticed a difference in his behavior and that you sense he is unhappy or struggling. With his help, try to determine the specific cause of his frustration or upset. This is the first step toward helping him change his behavior.

In response to your child's ongoing disobedience, you must examine your style and pattern of parenting, including your own background. How were you raised? How consistent are your disciplining efforts? Do you reward cooperation, or just react to disobedience and conflict? Are you and your spouse supportive of one another? Do the two of you agree about discipline?

If you react to your child's talking back by exploding or losing your temper, he will respond with disobedience and disrespect. By contrast, he will become more obedient when you remain calm, cooperative, and consistent. He will learn to be respectful if you are respectful toward him and others in the family. If he becomes disobedient and out of control, impose a timeout until he calms down and regains self-control.

Have your child apologize for any disrespect he shows toward you or others, as a way of demonstrating his regard for parental and adult authority.

When your child is obedient and respectful, compliment him for that behavior. Reward the behavior you are seeking, including cooperation and resolution of disagreements. These positive efforts will always be much more successful than punishment.

When to Seek Additional Help

For some disobedient children, you may need to obtain professional mental-health treatment. Here are some situations where outside counseling may be necessary:

- If there is a persistent, long-standing pattern of disrespect of authority both at school and at home

- If the patterns of disobedience continue in spite of your best efforts to encourage your child to communicate his negative feelings

- If a child's disobedience and/or disrespect is accompanied by aggressiveness and destructiveness

- If a child shows signs of generalized unhappiness—perhaps talking of feeling blue, unliked, friendless, or even suicidal

- If your family has developed a pattern of responding to disagreements with physical or emotional abuse

- If you or your spouse or child use alcohol or other drugs to feel better or cope with stress

If relationships within your family show signs of difficulty and a lack of cooperation, then family therapy may be indicated. By dealing with and resolving these problems at a young age, you can minimize and even prevent more serious struggles that may emerge as your children reach adolescence. The key is early identification and treatment.

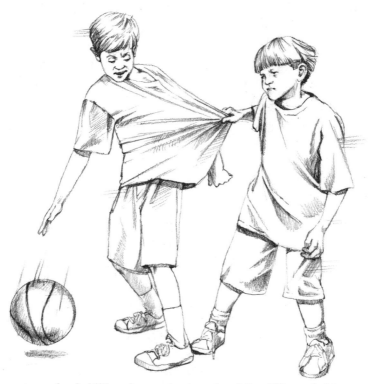

Some elementary-school children have not yet mastered the skills needed to manage their aggression effectively.

AGGRESSIVE BEHAVIOR

An aggressive child is one who hits, bites, bullies, demands, and/or destroys. Although aggression is a part of human nature, most people learn to manage and control their aggressive impulses and to channel them into appropriate and socially acceptable activities.

Aggression is particularly likely during times of threat, anger, rage, and frustration. As an important task of early childhood, youngsters must develop the ability to manage aggression and replace it with more socially acceptable responses. By the time most children reach school age, their coping skills are sophisticated enough, and their range of social skills broad enough, that they can generally remain calm and cooperative even in the face of stressful or unpleasant circumstances. Such appropriate behavior does not prevent them from competing and striving toward competence.

Some elementary-school children have not yet mastered the skills needed to manage their aggression effectively. Their behavior ranges from hitting to throwing to having tantrums. By kindergarten, children whose aggressive behavior is a threat to their peers and to themselves should receive professional help. Other children, usually between ages six and nine, occasionally regress and exhibit aggressive behavior when they are under extreme stress. By about a seven-to-one ratio, boys have more problems with aggression than girls; this is due to a combination of factors, from the innate aggressive tendencies of boys to the fact that our society encourages and accepts more aggressive behavior from them.

Socially immature children may express their negative and hostile feelings in destructive ways. They may have bouts of aggression that damage property (such as their own toys or the property of others), throw objects, turn over furniture, break lamps, or kick walls. These behaviors are usually triggered by frustration, anger, or humiliation. Some children who have failed to receive sufficient positive attention for their more socially desirable behavior develop a habit of resorting to negative behaviors to get parental attention.

Sometimes these children exhibit even more serious antisocial behavior—so-called *conduct disorders*—such as setting fires, being cruel to animals, hurting other people (physically and/or emotionally), or lying habitually. As youngsters grow older, this pattern may evolve to include vandalism and truancy and is often associated with alcohol and other drug abuse. These kinds of worrisome behavior occur only rarely in some children, but they have serious implications for later functioning, and their presence should prompt an evaluation by a specialist in child behavior and emotional problems.

What Causes Aggressive Behavior?

As with any kind of behavioral difficulties, there are many complicated reasons for aggressive and/or destructive behavior. Some children, because of inherited personality traits, are more predisposed to aggression. Children with "difficult" or intense temperaments experience more problems with aggression. (See the section on "Temperament," page 123, for a more complete discussion.) Others who are very active, strong-willed, or impulsive have more trouble learning to control their aggression.

Your child's environment—family, school, and peers—can shape his responses to stressful situations and greatly determine the way he handles anger and displays aggressive behavior. Imitation is one of the most powerful influences upon a child's development, and children learn to handle themselves by watching and copying how adults and other children control their own aggressive impulses. Thus, if you and your spouse act aggressively toward your children, toward each other, or toward others with whom you come into contact, or if you permit fighting and destructiveness by your youngsters, they will learn that this behavior is acceptable.

Sometimes a child is aggressive because he has failed to learn self-control. Children develop self-control by learning from their parents what are acceptable limits to their aggressive impulses. Typically, when children have little self-control, their parents are permissive, have set no limits, and have let their youngsters do whatever they wish. Sometimes parents use inappropriate means—physical punishment, for example—when responding to their children's negative behavior. These parents may erroneously believe that a spanking, or a similarly aggressive and abusive response, is a proper reaction when a child fights or misbehaves. However, physical punishment will not help a child learn to control his negative emotions or hostile behavior; rather, it teaches him to be aggressive when he is angry.

Physical punishment is rarely if ever effective. Rather, it usually occurs when a parent is unable to manage his or her own anger or frustration effectively and thus inappropriately resorts to aggression. When a child's aggressive behavior is met with more aggressive behavior from a parent, things usually get worse, not better.

Aggressive behavior can have other causes too. Children may become more aggressive and destructive when they feel overwhelmed by stress, including family problems like marital discord, divorce, unemployment, financial distress, parental illness, or a move to a new city. When a youngster has been abused physically, sexually, or emotionally, or has been neglected, his aggression may be a cry for help. Some children may lash out in frustration or anger if they feel they have not lived up to their parents' expectations. Sometimes, although rarely, aggressive behavior has its roots in medical problems such as head injuries or hyperactivity.

Child psychiatrists, when trying to deal with aggressive behavior, believe it is important to distinguish between children who have never learned to control their aggressiveness and those who previously had good self-control but have since regressed. The first situation is more difficult to treat, since the youngster has never developed any control over his aggression and so must learn new skills. In the second circumstance, the child's symptoms may be a sign of a new and powerful stress in his life. Treatment for these children is aimed at helping the child deal with the stress that may be provoking his aggressive behavior.

Aggressiveness with Peers

When a child exhibits aggressive behavior at home—perhaps throwing toys or screaming at siblings—his parents can intervene immediately and help the child learn better self-control. If the child has learned how to manage this aggression at home, he is better prepared to deal with the inevitable conflicts that arise with peers. Many youngsters, however, still struggle with their aggressiveness upon entering school. Parents find the situation more disturbing and more difficult to manage if their child is fighting or intimidating *other* children, either at school or on the playground, thus becoming a schoolyard bully.

In some families, however, parents encourage fighting as a way for a child to assert his manhood, settle conflicts, and "stand up for himself." This pattern of aggressive behavior and response becomes self-perpetuating and can lead to lifelong problems with relationships and social rules. Parents need to teach their youngsters socially appropriate ways to manage themselves in conflicts with peers.

What Parents Can Do

When your child is fighting with or bullying his peers, or exhibiting destructive behavior, he probably should be evaluated by a mental-health professional. Meanwhile, here are some strategies you should consider:

1. Express disappointment in the specific behavior you disapprove of, without implying that your child himself is bad. Discuss in depth the situation that occurred, giving other options for action.

2. Help your youngster see how it might feel to be bullied by others.

3. Help him understand that no one likes a bully. Explain how bullies develop reputations that can result in a loss of friends and difficulty making new ones. Tell him that the sooner he alters his behavior, the better, since long-standing reputations are hard to change.

4. For a child prone to fighting, insist that he learn to resolve conflicts without physical force. As a starting point, do not permit conflicts at home to be settled by physical means. Teach all of your children to use words, not fists, to resolve their differences. Work with them so that instead of acting out, they stop, consider what they are feeling, and then turn their feelings into words. Reward them for settling conflicts without fighting.

5. Do not become intimidated by your child's anger, nor avoid conflicts that may arise with him. Instead, take charge of these situations in a consistent way, aimed at helping him control his aggression.

6. Establish effective ways of promoting self-control in your child at home. Timeouts work for most youngsters—telling them they must stay in their room until they get themselves back under control. This will provide them with a safe environment as they learn to manage themselves better.

7. If any destruction of property has occurred outside the home, your child should be responsible for restitution. For example, if he destroys a neighbor's toys (or his own sibling's toys), he might need to increase the number of chores he does around the house, earning money to replace what he has broken. Don't forget to have him apologize.

8. Reward your child (with praise or star charts, for example) as he learns to express his anger and frustration in more acceptable ways. This will be the most important way to change his behavior.

9. Explore whether your child's school offers courses in conflict resolution, or if such opportunities exist with other community organizations.

10. Develop an attitude of hopeful expectation that your child can learn to manage his own frustration and anger. If you are doubtful that he can control himself, look within yourself to determine why. Remember, parental attitudes help shape your child's behavior.

11. Examine your family's style of expressing anger and resolving conflict. If the family exhibits a style similar to that of your child with his peers, the key to helping your youngster rests with changing these family patterns.

When to Seek Additional Help

If your own efforts at assisting your child or family to control aggressive behavior are not working or seem unlikely to do so, ask your pediatrician for a referral to a mental-health professional or behavioral pediatrician who can help. The earlier these professional interventions occur, the greater the likelihood of success.

TEMPER TANTRUMS

Some of a parent's most trying and embarrassing moments occur during a child's temper tantrums. The youngster who expresses her anger or frustration by screaming, throwing toys, or hitting a playmate, perhaps hurting others or even herself, the child who falls to the floor crying when she doesn't get her way, perhaps even swearing or destroying property—these children present a special challenge.

Occasional tantrums are quite normal for children from ages one or one and a half to four, and these outbursts subside for most children by the time they enter school. Normal psychological development tends to provide most youngsters with better self-control and make them considerably more cooperative and educable by school age. Even when they are upset, school-age children generally can express their frustration and anger in words, with reasonable control.

But that is not always the case. For some children, temper tantrums persist into the school years and occur with regularity. Their parents understandably become terribly frustrated and upset by this behavior. Why, they ask, hasn't my child developed more socially appropriate ways of communicating anger and frustration?

To answer this question, pediatricians often recommend that parents first evaluate what kind of role models they have been—how they themselves respond to anger, and how they have taught their children to react. When parents are prone to exaggerated, disruptive outbursts and fits of temper, their children often are too. When parents are explosive—having tantrums of their own in their relationships with others—that is the type of behavior they are teaching to their children.

Of course, other factors can come into play too. Some parents, especially those with little previous experience with children, may have unrealistic expectations of their children's behavior. Asking children to sit quietly for long periods of time, to do tasks beyond their physical or developmental abilities, or to accept responsibilities or parents' decisions that are clearly unfair are examples of situations that will be frustrating and can trigger an outburst.

Because of their temperament or constitution, some children have a lower threshold for feeling frustrated and a greater tendency toward intense negative expressions of displeasure. (See "Temperament," page 123.) Children with strong wills have more difficulty managing their anger and negative emotions and a harder time learning self-control. However, with proper guidance and support, they can learn to suppress their more explosive behavior.

In some situations, a tantrum is a way for a child to get attention from her parents, who respond to their youngster only when she is so provocative and demanding.

When a family is under continual stress and strain—perhaps because of financial troubles, alcoholism, marital conflict, poverty, physical or sexual abuse, or moves from friends and family—children may react with more frequent temper tantrums. Also, some parents report that children with chronic illnesses or learning disabilities are more prone to tantrums, perhaps because of the ongoing frustration created by their disorders; however, not all children with these problems have tantrums, and in fact, most do not.

Sometimes, school-age children have gone tantrum-free for several years—apparently with a high tolerance for frustration and an ability to cooperate well—only to develop tantrums later on. If this sounds like your child, consider whether these symptoms are being provoked by a new, overwhelming stress occurring at school, at home, or in the neighborhood. If your child is unable to handle the emotional tension of the stressful situation, she may express her anxiety, fear, or anger in this inappropriate way. As a parent, you need to pinpoint the source of this stress and try to help your child cope more effectively. If necessary, talk to teachers, babysitters, or your child's friends to help you discover the cause of the problem.

What Parents Can Do

Many parents have difficulty deciding just how to respond to a child's temper tantrums. Here are some suggestions to keep in mind.

- Recognize that some children are simply more intense than others, or have more difficulties to overcome.

- Avoid having unrealistic expectations of your child. Compare your expectations against those of the parents of your child's friends, especially those whose behavior you admire.

- When your child is out of control, ignore the temper tantrum so as not to create a "reward" for her inappropriate behavior. She may be trying to get attention and *any* response, positive or negative, can reinforce her outbursts. So instead, try ignoring her or walking away. This provides the child with an opportunity to learn self-control.

Sometimes, however, you may be unable to ignore her tantrums, perhaps because she comes running after you or is destroying toys or hitting a sibling. In cases like these, insist that she go to another room for a timeout away from others until she can bring herself under control. Physically escorting her to her room may be necessary. (See Chapter 14, "Changing Your Child's Behavior.")

In general, parents should remain as calm as possible and avoid becoming involved in the tantrum by controlling their own frustration and anger. They should also avoid physical confrontations, which can escalate to frightening levels and even end up with someone, usually the child, getting hurt.

After your child and you have calmed down, sit and talk with her about what provoked the outburst. Emphasize the importance of communicating her negative feelings through words, not actions, and discuss more positive ways to respond. You might find a reward system useful, offering praise or perhaps something more material when your youngster solves conflicts without throwing a tantrum.

When to Seek Additional Help

Some middle-years youngsters can benefit from consultation with a child psychiatrist or psychologist because of their temper tantrums, but most do not need this help. Your pediatrician usually can guide and support you through the resolution of this problem behavior. You should consider seeking professional help in any of the following situations:

- The tantrums become a pattern whenever your child feels frustrated or angry.

- The tantrums occur frequently, such as several times a day.

- Your child has tantrums outside the home, perhaps at school.

- The tantrums result in destruction of property or physical harm to your child or others.

- The tantrums are becoming unbearable for the parents and are interfering with a normal, happy parent-child relationship.

In any of these situations, address the problem at once. Temper tantrums do not necessarily go away on their own. You need to try to understand what your child is experiencing—and perhaps change your own response to the outbursts—so that she can learn to control her negative feelings effectively, with your guidance.

If these symptoms continue into adolescence, they can become even more of a concern. With the added pressures of the teenage years, and the expanded repertoire of behavior available to teenagers along with their increased physical size, tantrums can become increasingly worrisome, dangerous, and difficult to manage.

STEALING

Much to their dismay, parents often discover that during the middle years of childhood their youngsters are being dishonest and are stealing, lying, or cheating. This can be a real shock, and the first response of many parents is to be embarrassed, angry, and occasionally (and inappropriately) explosive.

However, these childhood behaviors, although unacceptable, are a normal part of the developmental process of young children. They are a part of learning about themselves and the world around them and developing their personal morals, ethics, and conscience.

From ages six to twelve, children are increasingly psychologically and physically independent from their parents. They are more heavily involved with school and their peers and are developing a new sense of themselves at a greater distance from the watchful guidance of their mother and father. They are facing new challenges to maintain friendships, compete with peers, and meet the demands of teachers and fellow students. Thus, at a time when pressures can be great, and when they have not yet fully adapted to the rules of society, they may find dishonesty to be an expedient way of coping.

Before age six, children may not have a clear sense of what belongs to them and what does not. Three- and four-year-old children take toys that others might be playing with, simply because they want them. If that behavior is not responded to by parents (or others), it may progress to taking toys that belong to other children when they are not looking. The behavior clearly then becomes stealing.

After age six, children are much more likely to be aware that they are doing something wrong when they take things they know are not theirs. Commonly, the first stealing incident occurs at about age seven.

In the preschool and kindergarten years children are occupied with learning about social order and, especially, the significant relationships within the family; these are times of family intimacy. However, by the time children reach ages six to eight, they have developed some sense of independence from their family and have a heightened feeling of being in charge of themselves. As they enter school and their peer relationships become more important, they have an increased desire to belong, to show off, and to compete with others.

At the same time, children develop feelings of possessiveness and an interest in their belongings and collections, their rooms, and their activities at home. All these needs intensify at about seven years old.

Children of this age often take an object from a teacher, a friend's home, or from the friend himself. Perhaps they feel deprived—they want something for themselves that they do not have—and they impulsively take it. Or they may steal money from home to share with their friends at school or to buy candy for themselves and their friends. Children may also secretly take something from a store.

The seven-year-old child who takes things often is a little less popular than many of his peers, and perhaps his stealing fills an emotional void. Stealing may also be a way of responding to feeling deprived, or a way of getting something a child wants that he feels would otherwise be unavailable. Sometimes stealing is an expression of anger or hostility. Child psychiatrists theorize that children who have stolen feel some sense of deprivation, envy, anxiety, or resentment.

There is another peak incidence of stealing at about age thirteen. Of course, this is also a period of rapid change—physically, psychologically, and so-cially—and stealing may again become a way to impress friends. Peer (and gang) pressure can also sometimes coerce children into acts like stealing. In particular, dares can lead to stealing.

Sometimes stealing occurs repeatedly or is associated with a multitude of other behavioral or emotional difficulties. In this context stealing is much more troubling and indicates that the child is in need of professional help.

What Parents Can Do

When you discover that your child has stolen something, it is important that your child understands that stealing is wrong. You may remember how ashamed you yourself felt if you were ever caught stealing as a child. Your youngster needs to learn the same lessons, although most experts say that in-tensely embarrassing or ridiculing him is not beneficial. Simple explanations are best.

In most cases it is probably best not to ask your child directly whether or why he has stolen something; this will only tend to prompt a series of lies as he tries to save face. Rather, be straightforward and acknowledge that you know the theft has occurred.

It is important to establish some restitution. Your child needs to return the object that was taken, either to the store, his friend, or the school. You might wish to accompany him and encourage him to apologize, stating that he will never do it again.

Thereafter, have a talk with your child. Rather than implying that he is a bad person, try to discover why he stole. Explain that while children understand-ably want things, they should not take the possessions of others. In most sit-uations, if the stealing incident is handled directly and immediately, it will not recur and your child will learn from it.

When an older child (approaching or entering adolescence) has stolen, again you should offer him an opportunity to explore and discuss his behav-ior, especially addressing stresses he is experiencing. In some situations you may respond to stealing episodes with a serious discussion about peer pres-sure and its influence upon his behavior. At this age stealing is often indicative of a personal or social difficulty and may require professional help.

When to Seek Additional Help

You should seek outside assistance through a child-guidance agency, child psychologist, or mental-health worker in the following situations:

- Your child repeatedly steals from home or school, from parents, or from others.

- Your youngster is "buying" his peer relationships by stealing.

LYING

Children younger than age six often have difficulty distinguishing between reality and fantasy. Hence, for them there is often an uncertain boundary between truth and fiction.

After about age six, however, children clearly can differentiate truth from fantasy. As a result, when a child lies she knows she is being deceitful.

Many pressures can cause a child to lie. Most frequently, when a youngster has been brought up in a loving and responsible home, she will first lie when she is confronted with having done something wrong and feels afraid of disappointing her parents or being punished by them. Already feeling guilty, she will try to protect herself from what she thinks will be harsh discipline.

In many cases, parents of children who lie have unusually high standards of behavior and expectations. These youngsters know right from wrong and, in what they view as a difficult situation, are trying to save face.

Sometimes children lie when they are under significant stress to meet impossible demands. Thus, youngsters who are struggling at school and cannot keep up with their studies may feel overwhelmed and lie about having completed all their homework. Because of circumstances like these, lying has to be interpreted in relation to the surrounding events.

Remember, *lying shows that a child is aware that she has done something wrong.* By attempting to protect herself from parental disappointment and disapproval, she is demonstrating that her conscience is working. Parents who overreact and become extremely negative may push their child into a position of feeling that she needs to lie again and again to protect herself.

Youngsters in middle childhood also might become confused in a home where there is a double standard about lying—that is, where she is forbidden to lie but her parents sometimes tell "white lies," distorting the truth for their own convenience. It gives confusing signals to a child who has always been told to be honest, to witness a parent stretching the truth on the phone or with neighbors with white lies. Children often have a hard time differentiating among the subtleties in situations like these.

What Parents Can Do

If you discover that your child has lied, let her know immediately that you are aware she is not telling the truth. Harsh punishment is usually not very effective. Instead, make the following points with both your words and your behavior:

- "I want you to tell me only the truth, and I will always tell you the truth, so that we can always believe each other."

- "You will get in much less trouble if you tell the truth instead of lying."

Also, remember that your own actions and your own style of telling the truth are probably the most important ways you can teach your child the importance of honesty.

When to Seek Additional Help

A child who has a history of chronic lying should be seen by a counselor, child-guidance clinic, or mental-health professional. Chronic liars often have had difficulty establishing a true conscience that can clearly differentiate between right and wrong. These children also may be crying out for help because of disturbances in their family life or outside the home.

CHEATING

Cheating is the result of competition. In our culture, with few exceptions, competitiveness is commonplace and in fact is rewarded. Children learn that losing is bad, and especially in the early school years, their wish to do well is very strong.

As children play games with one another, cheating will frequently occur. In the early years there is a lot of breaking of rules and conflicts in these peer struggles. Watch how children play board games or card games, and you will recognize the competitiveness, striving, and social learning taking place and sometimes digressing into cheating. As children become older and approach adolescence, however, this behavior is much less tolerated by peers, and thus some children become labeled as cheaters. A sense of fairness has a higher value in these older peer relationships.

If you are confronted with a situation where your child has cheated, you need to consider many factors, including the degree of pressure that he is under to win or do well, and his own background regarding competition. Children tend to cheat, or set their own rules, when they are engaged in games or schoolwork that is too complex for them to handle. If you or others in his life expect him always to perform exceedingly well, then cheating can become almost a self-defense mechanism under the strain of this tremendous pressure. He may feel he has no other outlet than to cheat as a means of achieving success. Thus, the end becomes much more important than the process.

Also, consider the example that your family environment is providing for your child. If you or your spouse cheat from time to time—perhaps declining to return too much change given to you at the supermarket, or maybe even talking about fudging on your income taxes—those are the moral values you are teaching. Be sensitive to the examples you set; you can be an important role model for the prevention of cheating. To a large degree, your child's willingness to cheat is related to the values with which he is being raised.

What Parents Can Do

For a child in the middle years, parents need to identify and deal with any cheating episodes in order to teach him right from wrong. For example, if he is caught cheating at school—a common phenomenon—sit down with him and discuss the seriousness of this infraction. Talk about the kinds of stresses and pressures he may be feeling, including your own expectations for success. Excessive punishment for these misdeeds is rarely helpful.

Playing family games where chance is involved can teach children to compete with one another without cheating. Under your watchful eye, your youngster can be guided toward appropriate conduct and healthy competition.

When to Seek Additional Help

A child who has a chronic cheating problem, or who gets so labeled at school, may need further help. Often cheating is a symptom of an internal emotional struggle or peer problems that should be addressed. You can find assistance from a mental-health counselor or a child-guidance clinic.

SWEARING

Swearing—the use of profanity or "dirty" words—is almost a developmentally normal behavior for children during middle childhood and early adolescence. For these youngsters, swearing is often a sign of being worldly-wise and unafraid to be a little "bad." Profanity is used to impress friends and can become a part of peer relationships. Quite frequently, younger children do not know the meanings of the words they are using, but they will say them anyway simply because they have heard others use them.

Fortunately, this phenomenon of cursing seems to lose its attraction and abate as children become more mature. Until then, however, youngsters often delight in shocking their parents with the swear words they have learned away from home. (Bear in mind that parents who swear in the home are teaching their children to do the same and should not be surprised when their youngsters copy their behavior.)

Clearly, there is a smaller group of "incorrigible" children who swear. In addition to cursing, they have many other difficulties, personally and socially. These youngsters may be more prone to swear and rage at other people—a different phenomenon than using a few swear words during times of frustration. Profanity directed at another individual should never be tolerated.

What Parents Can Do

Here are some suggestions to help you manage the problem of swearing:

- If you feel it is appropriate, establish a rule that "no swearing will take place in our home." Do not under any circumstances tolerate swearing that is aimed at someone in anger. If this occurs, a child may be sent immediately to her room for a timeout.

- Minor swearing in frustration is almost a natural human behavior. Although perhaps inappropriate, it is commonplace in some families. If that is your own personal style, you will find it hard to teach your child something different.

- When your youngster swears, do not overreact with your own outbursts of rage and cursing. Also, washing a child's mouth out with soap is clearly improper, extreme, and ineffective.

- On occasion, you may feel that your child is using profanity in an attempt to provoke a response from you. In these instances, ignoring her may be the most effective strategy.

- Reward your child for expressing her frustration appropriately without swearing. Star charts and money are helpful approaches. For example, use a jar of nickels that she can earn at the end of two weeks; for each day that she doesn't swear during this time, two additional nickels will be placed in the jar; but each time she swears, nickels will be removed. Your child will catch on quickly.

When to Seek Additional Help

In and of itself, swearing is not a sign of emotional disturbance. However, if there are other problems—chronic lying, chronic stealing, or difficulty with peers—then swearing may be just another symptom of a psychological or social disturbance. In this situation, talk to your pediatrician about counseling—either individual or family therapy.

RUNNING AWAY FROM HOME

In our culture running away has often been glorified in movies, TV, and books, as if it were an adventurous American tradition of seeking a better life. The reality is much more sobering. In most cases, children are not running *toward* a specific new situation but rather are running *away* from existing problems—and thus may be issuing a loud cry for help.

Not only do runaways leave anxious and worried parents behind, but they may enter a world of gangs, drugs, prostitution, AIDS, malnutrition, and truancy. They are quite vulnerable and at a much higher risk of becoming involved in early sexual behavior, sexual exploitation, or alcohol and other drug use. They may end up living on the street, in a homeless shelter, or in jail.

Most children who run away and are reported to the police as missing are between ages thirteen and fifteen. However, some younger children threaten to, or actually do, leave home.

When a child runs away, there has often been a crisis in the family. The child himself may be in some sort of trouble that he feels he cannot face for fear of severe punishment. Or there may be family stresses that can range from marital difficulties to alcohol-related problems to physical or sexual abuse—situations from which the child feels an overwhelming need to escape. Sometimes children are made to feel that they are a burden for their parents or the cause of the family's difficulties; children then run away to relieve their families, as well as to punish them.

On the other hand, some children run simply because they are looking for a good time. Impulsively and without planning, they will flee with a friend or two, seeking the thrill of life on the run. Often these children have already experienced various difficulties, perhaps conduct problems or substance abuse.

Some youngsters who run are loners, without many friends and with little support at home. Rather than running away with a friend, these loners often flee by themselves. They are driven by a feeling that there must be a better world out there.

When Your Child Threatens to Run Away

As a part of normal development, some children will talk of running away when they face conflicts with parents. If your child threatens to leave home, talk with him. Ask about any stresses and problems he may be experiencing. At the same time, be aware that these threats can sometimes be little more than a child's attempt to manipulate you. Perhaps he is trying to avoid chores or responsibilities. Or maybe he is attempting to relieve guilt feelings over having fought with you or having done something for which he is ashamed. If a situation has occurred in which the child and parents have been at odds, the youngster may feel that the only resolution is to hurt his mother and father by threatening to run away. Be aware of your own vulnerability to your child's manipulation, and remain in control of your emotions. In cases like these, the child will rarely leave home, but his threats should be heard as a last-ditch effort, one designed to turn the tide in the parent-child conflict, changing his parents' attitudes in a direction more sympathetic to his own.

If a child says he is going to run away, his parents should use their judgment on how to react. If he has never left home before, the threat may not be a serious one. Sometimes parents become very upset by their child's threats and try to talk him out of running away. However, arguments aimed at changing the child's mind are usually counterproductive. In effect, they acknowledge that the child is in control, something few children actually want. In addition, by focusing on the threat to leave, parents are ignoring the underlying issues and needs. Some parents wrongly "help pack their bags" or "wish them luck" on their running away as a way to defuse the conflicts with their children. This is likely only to heighten the child's sense of rejection and distrust. Sometimes parents and children contrive a pseudo-runaway, in which the parents know where the child is going and even encourage the behavior. Children can learn a lot from this experience, but their safety must be assured.

If your child lives in a divorced family and threatens to go live with his other parent, you might feel insecure about how you are faring as a parent or guilty over something you think you might have handled wrong. It is possible that your child may be trying to manipulate your thoughts and behavior. At some time, most children of divorced parents either threaten or request to live with the noncustodial parent. Try to understand your child's actions and appreciate his point of view. Talk over the situation with him, but let him know that until he's much older, the decision about where he will live remains his parents' decision. Do not make a hasty decision regarding living with the other parent, particularly during times of conflict. Consider these important decisions calmly and carefully. For your own peace of mind, remember that most of these conflicts eventually resolve themselves.

If Your Child Runs Away

What should you do if your middle-years child does actually run away? Of course, your most immediate efforts should be directed toward locating your youngster and returning him home. Runaway children often will wind up spending the night at a friend's or a relative's home, so check there first. Then enlist the aid of the police, school, friends, and family. Be prepared to tell the police the last time and place you saw your child, who he was with, and what he was wearing. Having a child missing is a frightening experience, so turn to a spouse, a friend, or a relative to help and support you through the ordeal.

Many, perhaps most, runaways return home. Some use a runaway hotline to contact their parents before the more stressful step of a face-to-face reunion (such as the National Runaway Switchboard at 800/621-4000 or 800/621-0394 (TDD)). After your child is found or returns, you need to aggressively seek out the reasons that led him to run away. What kinds of stresses has he been feeling at home or in school? What was making him frightened or unhappy? What kinds of negative peer pressure or threats has he had difficulty handling? The answers to these questions must be confronted and resolved, or running away may recur. When these issues are discussed and acted upon, you and your child may see some beneficial effects from his decision to run away, even if the overall experience was negative.

When to Seek Additional Help

If your child has threatened to run away but never has done so, he may not require outside help. However, if these threats have become an ongoing way in which he deals with conflicts, then he (and maybe the entire family) may benefit from an evaluation and, perhaps, treatment. Your pediatrician can refer you to the most appropriate type of help—whether from a child psychiatrist or psychologist, a behavioral pediatrician, or a social worker. This therapy should attempt to help you and your child understand and resolve the misunderstandings and conflicts in your household.

Any child who has actually run away—or who repeatedly threatens to do so—should be referred to a mental-health professional. It is a serious situation when a school-age child leaves home. The reasons for running away are often complex, and need to be fully explored by examining both internal personal distress and external threats. Crises must be resolved, and the family's lines of communication must be reopened. Running away is always a cry for help, and the underlying issues must be confronted and resolved. Treatment will often take time and commitment by the family to truly understand what their desperate child is experiencing in his world.

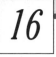

16

SEEKING
PROFESSIONAL HELP

A variety of specific kinds of behavior (or *symptoms*) usually indicate underlying behavioral, developmental, or emotional problems and require parents to take action. You should consider seeking professional help when problems are interfering with your child's or the family's ability to function well in day-to-day life. Problems that are persistent, severe, or cause significant stress to the family—or to your child's teachers or coaches—need attention.

WHEN TO SEEK HELP

Help is probably warranted when your child demonstrates:

- Behavior that you believe is very immature

- An inability or great resistance to respond to your initial, appropriate interventions, so that behavioral and emotional problems are repeated without resolution

- Worrisome changes, such as sleep problems, sudden alterations in mood or behavior, intense self-stimulation, sexual promiscuity, runaway behaviors, sudden interest in adult sexual topics, use of alcohol or drugs, complaints of chronic pain, poor school performance, poor relationships with peers or family members, repeated victimization, and diminished self-esteem

- Severe anxiety reactions, in which your child seems panicky and cannot be calmed down, including phobias and extreme separation difficulty

- Risky behavior that threatens the safety of the child or others; these might include intentionally harming an animal, setting a fire, or beating up a youngster in the schoolyard

- Suicidal actions, including talk about killing herself or especially where there has been an attempt at suicide

To find a competent professional and an appropriate treatment or therapy, start by talking to your child's pediatrician. Pediatricians are trained in the recognition of mental-health problems and can assist in the management of many common behavior problems. Discuss with him or her the problems your child is having and the reasons you are considering further evaluation and treatment. Because your pediatrician probably knows your family and your child and understands some of the difficulties you and your child are facing, he or she may be in a good position to either see your child him- or herself, or recommend the specific kind of help your youngster may need.

Because your pediatrician is probably also familiar with many of the mental-health professionals in your community, including their particular expertise and professional interests, he or she will be able to refer you to the most appropriate professional who can best deal with your child's problem.

School principals, clergy, teachers, or friends may also supply names of professionals. Reassurance from individuals who are satisfied with their experiences may make you feel more comfortable and confident that a professional is competent and trustworthy. Share such suggestions with your pediatrician when you discuss treatment options.

When making your decision, also consider the time and cost of the treatment and the distance you must travel to get there. Mental-health therapy concentrates on social, emotional, and behavioral problems and is usually provided on a weekly or every-other-week basis. Sessions typically last an hour and the fee is calculated on a per-hour basis.

Evaluate your insurance coverage to determine whether some or all of the cost of this care will be reimbursed by your insurer. Some insurance policies require prior authorization from your child's physician before it will cover mental-health treatment. If you belong to a health maintenance organization (HMO), you may have to use the HMO's own mental-health specialists. Some insurance companies have their own mental-health clinics; others allow patients to choose any professional they would like. Review your insurance coverage *before* you begin searching for a mental-health provider.

When you tell your child about your decision to seek counseling for her, she may resist the idea. She might feel there is a stigma attached to this type of care ("I'm not crazy, am I?"). Or she simply may not understand what will take place during the sessions.

Before your child begins seeing a mental-health professional, talk with her about the reasons for this care. Share with her that you are aware of the struggles she is having and the pain she is experiencing because of her symptoms. Emphasize that counseling is to help make things easier for her. Tell her that the therapist will help her get along better with her classmates, conquer her phobias, or whatever the specific problem and goals may be. Emphasize that the entire family will be getting help to deal with any family issues that may be involved. Assure her that any individual counseling will be confidential within appropriate limits. Do not make her feel as though she alone is to blame, or that she alone has a problem or is the "sick" one.

As the treatment process begins, your child should undergo a medical evaluation to ensure that she has no associated or contributing medical problems.

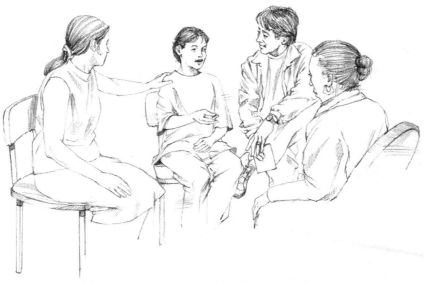

Successful therapy requires that children feel safe and respected.

APPROACHES TO COUNSELING AND THERAPY

Treatment should begin with at least one or two assessment sessions in which the therapist gathers background information and meets you and your child. During this time additional information may be acquired from the

Types of
Mental-Health Professionals

Many types of professionals and agencies are available for mental-health consultation and treatment. Here are those you are most likely to encounter:

Psychiatrists. General psychiatrists are physicians (M.D.'s) who have gone to medical school for four years and then have had four years of training in general psychiatry. Child psychiatrists specialize in the mental health of children and have had two additional years of special training after the four years of general psychiatry. They have also been trained in neurology and child development.

If there is no child psychiatrist available, your pediatrician may know of a general psychiatrist with a special interest in working with children. All psychiatrists, and especially child psychiatrists, have had experience providing psychotherapy to individuals and, to varying extents, to families.

Psychiatrists are able to prescribe medications that may be helpful for particular kinds of disorders, including attention deficit hyperactivity disorder, depression, anxiety, and obsessive-compulsive disorder.

Psychologists. They may have either a master's degree (M.S.) or a doctoral degree (Ph.D., Ed.D., Psy.D.) in psychology or education. They are not medical doctors. They have been trained in human development and behavior, and the treatment of learning, behavioral, and emotional difficulties. Part of their training included supervised work providing therapy for children or adults. Psychologists have

schools or other people who know your child. Thereafter, recommendations and a treatment plan should be discussed. Following that will be several sessions devoted to helping you and your child solve specific difficulties. After that, you and your child may be seen less frequently to monitor his progress and to help deal with anticipated or unforeseen problems that may occur. In the initial evaluation of your child's behavioral problems, his teachers may be of help, since behavioral difficulties often occur in school and sometimes stem from problems with learning or attention and the frustrations they can cause.

special skills in evaluating and treating emotional problems and learning disorders. Some have had special training in family or marital counseling.

Behavioral and Developmental Pediatricians. They are pediatricians (medical doctors) who have had four years of medical school, three years of pediatric training, and additional training in child development and the emotional and educational problems of children. They treat children with behavioral and emotional problems, and a wide range of developmental difficulties, from attention problems to mental retardation. Pediatricians can also prescribe medications for a variety of disorders.

Mental-Health Counselors. Several types of practitioners fall into this category. *Licensed clinical social workers* with master's degrees in social work (M.S.W.) are among the most common; they have had four years of college and two years of postgraduate training in counseling children and families. *School counselors* are educators who work directly with children in school settings, providing guidance and counseling, and making referrals when necessary. They have had four years of college and additional training in counseling children with behavioral problems.

Community Mental-Health Resources. Many community agencies provide mental-health services or can make appropriate referrals. They often are associated with county health departments, religious organizations (such as Catholic Family Services), or nonprofit counseling agencies. Colleges and medical centers also may offer a variety of mental-health services available to the public.

Depending on the type of problem, one or more methods may be used:

- The counselor works directly and only with the child. This child-centered treatment is what most parents expect, but it is often not completely effective.

- The counselor works with the child and the parents, sometimes together, sometimes individually, to better understand the potential causes of the behavior, the nature of the problems, and parenting techniques, and to implement new strategies.

- The counselor works with the parents to help them understand and resolve personal problems such as marital stress, financial difficulties, and emotional problems that may be causing or contributing to the difficulty.

- The counselor works with the entire family in a family-systems or family-centered approach that seeks to deal with behavior problems and improve communication.

The duration of the therapy may range from weeks to over a year, depending on the needs of the child and family, the therapist's skill, the response to therapy, and its costs.

Therapies for children can be grouped into the three general categories that follow. Each has a distinctive aim and perspective of the child, and there are many variations within each of them. Some therapists employ and blend parts of different therapies into their own individual therapeutic style.

1. **Psychodynamic therapy** helps the child look inward, to reflect on his experiences, feelings, and reactions. Its aim is for the youngster to gain insight into and understanding of his behavior and emotions, especially those of which he may not have been conscious, and to change them in some fundamental way. Some therapists are *nondirective,* meaning that they may encourage a child to play and talk about whatever comes to mind while they listen for clues as to what may be at the root of the youngster's difficulties. This type of therapy is sometimes necessary to understand a child's deeper and more personal problems. Central to this approach is providing the child with an opportunity to form a relationship with the therapist. In this context the therapist can observe the child's problems firsthand and work with the youngster to overcome them.

   Other therapists are more *directive* and guiding, leading youngsters into discussions of specific problematic issues.

   Psychodynamic treatment may be lengthy and expensive and requires a highly skilled therapist such as a child psychiatrist, psychologist, or trained social worker. It may be more effective with older children who are reflective and insight-oriented.

2. **Family-system therapy** looks at the family structure and its subunits (marital, sibling, parental). In this approach a child's behavioral problem is seen as a reflection of a dysfunction or stress within the family. The child's behavior is considered to be the symptom of a larger problem within the family. While the child is identified as the patient, in fact the whole family is the patient. The aim is to change and improve the child's and the family's relationships, communication, and behavior. Therapy can last several sessions or many years and requires a trained family therapist.

3. **Cognitive-behavioral therapy** helps the child look outward and develop better ways of acting and reacting. Its aim is to change the child's behav-

ior, to allow him to see the world differently and think about and be aware of his actions and how they affect him and others. It uses behavior-modification techniques to change his expectations and responses, and it uses rewards and punishment. Role playing, storytelling, interactive games, talking, thinking, and problem-solving are used to help the child explore his feelings and perceptions, consciously think about his behavior, and then devise more effective behavior. This type of therapy also requires a change in parental behavior. It is usually carried out by pediatricians, psychiatrists, psychologists, or social workers and can last for varying lengths, but usually several months.

4. Because school failure or underachievement is such a common concern, an additional category of treatment might be called *school problem therapy.* Learning disabilities or difficulties usually have several causes, and a complete assessment may require the skills of a psychologist, an educator, and a pediatrician. They may find that emotional and behavioral problems have contributed to learning difficulties; or conversely, learning problems may have caused emotional and behavioral troubles. (See Chapter 52, "Learning Disabilities.")

Which style of treatment is best for your youngster? It depends primarily upon his particular problem and diagnosis. Certain children, perhaps because of their personalities, fare better in particular settings—maybe making more progress with a practitioner who directs and structures the sessions thoroughly. In some instances youngsters may feel most comfortable working with a therapist of the same sex. Successful therapy requires that children feel safe and respected.

Your pediatrician can help direct you toward the most appropriate style of therapy for your child.

WHAT ABOUT YOUR OWN ANXIETIES?

If you are like many parents, you may have to overcome some personal obstacles that make you reluctant to seek mental-health care for your youngster. Many parents feel anxious and uncertain about seeking out this kind of help.

These doubts are often fueled by feelings of parental guilt and responsibility for the child's difficulties. Sometimes parents may be reluctant to seek therapy because their child's behavior reminds them of their own difficulties growing up. Other times parents may recognize that the child's symptoms are really in response to discord between the parents, or to violence or alcoholism in the home, and they prefer not to confront these problems. They may also fear being lectured to or criticized as inadequate or incompetent parents.

Keep in mind that in most situations, the main focus of the therapy is to solve the problem at hand, not necessarily to determine its root cause. The job of the therapist is to help the child and his family overcome the difficulty, not to place blame.

Approaching a Treatment Program Realistically

Before beginning any kind of treatment plan—whether it is your own plan or that of professionals—keep these important points in mind:

1. No single theory of child development or behavior management has all of the explanations or answers.

2. No single treatment plan works for all children.

3. There are seldom simple solutions to complex problems. Things may initially get worse before they get better. Be patient, and be willing to modify goals and expectations according to the progress being made.

4. Beware of treatments or interventions that make you feel guilty or inadequate or that do not make sense to you.

5. Beware of becoming a clinical "expert" with your own youngsters, particularly if you work in one of the helping professions. It is not necessary—and in fact may even be harmful—to analyze and discuss every detailed aspect of your child's behavior.

6. Be careful of statistics or dogma that claims to explain everything or create broad generalizations or truths.

7. Be wary of therapies that discourage parents from doing their own problem-solving or using informal, commonsense approaches. On the other hand, don't try to do it all alone; keep in touch with the professional, even as you assume more responsibility yourself.

8. Ask your pediatrician for advice, or for a referral, in sorting out whether a treatment program is right for you and your child. If the program doesn't seem right, discuss it with the therapist. If you decide to stop treatment, talk it over *in advance* with both your child and the therapist so the last few sessions can be structured in a supportive way for your youngster.

PART V

EMOTIONAL PROBLEMS AND BEHAVIOR DISORDERS

17

STRESS AND YOUR CHILD

During the middle years of childhood, youngsters experience rapid social, emotional, and intellectual growth, along with pressures to achieve, succeed, and conform. Some children adjust better to these challenges than others, and as all of Part V will emphasize, emotional and behavioral problems can develop from time to time. In this and the ensuing chapters, the most common problem areas will be described. These chapters will help you identify causes of these problems, possible solutions, and when and how to get help for these problems.

This opening chapter specifically examines the stresses that your youngster may encounter during these middle years. In middle childhood, pressures may come from a number of sources—from within the child herself, as well as from parents, teachers, peers, and the larger society in which the child lives. Pressure can take many forms that challenge children and to which they must respond and, often, adapt. Whether these are events of lasting consequence like the divorce of their parents, or merely a minor hassle like losing their homework, these demands or stresses are a part of children's daily existence.

Children welcome some events and are able to adapt to them with relative ease. They perceive other events as threats to their own or the family's daily routines or general sense of well-being, and these stresses are more troublesome. Most stress faced by children is in the middle, neither welcomed nor seriously harmful, but rather a part of accomplishing the tasks of childhood and learning about themselves.

Youngsters may also worry about making friends, succeeding in school, combating peer pressure, or overcoming a physical impairment. Whatever its form, if stress is too intense or long-lasting, it can sometimes take a toll on children. Clusters of stressful events seem to predispose children to illness. Major events, especially those that forever change a child's family, like the death of a parent, can have lasting effects on children's psychological health and well-being. Minor daily stresses can also have consequences. They can contribute to loss of sleep or appetite. Children may become angry or irritable, or their school grades may suffer. Their behavior and their willingness to cooperate may change.

Children's temperaments vary and thus they are quite different in their ability to cope with stress and daily hassles. Some are easygoing by nature and adjust easily to events and new situations. Others are thrown off balance by changes in their lives. All children improve in their ability to handle stress if they previously have succeeded in managing challenges and if they feel they have the ability and the emotional support of family and friends. Children who have a clear sense of personal competence, and who feel loved and supported, generally do well.

Certainly, a child's age and development will help determine how stressful a given situation may be. Changing teachers at midyear may be a major event for a child in the first grade and merely an annoyance for a sixth-grader. Being short may be a minor issue for a five- or six-year-old boy but a source of daily embarrassment for an adolescent. How a child perceives and responds to stress depends in part on development, in part on experience, and in part on a child's individual temperament.

Ironically, many parents believe that their school-age children are unaware of the stresses around them and are somehow immune to them. After all, their children not only have all their basic needs met, but perhaps they also have a roomful of toys, friends to share them with, plenty of playtime, and a full schedule of extracurricular activities.

Yet children are very sensitive to the changes around them, especially to the feelings and reactions of their parents, even if those feelings are not communicated directly in words. If a parent loses a job, children will have to adjust to their family's financial crisis; they must deal not only with the obvious family budgetary changes but also with the changes in their parents' emotional states. Children may have to cope with a bully on the playground, a move to a new neighborhood, a parent's serious illness, or the disappointment of a poor sports performance. They might feel a constant, nagging pressure to dress the "right" way, or to achieve the high grades that can put them on the fast track toward the "right" college.

Some psychologists believe that today's middle-years youngsters actually are faced with more stress than the children of previous generations were and have fewer social supports available. The change in family structure from the large, supportive, extended families (including both parents, aunts, uncles, and grandparents) of previous generations, to the present high incidence of divorced families, single-parent families, and stepfamilies has drastically altered the experience of childhood. Millions of youngsters must adjust to such changes.

Even in intact and stable families, the growing number of households with two working parents often forces children to spend more time in after-school programs or at home alone. For some children this loss of time with their parents is quite stressful. So, too, is the responsibility for caring for themselves and the family home and sometimes for overseeing a younger sibling after school.

Many children and their families are stressed by the multiple activities that fill children's "free time." Overscheduled children with inadequate "down time" can become exhausted.

Today's children are also being raised in an era in which they are exposed to violence and peer pressure about sexual activity and drug use and are warned to be cautious about kidnapping, sexual abuse, and other crimes. This sense that they are living in an unsafe world is a constant source of stress for some children. In short, today's youngsters are regularly confronted with challenges to their coping skills and often are expected to grow up too fast.

Even so, not all stress is bad. Moderate amounts of pressure imposed by a teacher or a coach, for example, can motivate a child to keep her grades up in school or to participate more fully in athletic activities. Successfully managing stressful situations or events enhances a child's ability to cope in the future.

What Your Child Worries About

In a research study, fifth- and sixth-graders were asked about the life events that had made them (or would make them) worried or feel bad. Here are the circumstances most commonly mentioned, with the most frequent ones listed first.

- Feeling sick

- Having nothing to do

- Not having enough money to spend

- Feeling pressure to get good grades

- Feeling left out of a group of peers

- Not spending enough time with parents

- Not having homework done

- Not being good enough at sports

- Not being able to dress as desired

- Experiencing body changes

- Being late for school

- Being smaller than other children of the same age

- Having parents argue in front of them

- Not getting along with teachers

- Being overweight or bigger than other children of the same age

- Moving

- Changing schools

- Arguing with parents about rules in the family

- The separation of parents

- Being pressured to try something they didn't really want to (e.g., smoking)

When the stress is continuous or particularly intense, it takes a toll on both the psyche and the body. Sudden stressful events will accelerate your child's breathing and heartbeat, constrict her blood vessels, increase her blood pressure and muscle tension, and perhaps cause stomach upset and headaches. As stress persists, she might be more susceptible to illness and experience fatigue, nightmares, teeth-grinding, insomnia, tantrums, depression, and school failure.

The way children show they are overloaded and are having difficulty coping with stress is different at different stages of development. During the preschool years you may have noticed that under stress, your child regressed a little. Perhaps she had trouble separating from you, was especially clingy, or even temporarily lost some skills associated with growing up, such as potty training.

Young school-age children also openly act out their feelings; however, they may be more likely to internalize their stress. They might express stress through sadness, depression, or withdrawal. Other children will externalize stress by overactivity, anger, or creating conflicts. Parents should be attuned to these and other signs of overload.

Signs of Overload

Although stress is a part of life and growing up, you need to intervene when you sense that it is undermining your child's physical or psychological well-being. Here are some clues that stress may be having too negative an effect.

- Your child develops physical symptoms like headaches and stomach pains.

- He seems restless, tired, and agitated.

- He appears depressed and is uncommunicative about how he feels.

- He gets irritable, negative, and shows little excitement or pleasure in his activities.

- He seems less interested in an activity that was once extremely important to him and prefers to stay at home.

- His grades at school begin to fall, and he has less interest than usual in attending classes and doing homework.

- He exhibits antisocial behavior such as lying and stealing, forgets or refuses to do his chores, and seems much more dependent on you than in the past.

Are You Pushing Your Child Too Hard?

Much of the stress in your child's life comes from outside the family and may be beyond your control. Yet many youngsters may feel pressure because their parents, with the best of intentions, are overscheduling them with music lessons, sports activities, computer courses, and art classes.

At first glance it might seem advantageous to expose your child to as many educational, cultural, and athletic experiences as possible. For some parents, this seems to be a way to give him a little edge over his peers in our very competitive society. But experts believe that when children are driven to be overachievers—when nearly the entire day is structured for them—it can have negative effects. Many children find it stressful to race from activity to activity without any time to relax, to play, to "hang out" and just "be a kid."

You and your child together need to find a balance between structured and unstructured activities. Don't worry about his becoming bored; he can actually benefit from some unplanned time, when he can use his imagination and pursue interests of his own. As for his structured activities, limit them to those he truly enjoys, and in which he is able to succeed, gain new skills, or see improvement. Solicit your child's suggestions and opinions before making any plans for him.

Once your child has become engaged in activities, be supportive (but not pushy), offering praise and showing your interest by attending his baseball games and piano recitals. Sometimes, your child may complain about losing interest in an organized program, or of feeling anxiety about his inability to perform as well as his peers or teammates. Explore the reasons for and realities of his complaints. There may be problems to resolve together, or it may be time to discontinue the current activity. As a parent, keep in mind that in these middle years your youngster is still very much a child. Particularly as children approach adolescence, they often feel pressure to be more grown-up. Parents and peers alike may encourage more adult actions or dress. Help your youngster enjoy his childhood without unnecessary stressors like these. As he matures, let him set his own pace of discovery. Talk with him about issues like individuality and peer pressure.

Helping Your Child Cope

When your child is facing a lot of stress, she may benefit from your help in figuring out how best to cope. Take the time to talk with her about the pressures she is feeling and the anxiety in her life. School-age children often find it difficult to sit down and discuss these matters. But let her know that you are interested and care, and that you would like to help. Approach each situation as a problem to be solved.

You may need to put yourself in your child's place and imagine what she may be feeling. Talk about some of her behavior and displays of emotion you have noticed recently, which suggest to you that she may be struggling with some issues. Gradually, your efforts may help her put her feelings into words. (See Chapter 13, "Communicating with Your Child," for a discussion of this subject.)

Help your child understand her own temperament (see Chapter 8). Use some guiding statements about observations that you have made about her. Say things like "I know you react pretty strongly to stress." Or, "You seem to prefer to take your time making decisions." This can help foster insight and help your child cope.

Together, you and your child should evaluate the situations or activities that are producing problems. Are there issues with friends that need to be resolved? Does she need to be reassured that, despite a divorce or other family disruption, she is still loved by both parents? Do you need to cut back her schedule of extracurricular activities or choose them more carefully?

Clarify the problems together, and identify a number of possible solutions. Look at the influences that might be adding to the difficulty your child is having in adjusting to or managing the situation, and find ways in which she can change them.

If your youngster seems to have too little free time, help her modify her schedule so she can relax and play. She will probably increase her creativity and devise her own forms of recreation. Encourage her to use her imagination and skills to create play and pleasure. Remember, your job is *not* to keep her entertained; in fact, most children enjoy playtime free of the frenetic pace and the tension that usually accompany formal overscheduling.

You may also wish to protect ten to fifteen minutes of time each day to devote solely to your child in an activity that she chooses and directs. This can promote family closeness while offering some stress-free time.

If you feel you need additional help in the area of stress management, discuss this issue with your child's pediatrician, who can talk to you and your child and help the family develop less stressful avenues for your youngster to pursue. In some cases, when your child is coping especially poorly and the stress is interfering with her day-to-day functioning, the doctor might refer you to a professional counselor.

You also may need to examine your own life. Children under stress often have parents under stress, and some of the resulting anxiety is transferred from parent to child. If you are undergoing a personal crisis—a divorce, for example—or have filled your child's day with activities because you yourself are overcommitted, it may be time to make changes in your own life, easing the personal stress that might have an indirect impact on your child as well.

18

HABITS

Children often exhibit behavior and habits that parents find annoying—fingernail biting, thumb-sucking, nose picking, and twirling the hair. Children often resort to these repetitive activities during times of tension, idleness, fatigue, or boredom. Many of the habits begin during the preschool years and continue as the child grows to school age, or they reappear at various intervals. Children are frequently unaware of the behavior in which they are engaging and are thus not using these habits to defy their parents.

The causes of these habits remain unknown. Their repetitive nature suggests that they serve a soothing or calming process for the brain. Interestingly, even in adulthood many people cling to some of these self-comforting traits during times of stress: sucking on pencil tips or their fingers, pulling their earlobes, fingering their hair.

The Evolution of Habits

Some self-comforting habits—such as thumb-sucking and body rocking—begin in infancy and gradually fade in middle childhood. During these middle years, most thumb-suckers will confine their sucking to the privacy of their home, at bedtime, while watching TV, or when they are upset.

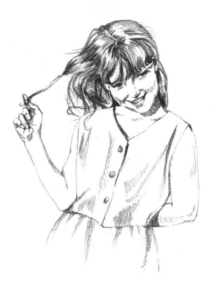

Often, this behavior is accompanied by other vestiges of earlier years, such as cuddling with a blanket.

As children mature and develop greater self-control and self-understanding, their thumb-sucking usually disappears, most often by ages six to eight. Also, with increases in peer pressure, children tend to assume greater mastery over their behavior.

Similarly, a small number of middle-years children exhibit the normal behavior of rocking themselves to sleep in bed. They may curl into a knee-to-chest position and rock with such vigor that the bed shakes and even bangs the walls until they are fast asleep. A few children roll their head back and forth, at times banging into the wall.

Common Childhood Habits

Here are some of the most common self-comforting habits of middle childhood that concern parents.

- Thumb-sucking
- Body rocking
- Head banging
- Fingernail biting
- Cuticle picking
- Hair twirling
- Masturbating

Still others sit up and rock. As unsettling as parents may find these unusual habits, children may exhibit them every night in order to settle into sleep. The rhythmic motion seems necessary to soothe or calm the central nervous system in the transition from wakefulness to sleep.

Fingernail biting, cuticle picking, hair twirling, and nose picking are also very common—and annoying—habits of childhood, developing between ages three and six. This behavior may continue throughout middle childhood and perhaps longer. Like other self-comforting habits, they are tension reducers, "time-wasters," and seem to be outside of consciousness or awareness.

The frequency and intensity of these habits tend to ebb and flow, often without apparent explanation or parental intervention. Some observers have noted that the child who bites his fingernails or picks his cuticles often causes bleeding or pain; perhaps this natural consequence plays a significant role in the eventual disappearance of the habit. In any case, these habits frequently fade with time.

Management of Self-Comforting Habits

As a first step in the simple management of your child's self-comforting habits, ignore them! Most commonly, they will disappear with time. When you call attention to them with harsh words, ridicule, or punishment, the tension that the habit presumably relieves will increase, and the habit will get worse. Punishment is not an effective way to eradicate habits.

Ignoring these habits, however, can be a difficult process for most parents. After all, if the mother or father finds a habit irritating or frustrating, ignoring it does not make the feelings disappear. Even so, try to withhold your negative comments and wait for the habit to pass.

If your child sucks her thumb or bites her fingernails, she may be interested in overcoming the habit and thus will cooperate with your own efforts toward that goal. Try using these techniques:

- When you notice that your child is *not* doing the behavior for extended periods, reward her in some agreed-upon way.

- Use over-the-counter agents, such as bitter-tasting compounds that can be placed on the fingers or the cuticles, to remind your child when she begins to bite or suck her thumb. This approach has a relatively low rate of success, but it is simple and, with your youngster's cooperation, may be an effective strategy. Ask your pharmacist about these products.

- Positive reinforcement is the most successful way to produce a change in behavior. Accentuate and reward the new behavior you want to see adopted. Star charts and daily rewards are very helpful. (For a complete discussion on this subject, see Chapter 14, "Changing Your Child's Behavior.")

19

TICS

Tics are rapid and repeated involuntary movements. Children who experience them may be embarrassed and teased by their peers. Tics usually affect the face and neck and take the form of eye blinking, shoulder shrugging, facial grimacing, neck twisting, throat clearing, sniffing, and dry coughs. Sometimes these movements occur frequently throughout the day; at other times, they occur only occasionally.

Tics occur in about 20 percent of school-age children, beginning most often between ages seven and nine, although they sometimes start as early as age two or three. Tics are irregular in their pattern, but they often appear suddenly after some type of physical or social stress, and they tend to increase when a child is tense, anxious, tired, or idle. Tics become less frequent when a child is able to relax and are never present during sleep.

Many parents find tics extremely irritating. They may urge their child to stop them, forgetting or unaware that the mannerisms are not totally under the child's conscious control. Sometimes they may feel that the child is purposely defying them as the tics continue.

Researchers are investigating the biological basis of tics. Since they are common in school-age children—whose brains are still developing and are not yet mature—tics may be a transient phenomenon of normal brain development and organization. Tics also seem to run in families, suggesting that they have a genetic component. The

Types of Tic Disorders

Simple tics are single facial twitches that are persistent but do not change in character. By contrast, multiple motor tic disorders have ever-changing patterns of different visible physical tics.

The most severe tic disorder is Tourette's syndrome, which is characterized by multiple motor and vocal tics. The motor tics begin in the face but later involve all parts of the body. The vocal tics are vocalizations like snorts, coughs, or hiccups. This syndrome is often associated with learning disabilities, obsessive thoughts, hyperactivity, and attention deficit hyperactivity disorder. The frequency of tics in this syndrome varies: Sometimes they can be relieved with the use of medications.

physical, organic origin of tics is just beginning to be understood.

Fortunately, most tics disappear on their own within several months. They may last longer when parents create stress for the child by pressuring him to stop the repetitive movements.

Management of Simple Tics

Scolding your child or calling attention to her unusual mannerism is not helpful, and usually makes it worse. Since the more attention is called to the tics, the worse they are likely to become, tics are best ignored.

On the other hand, since your child is likely to have questions about why her body is acting this peculiar way, silence about them might increase her anxiety. It is best to talk with her sensitively and supportively, letting her know there is nothing wrong with her and there is no reason to feel ashamed. Help her develop strategies for explaining the tics to friends who may ask about them.

Seek ways to decrease any stress and conflict in your child's life. If she feels pressured and overscheduled, lighten her commitments. Discuss with her other sources of stress and worry, and together find ways to deal with them. Sometimes tics may have started under times of stress or conflict but persist long after those situations seem to have passed. (See Chapter 17, "Stress and Your Child.")

In some situations, you and your child may benefit from some outside help or advice. Talk with your pediatrician in the following situations:

- The tics interfere with schoolwork or friendships and cause your child embarrassment, anxiety, or emotional problems.

- There are multiple tics or vocalizations, such as sniffs, snorts, throat clearing, chewing, and tongue thrusting. These may indicate the condition called Tourette's syndrome.

- The tics are intense and frequent.

- The symptoms are present for longer than a year.

- There is a strong family history of tic disorders, including Tourette's syndrome.

- Your child is on medication for attention deficit hyperactivity disorder (ADHD).

- Your efforts to identify the source of your child's tension or your efforts to help her reduce the stress are unsuccessful.

20

STUTTERING

Almost everyone has encountered a child who stutters. Stuttering or stammering (also called *dysfluency*) is a disorder of communication in which sounds or whole words are repeated as the youngster speaks, interrupting the flow of his communication. Sometimes these children make sounds that are prolonged, or their speech may actually stop momentarily.

Stuttering first becomes apparent during the preschool years. About 90 percent of children between the ages of eighteen months and four years have some degree of "normal dysfluency." This stuttering appears to be related to the development of language, perhaps occurring because the child's thought processes move much more rapidly than his ability to put those ideas into words. Without undue attention from parents or stress from the environment, this stuttering disappears on its own, usually in just two to three months.

At any age, children can develop stuttering as a manifestation of severe stress and social pressures. When a school-age child stutters, he can become more self-conscious, thus increasing his anxiety and making his speech dysfluency even worse. Pressure from teachers trying to be helpful or from peers can aggravate his stuttering too.

In some cases people who interact with a stuttering child—perhaps friends or relatives—notice the difficulties the child is having with his speech, feel uncomfortable, and change their behavior toward him. The child usually is aware that his speech patterns have produced this altered response, and thus he may become even more uncomfortable with the way he talks, perpetuating the stuttering. Some children try to deal with this by avoiding social contact and conversation.

Although the youngster may try to stop stuttering, this attempt will inevitably fail, only intensifying his negative self-image and perhaps making the symptoms even worse. Nevertheless, once stress is relieved, the stuttering usually will begin to subside. (See Chapter 17, "Stress and Your Child.")

A small number of middle-years children—only about 1 percent—have what is called *true stuttering*. They seem to have inherited a tendency for this disorder, rather than developing it in response to environmental factors or social pressures. In children with this "true" form of the condition:

- The stuttering becomes worse with time.

- There is a consistent pattern in their speech prolongations, pauses, grammatical forms, and repetition of words.

- They may demonstrate additional actions—called *starters*—which occur during stuttering, including knee-slapping, foot-tapping, or tics.

Management of Stuttering

If you have a child who stutters, you can help him by approaching his problem with some simple rules:

1. Encourage periods of conversation that your child will not find stressful.

2. Do not correct his speech.

3. Do not interrupt him.

4. Do not finish his sentences.

5. Do not ask him to repeat sentences or phrases.

6. Do not ask him to practice certain words or sounds.

7. Do not ask him to slow down his speech.

8. If he wishes, let him choose to avoid certain problematic words or sounds, finding alternative ones to use in their place.

9. If he finds it helpful, encourage him to pause, inhale a full breath, and then exhale while speaking.

10. Listen, offer encouragement, and provide support.

When to Seek Additional Help

If your child's stuttering pattern continues, find him some professional help. When a stuttering problem begins during middle childhood, or if an earlier stuttering condition persists or resurfaces, ask your pediatrician for a referral to a specialist—most likely, a speech and language therapist experienced in treating children with stuttering difficulties. Some children can also benefit from psychological counseling to address issues, like poor self-esteem, that may be contributing to the dysfluency.

You also should seek help if:

- Your child's stuttering becomes more severe.

- He becomes extremely self-conscious and fearful of communication.

- He develops new facial grimaces or tics.

The prognosis for children who stutter is excellent. About 80 percent outgrow their stuttering by adolescence. In a small number of individuals, however, it persists into adulthood, and they require continuous support and intervention.

To help a child who stutters, you can obtain the names of resources in your community from the American Speech-Language-Hearing Association, 10801 Rockville Pike, Rockville, Maryland 20852 (phone: 1-800-638-8255).

21

SLEEP DISTURBANCES

From the ages of five to twelve, the average youngster sleeps eight to ten hours a night. However, the sleep habits of children can vary considerably and still be within the range of "normal." Some children need significantly more or less sleep than others.

During these middle childhood years, sleep problems are relatively uncommon, although most youngsters experience nightmares or other sleep disturbances from time to time. Sometimes sleep problems have an emotional basis. For instance, insomnia (the inability to fall or stay asleep) can be caused by stress and anxiety. If a child is afraid of the dark or fearful of being alone at night, she may be unable to relax and go to sleep.

Here are some of the most common sleep disturbances, and the kind of treatment (if any) they require.

Bedtime Difficulties

Does your child fight going to bed at night? Does he take several hours to settle down and go to sleep?

Some families struggle for years in an attempt to establish a pleasant and amicable bedtime. For them, each night is a battle, with many "curtain calls" until their youngsters finally fall asleep.

There can be many causes for these nighttime difficulties, including:

- General problems with negative and oppositional behavior, in which he has difficulty following and adhering to rules and routines, including going to bed when he would rather keep playing. Most sleep problems are of this sort.

- Separation anxiety. Many children who have little contact or time with their parents will have difficulty separating again from them at bedtime. Some children will even have separation problems during the day at school.

- Wanting private time with parents when siblings are not around.

- Too early of a bedtime. Many a child has a disturbance of his sleep-wake cycle. He may be an "owl," with a body clock set for falling asleep late at night and waking up in the late morning; or he may be a "lark," falling asleep early or waking up very early. Ask your doctor about making some gradual adjustments of your youngster's sleep-wake patterns to fit in with the family's daily schedule.

- Habits and learned behavior. Some children simply get used to being up late, when the household settles down and the pace slows.

- Attention deficit hyperactivity disorder (ADHD). Some children with hyperactivity and impulsivity need less sleep than their peers. These youngsters may also have great difficulty settling down to sleep at bedtime.

If sleep struggles like these persist, talk them over with your pediatrician.

Sleepwalking

About 15 percent of all children between ages five and twelve have at least one sleepwalking episode. This disorder (also called *somnambulism*) tends to affect boys more often than girls, and in a small number of children, episodes take place several nights a week.

Sleepwalking usually occurs during the second or third hour of nighttime sleep. The child sits up and, without totally awakening, leaves his bed, usually walking awkwardly, with his eyes open and a blank look on his face.

For several minutes he may wander through the house, even opening doors along the way, but his actions are purposeless. If spoken to, he may seem to respond, but the words are usually unintelligible. He will probably return to his bed on his own and go back to normal sleeping, recalling nothing of this nighttime activity when he awakens in the morning.

If your child sleepwalks, you need to minimize his chances of hurting himself. Make sure he has a safe environment—that is, outside doors should be locked so that he cannot leave the house, stairways should be blocked so he cannot walk up or down them, and hazardous objects should be moved to a less dangerous location. When you find him walking in his sleep, gently lead him back to bed.

Sleepwalking tends to run in families. In most children this unusual habit disappears on its own, generally by early adolescence. For the frequent or troublesome sleepwalker, your pediatrician may prescribe medications to reduce the number of episodes.

Sleep Talking

Sleep talking (or *somniloquy*) occurs more often than sleepwalking. During sleep, the child begins speaking, often unintelligibly and in a monotone voice, and usually for no more than thirty seconds. Most episodes take place during nondreaming sleep.

Treatment is rarely needed or prescribed. However, when sleep talking occurs in combination with sleepwalking, pediatricians sometimes recommend medication.

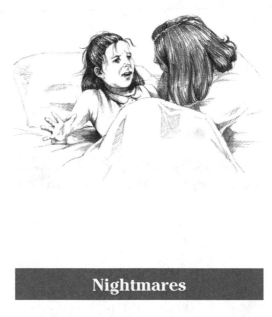

Nightmares

Nightmares are common in middle childhood. In a typical episode a child will have a scary dream, filled with monsters or other frightening beings. She may awaken, become anxious, breathe heavily, and begin crying. Sometimes the experience is so terrifying that the child may resist going back to sleep, needing close and constant reassurance. Hug your child and speak calmly, reassuring her that it was only a bad dream. Often she will vividly describe the details of the scary dream in an effort to calm herself, helped along by her parents' reassurance. She may also remember the dream the next day and want to discuss it further.

In most children nightmares occur only occasionally, usually in the early morning hours. If they happen often—or if the same frightening dream recurs—talk to your physician about them. Nightmares seem to occur with increasing frequency during times of stress, so if these dreams are recurrent, evaluate the stress in your youngster's life. On rare occasions your pediatrician may suggest that your child receive some professional counseling.

Night Terrors

Night terrors are a different phenomenon from nightmares and can be quite upsetting for a parent to watch. About 90 to 180 minutes after falling asleep, the youngster will abruptly sit up in bed, open his eyes, and scream loudly or cry out for help. For the next few minutes he may gasp, moan, mumble, thrash about, and seem to be in a confused, agitated state. His breathing and heart rate will accelerate significantly. He will be unresponsive to his parents' attempts at comforting him and may even push them away. These episodes can sometimes last for 30 to 60 minutes before the child rather quickly returns to a peaceful sleep, remembering nothing about it the next morning, and leaving parents baffled and terrorized—hence, the name "night terrors."

Night terrors (or *pavor nocturnus*) occur in a relatively small number of children (1 to 5 percent), taking place during a non-dreaming, deep stage of sleep. As frightening as they may be for parents, they are *not* a reflection of a psychological disturbance. They are a normal, although infrequent, part of the body's transition between sleep states. Sometimes physical exhaustion can contribute to a child's having night terrors. Most children outgrow night terrors without treatment, and parents can do nothing to resolve their occurrence. Parental patience and understanding are important, although these night terrors tend to be much more stressful for mother and father than for their children.

Daytime Sleepiness

Some children are excessively sleepy during the daytime hours. The most frequent cause of this daytime sleepiness is insufficient sleep at night. Some medications also interfere with children's normal alertness.

Narcolepsy

Children with narcolepsy are overpowered by strong, uncontrollable urges to sleep. They may fall asleep immediately for several minutes to an hour at a time, often in inappropriate places like a classroom. As this occurs, the body may relax and they may fall to the floor. They awaken refreshed but may become sleepy again in another hour or two, whereupon the process repeats itself.

Narcolepsy usually first occurs during adolescence and tends to run in families. Although it is a lifelong condition, it can usually be successfully treated with medication.

Sleep Apnea

Children with sleep apnea briefly stop breathing many times during the night due to an obstruction in the respiratory tract, perhaps related to enlarged tonsils and adenoids or to obesity. As the child instinctively gasps for breath, she awakens for a few moments, her normal breathing pattern returns, and she immediately goes back to sleep, probably with no recollection that this episode has occurred. Because these brief awakenings can occur dozens and even hundreds of times a night, the youngster is sleep deprived, creating sleepiness the following day. Occasionally, these children will snore in their sleep as a symptom of the obstruction of the respiratory tract.

The underlying cause of this airway obstruction must be determined and treated to cure the apnea. Once it is relieved, the child can enjoy normal sleep again.

Bed-Wetting

Bed-wetting may be related to a child's stage of sleep, but is not ordinarily considered a sleep disorder. For information, see Chapter 29, "Bed-Wetting."

22

ATTENTION DEFICIT HYPERACTIVITY DISORDER

Attention deficit hyperactivity disorder (ADHD) is a developmental disorder that affects the behavior, attention, and learning of children. If it is unrecognized, these children can face excessive criticism, failure, and disappointment, while their parents struggle with what to do.

ADHD youngsters are easily distracted and have trouble concentrating. They may be impulsive and seem to act without thinking, touching objects that are off limits or running into the street to chase a ball without apparent regard for their own safety. In calm moments, they might know better. They may not cope well with frustration and can have dramatic mood swings. At school they may be fidgety and brimming with energy, finding it difficult to sit still, jumping out of their seat constantly, as if unable to control their perpetual motion. They often have difficulty with sequencing and organizational skills. Others who cannot concentrate may sit quietly, daydreaming and appearing "spaced out." Because of their behavior they may be rejected by other children and disliked by teachers; in the process, their report cards may be disappointing and their self-esteem may suffer, despite the fact that they are often as bright as their peers.

Over the years a variety of labels—minimal brain dysfunction, hyperkinetic/impulsive disorder, hyperkinesis, hyperactivity, and attention deficit disorder with or without hyperactivity—have been used to describe children with some or all of these behavioral problems. Now, most experts are using the term *attention deficit hyperactivity disorder* as a diagnosis for children whose behavior tends to be characteristically impulsive, inattentive, or a combination of both. Since all children have these traits some of the time, the diagnosis usually requires that the symptoms be present for at least six months by age seven, be evident in various situations, and be more intense than usually seen in other children of the same age and gender.

More than 6 percent of school-age children have ADHD. Boys outnumber girls. Researchers are examining multiple causes of the disorder, including heredity, brain chemistry, and social factors. Some researchers believe that children with ADHD have abnormally low levels and imbalances of certain neurotransmitters, the chemicals that convey messages between brain cells. Recent studies suggest that various parts of the brain may be functioning differently than in the majority of children.

Many ADHD children also have reading disabilities and other specific learning problems, which further interfere with their success at school. (Most children who have specific learning problems do not have ADHD.) Children with difficulties

Does Your Child Have ADHD?

Only a physician or psychologist can properly diagnose attention deficit hyperactivity disorder. If your school-age child exhibits several of the following symptoms, which are associated with ADHD, and they are interfering with his ability to achieve academically and socially, as well as diminishing his motivation and self-esteem, have him evaluated by a physician, child neurologist, child psychiatrist, child psychologist, or a pediatric specialist in child behavior and development.

Inattention

- Produces careless work at school
- Exhibits an inability to pay attention
- Does not seem to listen
- Is disorganized
- Avoids tasks requiring sustained effort
- Loses things
- Is easily distracted
- Is forgetful

Hyperactivity-Impulsivity

- Squirms and fidgets
- Is restless
- Is excitable
- Lacks patience
- Displays uncontrollable energy
- Interrupts others
- Has trouble waiting his turn

with language and memory have problems with schoolwork that are compounded when ADHD characteristics like distractibility and impulsiveness are present.

A child with ADHD can affect his family in many ways. Normal family routines may be hard to maintain because the child's behavior has been so disorganized and unpredictable, often for a number of years. Parents may not be able to comfortably plan outings or other family events, not knowing what their child's behavior or activity level is likely to be. Children with ADHD frequently become "overexcited" and out of control in stimulating environments. They may also exhibit angry and resistant behavior toward their parents or have low self-esteem. This may be the result of the child's exasperation at failing to meet their parents' expectations or to manage day-to-day tasks due to ADHD symptoms.

School performance also suffers, and teachers complain to parents, who also must struggle with their child's difficulties with peers—conflicts, inappropriate behavior, and having few friends. The condition may produce enormous stress for families, who often search for physicians and others able to provide the care they need.

Diagnosing ADHD

ADHD is often diagnosed shortly after a child enters school. If you suspect ADHD in your child, discuss it with your pediatrician. Unfortunately, there are no specific medical or blood tests that can make the diagnosis. Instead, the diagnosis is made by a complete evaluation of a child's health, combining information obtained from a history and a physical examination, the observations of parents and others, and previous psychological testing, if available. The doctor may administer or arrange for further educational, psychological, and neurological tests and will talk at length not only with you and your child but also with your child's teacher. Your pediatrician will want reports on how your child does at play, while doing homework, and while interacting with both you and with other children and adults.

During these evaluations your pediatrician will rule out other conditions whose symptoms can sometimes mimic ADHD. Poor concentration, poor self-control, and overactivity can be signs of many other conditions, including depression, anxiety, child abuse and neglect, family stress, allergies, hearing and vision problems, seizures, or responses to medication.

In many cases, there is a strong family history of difficulty with attention, impulsivity, concentration, or learning difficulties. Often the child's mother, father, or another close relative has a history of similar struggles when they were young. Gathering this information is helpful for the pediatrician in this evaluation process.

Treatment of ADHD and Related Disorders

Although symptoms can be reduced, there are no cures and usually no easy solutions to ADHD and the problems it creates. However, early diagnosis and treatment can prevent the longer-term impacts the disorder may have if left untreated. The disorder is chronic and requires ongoing management as well as great patience and persistence on the part of family, school, and the child himself. Treatment is always multimodal, necessitating the cooperation of child, parents, pediatricians, teachers, and sometimes psychologists, psychiatrists, and social workers.

For true ADHD, medications remain an important component of treatment. ADHD can be improved with medications that correct the attentional dysfunction and impulsiveness.

Medications have received considerable attention in recent years for the management of attentional and activity symptoms. Additional treatment options, including educational efforts, psychological counseling, and behavioral management, may, in conjunction with medication, be helpful in dealing with the child's learning, emotional, and behavioral difficulties. For example, your doctor may recommend that your child participate in group therapy and social-skills training for peer difficulties; individual psychotherapy for his struggles with low self-esteem, anxiety, or depression; parent training and parent support groups so that mothers and fathers can learn better management of their child's behavioral difficulties; and family therapy so the entire family can discuss the effect of ADHD on their relationships.

A structured daily schedule, with routines, consistency, and predictability, can be very helpful for an ADHD child. Your pediatrician may be able to give you some specific ideas about how you can structure your child's environment to help him function better. Establishing consistency in the time that the child eats, bathes, leaves for school, and goes to sleep each day is a good way to start. Reward him (with kind words, hugs, and occasional material gifts) for positive behavior and for adhering to rules. To keep him focused on the task at hand (for example, dressing in the morning), you may need to be present. Also, before going into situations with lots of stimulation (parties, large family gatherings, shopping centers), review with your child your expectations for his behavior.

A learning or educational specialist may work with your child's school to assist the teacher in helping the youngster experience academic success. As the teacher better understands the child's struggle, he or she may be better able to help him become organized. The teacher also might establish a reward system for proper attention to the task at hand, while also avoiding humiliating the child because of his inattention behaviors. Working in small groups is helpful, since ADHD children tend to become easily distracted by those around them. Private tutors often work well, too, with ADHD youngsters sometimes accomplishing much more in thirty minutes or an hour of one-to-one instruction than during an entire day at school.

As you relate to your child, be realistic. Keep in mind that he has difficulty establishing control over his impulsiveness and restlessness.

Children diagnosed with ADHD are entitled to various supports from their school. Federal legislation specifies that under the category of "Other Health Impaired" (OHI), a child may receive such assistance as preferential seating in the classroom, extended time on tests, reduced homework, and flexible teaching methods. To receive such supports, a qualified pediatrician or other professional must make the ADHD diagnosis, and the child's teachers must confirm that the ADHD is having a significant impact on the child's learning.

What About Medication?

ADHD is best treated with medication, particularly when it interferes with a child's learning, home life, socialization, or the development of self-confidence and competence. There are some mild ADHD cases where the symptoms do not interfere with function and well-being, and thus no medical interventions are necessary. But most cases of ADHD require medication along with psychological care, teaching, and guidance.

The most frequently prescribed drugs are central-nervous-system stimulants, including methylphenidate (Ritalin), dextroamphetamine (Dexedrine), and pemoline (Cylert).

For most parents the decision to place their child on daily medication—particularly a drug that may have to be taken for many years—is difficult. Most, however, decide that the negative effects of ADHD—academic frustration and poor performance, rejection by peers, impaired self-esteem, parental frustration, and parent child tensions—are even more troubling than having their youngster reliant on medication.

Medication is only one part of a child's treatment plan, which must be individualized for her needs and include therapies for her behavioral, educational, social, and emotional difficulties. Your child's medication should be monitored and reevaluated regularly by her doctor to determine its effectiveness, what side effects (if any) may be present, whether dosage adjustments are necessary, and when it can be discontinued.

Critics of medication as treatment for ADHD have raised a number of concerns about methylphenidate (Ritalin), the drug most commonly prescribed for this condition. However, there is a scarcity of scientific data to substantiate their concerns. Here are some of the issues most frequently raised by people opposed to drug therapy for ADHD:

- *Methylphenidate causes severe side effects.* In more than 800 studies, this has been shown to be untrue. Some children do experience *mild* side effects with methylphenidate, such as a reduction in appetite, sleep disturbances, and minor weight loss. Over time, children on these medications seem to attain normal height and weight. When adverse effects occur, however, doctors are usually able to adjust the dosage to minimize these problems or change to another medication. The claims that methylphenidate occasionally leads to stunted growth and severe depression are untrue when children are properly diagnosed and are using the medication in properly prescribed dosages.

- *Children who take methylphenidate for long periods of time often become abusers of illegal drugs during adolescence.* A few ADHD children have such impulsive personalities with conduct problems that they may experiment with drugs in their teenage years; but that has nothing to do with methylphenidate, and is a rare problem. To the contrary, when this medication is most effective—helping children achieve in school and in life—their self-esteem is better and thus they may be *less* inclined to try drugs.

  Some children with *conduct disorders* are misdiagnosed as having ADHD and thus are inappropriately treated with methylphenidate. If their conduct problems are not effectively dealt with by the time they enter adolescence, their behavior will often become worse and include the abuse of drugs and trouble with the law.

- *Children might become addicted to methylphenidate after taking it for so many years.* There are no addictive properties in methylphenidate; nor do ADHD youngsters experience withdrawal symptoms when they ultimately go off the medication. They do not crave the drug when they stop taking it.

- *Methylphenidate is nothing more than a tranquilizer that makes it easier for teachers to control their students.* Methyl-

phenidate does not sedate or tranquilize children. Rather, it is a stimulant that may remedy the biochemical imbalances in the brain, thus improving the concentration abilities of these youngsters.

- *Methylphenidate masks and covers up real behavioral problems, which are never dealt with as long as the child is on medication.* On occasion a youngster may be improperly diagnosed as having ADHD; if, for example, she actually suffers from clinical depression, not an attention deficit, then methylphenidate is a poor treatment option and may worsen the child's social withdrawal and depressed mood. However, for a youngster with properly diagnosed ADHD, methylphenidate is one of the most effective treatment choices available, allowing her to have a positive experience in the classroom while effectively managing her behavioral difficulties.

Controversial Treatments

Over the years, parents and even some physicians have promoted a variety of other approaches for ADHD management. Although they have claimed some success, close scientific scrutiny has proven that most of these therapies are ineffective for the majority of youngsters.

Probably the most famous of these treatments involves dietary adjustments, based on the theory that artificial colors and flavors may trigger ADHD symptoms. However, studies have concluded that except in very rare instances, food additives are not responsible for ADHD symptoms. Most of the claims of success with dietary changes have been exaggerated, and the children seem to be responding more to the extra attention they receive from their parents than to the dietary changes themselves.

Other unconventional therapies have fared no better for the overwhelming majority of ADHD children, including sugar-restricted diets, large doses of vitamins, and eye-training exercises. Nevertheless, a few recent rigorous scientific studies suggest that a *very* small group of young children with ADHD may have more trouble concentrating when their diets include red dyes, and thus they might be helped by special diets. A small percentage of children also seem to have ADHD symptoms when exposed to foods that commonly trigger allergic reactions (chocolate, nuts, eggs, and milk). Parents can readily identify these reactions when they occur and should report them to their child's pediatrician. These children are by far in the minority, and dietary management alone is not a recommended therapy for ADHD.

Do Children Outgrow ADHD?

Some adolescents still have symptoms and continue to need medication and/or other treatment throughout their teenage years.

Studies show that 50 to 70 percent of children diagnosed with ADHD between ages six and twelve continue to exhibit symptoms of the disorder at least until middle adolescence. Often, although the hyperactivity may have been resolved, problems with inattention and distractability may persist. Particularly in middle school, when the demands for cognitive and organizational skills increase, these symptoms can interfere with academic achievement. In less than 3 percent of cases, classic ADHD signs like impulsiveness and poor concentration, and underachievement and the resultant frustration, continue into adulthood, although they may become less severe with time.

ADHD is a true neurodevelopmental disability that, if unmanaged, can result in the impairment of a child's future success and strain his relationships with others. But with careful monitoring, family education, and psychological help, your child can achieve success both academically and socially.

23

DEPRESSION

Everyone feels sad or blue once in a while. However, when that sadness turns into despair and persists for weeks and even months, then it becomes a worrisome emotional disorder called depression.

Depression is a syndrome in which an individual feels discouraged, hopeless, miserable, and despondent. Not too many years ago psychiatrists disagreed over whether children could in fact become depressed. Now, however, almost all concede that depression can occur at any age.

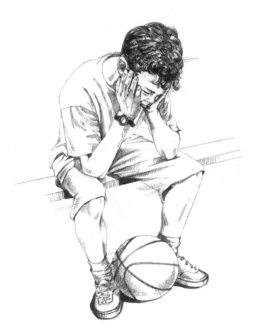

Children become depressed for a variety of reasons. Genetic factors play an important role, but having a parent who is depressed is the single most important risk factor for a child becoming depressed. Depressed parents' behavior can be a factor in children's depression, as these parents may be less able to respond appropriately to their children's emotional needs. Children feel less supported and parent-child conflict may be more common. Other highly stressful events, such as physical or sexual abuse or the loss of a family member or close friend, may contribute to children becoming depressed. Less stressful but important events such as family discord, school failure, or difficulty with peers can produce depressive symptoms. Sometimes it is not possible to identify a cause of depression.

In middle childhood most youngsters will not label themselves as depressed. Instead, they might use words like *sad, low, down in the dumps, blue,* or *bored*. In many cases they will not even speak of feeling any different from the way they did before.

Thus, as a parent, you need to be sensitive to the signs of childhood depression. A depressed youngster might say she is sad or unhappy. She may say, "No one likes me"; "I'm dumb and stupid"; "I wish I was dead."

A depressed child may spend more time alone in her room and stop playing with her friends. Her grades at school may noticeably decline. She may become more quiet and less talkative than usual, may eat slowly or lose her appetite altogether. She may have trouble falling or staying asleep, become fatigued easily, and, often, stop showing concern about her grooming and dress. She may complain of headaches, stomachaches, or chest pains.

Often a depressed child's symptoms are more subtle than you might expect. For instance, she might make less eye contact than in the past. Her mood and behavior may turn from being good-natured to irritable and angry. She may become harder to get along with, and fights and arguments with siblings and parents might become more of a problem.

If you suspect that your child is depressed, you need to do more than tell her to "cheer up" or "snap out of it." Instead, get her some professional attention—as early as possible. If treatment is delayed or avoided, the child's functioning in everyday life will continue to erode, as will her self-esteem, her schoolwork, and her relationships with friends and family. Also, the longer the depression persists, the more difficult it may be to treat.

Is Your Child Depressed?

Here are some questions to ask yourself to help determine whether your child should be evaluated for depression. If you answer yes to several of these questions, your child may be depressed.

- Does your child cry more often than in the past?

- Does he complain of feeling blue or empty inside?

- When things do not go your child's way, does he tend to view his life as hopeless?

- Does he have difficulty keeping his attention focused on his homework?

- Has your child had difficulty falling asleep at bedtime, or does he awaken in the middle of the night and have trouble going back to sleep?

- Does your child have a limited number of activities he enjoys, or has he lost his enthusiasm for the activities that used to occupy his time?

- Does he spend more time alone, away from friends and family?

- Has your child gained or lost weight in recent weeks?

- Does he seem more fatigued and tired than in the past?

- Does he sometimes talk about hurting himself?

Where to Get Help

If you suspect depression in your child, talk to your pediatrician. Before referring you to a child psychiatrist or psychologist, he or she will rule out medical conditions whose symptoms can cause or mimic those of depression.

Once under the care of a psychiatrist or psychologist, your child may undergo a number of tests to assess whether she is, in fact, clinically depressed. The therapist will also talk extensively to both you and your child, reviewing her history to determine your youngster's moods and feelings. Without careful evaluation, children with depression may be misdiagnosed as having a conduct disorder or an attention deficit disorder.

Once the diagnosis of depression has been made, treatment can begin. Psychotherapy (or "talk," play therapy, and cognitive-behavioral therapy) will probably be part of the treatment program, during which your child will be encouraged to discuss and to play out what is occurring in her life. She will be asked to describe her anxieties, worries, sadness, and other emotions. If there are particular negative events that she is dwelling on, the therapist will try to help her resolve them. While achieving a better understanding of her own life situation, your child will be able to relate in more positive ways to the people around her and the troubling circumstances in her life.

Throughout the treatment process, the therapist will also involve you as much as possible, scheduling regular conferences with you and your spouse, suggesting ways to help your child meet her own needs and adjust to the world around her. You might also be asked to participate in family therapy, in which you, your spouse, your child, and her siblings together will explore how all of you can function more positively as a family unit.

At home, you should give your child some extra attention, spending additional time with her apart from other family members. Provide her with special times to talk with you about the day's events. Let her know that you are available to discuss any problems or concerns she may have.

Sometimes your doctor may recommend not only psychotherapy for your child, but also medication as part of the treatment regimen. Particularly when the depression is severe—with major weight loss, sleep problems, and school difficulties—medication may be advisable. The class of drugs called selective serotonin reuptake inhibitors (SSRI) is most often prescribed for depressed children. Other types of medications (tricyclic antidepressants, monoamine oxidase inhibitors, lithium carbonate) might be used instead. SSRI drugs are also used to treat anxiety and obsessive-compulsive disorders.

Unless the depression is severe, most cases can be resolved after two to six months of treatment. Particularly when therapy has begun in the early stages of depression, this disorder is rapidly treatable. However, depression symptoms recur in a large proportion of children.

Suicide Prevention

Occasionally, during times of anger and upset, youngsters in middle childhood make provocative statements like "I'm going to kill myself." More than anything, these threats are designed to agitate parents and get their attention, and children usually have no serious intention of doing themselves real harm. Nevertheless, if frequent, these statements are messages of a very unhappy child, and parents need to be sure that the child is, in fact, in no jeopardy.

Youngsters in the six-to-twelve age range rarely commit suicide, but there is an increasing trend for them to make suicide attempts. Nevertheless, a small number of them who are severely depressed do think about killing themselves. Overwhelmed by despondent and hopeless feelings, a few actually do try to end their lives.

Children who attempt suicide often first display warning signs, including withdrawal, sadness, loss of appetite, and sleep disturbances. They may give away some of their most prized possessions, such as a baseball card collection. Sometimes the suicide of a friend or classmate can prompt children to consider killing themselves to reduce the psychological pain they are feeling.

If you sense that your child is troubled, you need to talk with him about it. Listen and share feelings. Do not hesitate to use the word *suicide*. Despite the myth that talking about suicide might give your child the idea of killing himself, that will not happen. Instead, your concern will show your child that you really care about him and his well-being and are willing to help him with his problems.

You should obtain some professional help for a seriously troubled child. If your pediatrician has developed a good relationship with your child over the years, he or she may be the best person for your youngster to talk to in the beginning. The doctor might then refer your youngster to a child psychiatrist or psychologist. If a child is truly suicidal and cannot be constantly monitored by the family, he may need to be hospitalized.

For emergency situations, most communities have suicide hotlines that can provide immediate advice and help. Check the telephone directory for these crisis hotlines, as well as for local mental-health centers to which you might turn for support.

For additional information about suicide, contact:

The American Association of
Suicidology
2459 South Ash
Denver, Colorado 80222

National Committee for Youth
Suicide Prevention
230 Park Avenue, Suite 835
New York, New York 10169

National Mental Health Association
1021 Prince Street
Arlington, Virginia 22314

American Psychiatric Association
1400 K Street N.W.
Washington, D.C. 20005

24

SCHOOL AVOIDANCE

With the start of school, youngsters begin to regularly spend a considerable amount of time away from the family. This time brings new experiences and many personal challenges. Much of their time is spent at school—a place where pressures in the classroom and relationships with other children can be quite stressful. While some youngsters naturally greet new situations with enthusiasm, others tend to retreat to the familiarity of their home. For some children, merely the specter of being at school away from home and apart from their parents causes great anxiety. Such children, especially when faced with situations they fear or with which they believe they cannot cope, may try to keep from returning to school.

This school avoidance—sometimes called school refusal or school phobia—is not uncommon and occurs in as many as 5 percent of children. These youngsters may outright refuse to attend school or create reasons why they should not go. They may miss a lot of school, complaining of not feeling well, with vague, unexplainable symptoms. Many of these children have anxiety-related symptoms over which they have no conscious control. Perhaps they have headaches, stomachaches, hyperventilation, nausea, or dizziness. In general, more clear-cut symptoms like vomiting, diarrhea, fever, or weight loss—which are likely to have a physical basis—are uncommon. School refusal symptoms occur most often on school days, and are usually absent on weekends. When these children are examined by a doctor, no true illnesses are detected or diagnosed. However, since the type of symptoms these children complain of can be caused by a physical illness, a medical examination should usually be part of their evaluation.

Most often, school-avoiding youngsters do not know precisely why they feel ill, and they may have difficulty communicating what is causing their discomfort or upset. But when school-related anxiety is causing school avoidance, the symptoms may be ways to communicate emotional struggle with issues like:

- Fear of failure

- Problems with other children (for instance, teasing because they are "fat" or "short")

- Anxieties over toileting in a public bathroom

- A perceived "meanness" of the teacher

- Threats of physical harm (as from a school bully)

- Actual physical harm

For some youngsters the school environment can increase preexisting tension. For example, if children tend to be overly conscientious and expect excellent performances from themselves, their fear of failure can gradually create overwhelming and paralyzing anxiety.

In some cases children have experienced the loss of a loved one through death, divorce, or moving to another locale. Especially when they are young, they may fear that in their absence from home another loss will occur.

In addition to the school environment itself, school avoidance may be related to a child's difficulty in separating from her parents and feeling safe while assuming more independence. These youngsters tend to be unsure of themselves and less independent than most of their peers. They may be less socially involved. They may be reluctant to go on overnight stays at friends' houses, preferring to be home with their own parents. Some children who have disabilities or chronic illnesses may struggle more with entry to school and being away from the shelter and care of home.

While the parents of these children are very loving and conscientious, they also may be somewhat overprotective. In some cases parents are depressed or physically ill and may unconsciously desire the company of their children. The youngsters are often the only child in the family or are special in some other way—for example, they may be the first or the last child of a larger family.

As children approach adolescence, the incidence of school phobia decreases significantly; however, when it does develop in a pre-adolescent, it is of much greater concern. Phobic young adolescents often fear growing up. They also may be overwhelmed by stresses at home that shake their sense of security or personal confidence, leaving them even less able to face academic and social challenges.

Managing School Avoidance

As a first step, the management of school avoidance involves an examination by a doctor who can rule out physical illness, and who can assist the parents in designing a plan of treatment. Once physical illness has been eliminated as a cause of the child's symptoms, the parents' efforts should be directed not only at understanding the pressures the youngster is experiencing but also at getting him back in school.

Here are some guidelines for helping your child overcome this problem:

- Talk with your child about the reasons why he does not want to go to school. Consider all the possibilities and state them. Be sympathetic, supportive, and understanding of why he is upset. Try to resolve any stressful situations the two of you identify as causing his worries or symptoms.

- Acknowledge that you understand your child's concerns, but insist on his immediate return to school. The longer he stays home, the more difficult his eventual return will be. Explain that he is in good health and his physical symptoms are probably due to concerns he has expressed to you— perhaps about grades, homework, relationships with teachers, anxieties over social pressure, or legitimate fears of violence at school. Let him know that school attendance is required by law. He will continue to exert some pressure upon you to let him stay home, but you must remain determined to get him back in school.

- Discuss your child's school avoidance with the school staff, including his teacher, the principal, and the school nurse. Share with them your plans for his return to school and enlist their support and assistance.

- Make a commitment to be extra firm on school mornings, when children complain most about their symptoms. Keep discussions about physical symptoms or anxieties to a minimum. For example, do not ask your youngster how he feels. If he is well enough to be up and around the house, then he is well enough to attend school. Err on the side of sending your child to school. Once your youngster begins to attend school regularly, his physical symptoms will probably disappear.

- If your child's anxieties are severe, he might benefit from a step-wise return to school. For example: On day one he might get up in the morning and get dressed, and then you might drive him by the school so he can get some feel for it before you finally return home with him. On day two he might go to school for just half a day, or for only a favorite class or two. On day three he can finally return for a full day of school.

- Your pediatrician might help ease your child's transition back to school by writing him a note verifying that he had some symptoms that kept him from attending school, but though the symptoms might persist, he is now able to return to class. This can keep your youngster from feeling embarrassed or humiliated.

- Request help from the school staff for assistance with your child while he is at school. A school nurse or secretary can care for him if he becomes symptomatic, and encourage his return to the classroom.

- If a problem like a school bully or an unreasonable teacher is the cause of your child's anxiety, become an advocate for your youngster and discuss these problems with the school staff. The teacher or principal may need to make some adjustments to relieve the pressure on your child in the classroom or on the playground.

- If your child stays home, be sure he is safe and comfortable, but he should not receive any special treatment. His symptoms should be treated with consideration and understanding. If his complaints warrant it, he should stay in bed. However, his day should not be a holiday. There should be no special snacks and no visitors, and he should be supervised.

- Your child may need to see a physician when he has to stay home because of a physical illness. Reasons to remain home might include not just complaints of discomfort but recognizable symptoms: a temperature greater than 101 degrees, vomiting, diarrhea, a rash, a hacking cough, an earache, or a toothache.

- Help your child develop independence by encouraging activities with other children outside the home. These can include clubs, sports activities, and overnights with friends or relatives.

When to Seek Help

While you might try to manage school refusal on your own, if your youngster's school avoidance lasts more than one week, you and your child may need professional assistance to deal with it. First, your child should be examined by your pediatrician. If her school refusal persists, or if she has chronic or intermittent signs of separation difficulties when going to school—in combination with physical symptoms that are interfering with her functioning—your doctor may recommend a consultation with a child psychiatrist or psychologist.

Even if your child denies having negative experiences at school or with other children, her unexplainable physical symptoms should motivate you to schedule a medical evaluation.

25

FEARS AND PHOBIAS

From time to time, every child experiences fear. As youngsters explore the world around them, having new experiences and confronting new challenges, anxieties are almost an unavoidable part of growing up.

According to one study, 43 percent of children between ages six and twelve had *many* fears and concerns. A fear of darkness, particularly being left alone in the dark, is one of the most common fears in this age group. So is a fear of animals, such as large barking dogs. Some children are afraid of fires, high places, or thunderstorms. Others, conscious of news reports on TV and in the newspapers, are concerned about burglars, kidnappers, or nuclear war. If there has been a recent serious illness or death in the family, they may become anxious about the health of those around them.

In middle childhood, fears wax and wane. Most are mild, but even when they intensify, they generally subside on their own after a while. Sometimes, however, these fears can become so extreme, persistent, and focused that they develop into phobias. Phobias—which are strong and irrational fears—can become persistent and debilitating, significantly influencing and interfering with a child's usual daily activities. For instance, a six-year-old youngster's phobia about dogs might make him

so panicky that he refuses to go outdoors at all because there could be a dog there. A ten-year-old child might become so terrified about news reports of a serial killer that he insists on sleeping with his parents at night.

Some youngsters in this age group develop phobias about the people they meet in their everyday lives. This severe shyness can keep them from making friends at school and relating to most adults, especially strangers. They might consciously avoid social situations like birthday parties or Scout meetings, and they often find it difficult to converse comfortably with anyone except their immediate family.

Separation anxiety is also common in this age group. Sometimes this fear can intensify when the family moves to a new neighborhood or children are placed in a child-care setting where they feel uncomfortable. These youngsters might become afraid of going to summer camp or even attending school. (See Chapter 24, "School Avoidance.") Their phobias can cause physical symptoms like headaches or stomach pains and eventually lead the children to withdraw into their own world, becoming clinically depressed.

At about age six or seven, as children develop an understanding about death, another fear can arise. With the recognition that death will eventually affect everyone, and that it is permanent and irreversible, the normal worry about the possible death of family members—or even their own death—can intensify. In some cases, this preoccupation with death can become disabling.

Treating Fears and Phobias

Since fears are a normal part of life and often are a response to a real or at least perceived threat in the child's environment, parents should be reassuring and supportive. Talking with their children, parents should acknowledge, though not increase or reinforce, their children's concerns. Point out what is already being done to protect the child, and involve the child in identifying additional steps that could be taken. Such simple, sensitive, and straightforward parenting can resolve or at least manage most childhood fears. When realistic reassurances are not successful, the child's fear may be a phobia.

Fortunately, most phobias are quite treatable. In general, they are *not* a sign of serious mental illness requiring many months or years of therapy.

The techniques in this chapter may help your child conquer her everyday fears. However, if her anxieties persist and interfere with her enjoyment of day-to-day life, she might benefit from some professional help from a psychiatrist or psychologist who specializes in treating phobias.

As part of the treatment plan for phobias, many therapists suggest exposing your child to the source of her anxiety in small, nonthreatening doses. Under a therapist's guidance a child who is afraid of dogs might begin by talking about this fear and by looking at photographs or a videotape of dogs. Next, she might observe a live dog from behind the safety of a window. Then, with a parent or a therapist at her side, she might spend a few minutes in the same room with a friendly, gentle puppy. Eventually she will find himself able to pet the dog, then expose herself to situations with larger, unfamiliar dogs.

This gradual process is called *desensitization,* meaning that your child will become a little less sensitive to the source of her fear each time she confronts it. Ultimately, the child will no longer feel the need to avoid the situation that has been the basis of her phobia. While this process sounds like common sense and easy to carry out, it should be done only under the supervision of a professional.

Sometimes psychotherapy can also help children become more self-assured and less fearful. Breathing and relaxation exercises can assist youngsters in stressful circumstances too.

Occasionally, your doctor may recommend medications as a component of the treatment program, although never as the sole therapeutic tool. These drugs may include antidepressants, which are designed to ease the anxiety and panic that often underlie these problems.

Helping the Fearful Child

Here are some suggestions that many parents find useful for their children with fears and phobias.

- Talk with your youngster about his anxieties, and be sympathetic. Explain to him that many children have fears, but with your support he can learn to put them behind him.

- Do not belittle or ridicule your child's fears, particularly in front of his peers.

- Do not try to *coerce* your youngster into being brave. It will take time for him to confront and gradually overcome his anxieties. You can, however, encourage (but not force) him to progressively come face-to-face with whatever he fears. If he is afraid of darkness, hold his hand as you spend a few seconds together in a dark room.

If he is fearful of water, accompany him as he wades into a children's pool, with the water reaching up to his knees. Praise every small success, and the next step will be easier. Focus most of your attention on what he has accomplished, not on the anxiety itself.

26

OBSESSIVE-COMPULSIVE DISORDERS

A small number of children are preoccupied with repetitive thoughts or actions that, to the outsider, seem foolish and illogical. These recurring ideas (obsessions) and repeated actions (compulsions) are uncontrollable, and can upset their lives and ultimately disrupt the normal functioning of their families. In about one-third to one-half of all affected individuals, obsessive-compulsive disorder begins in childhood and adolescence.

Children with obsessive-compulsive behavior may excessively wash their hands or brush their teeth. They may be driven to check things repeatedly, making sure they have packed their homework assignments or their lunch in the morning. They may repeat certain rituals, perhaps entering and exiting a room a particular number of times. They may arrange and rearrange a table setting meticulously, or become concerned with germs, dirt, crime, violence, disease, or death in an overly dramatic manner.

One doctor treated an obsessive-compulsive child who was preoccupied with thoughts of a devastating tornado. From the age of six, this youngster would check radar weather maps on television and continuously ask his mother about whether she had heard of any tornado warnings.

An eight-year-old boy's obsessive-compulsive behavior began with frequent hand-washing and soon escalated to constant anxiety about fires and accidents. He would spend six to eight hours a day monitoring the electrical outlets and the light switches in his house, as well as scrubbing his hands and indulging in other compulsive behavior.

Even at their young ages, these children often recognize that their behavior is bizarre. However, if they attempt to control it, they are usually overcome with anxiety and revert to their peculiar rituals for relief. Knowing that their behavior is not normal, they often try to hide it from family and friends. Many children have these unusual behaviors for many months before they are discovered.

Why do these youngsters go through such rituals? Most children say they simply do not know. Researchers investigating the causes of obsessive-compulsive disorder describe it as a neurobiological disturbance that seems to run in families.

What Is the Treatment?

If your child is exhibiting compulsive behavior, talk with your pediatrician, who may refer you to a child psychiatrist or psychologist.

Behavioral therapy works for many children, often by desensitizing them to their rituals. For example, a child overly concerned or repelled by dirt, one who washes her hands many times a day, might have dirt placed on her hands while being denied the opportunity to clean them. Initially, this is very frightening and difficult for the child. Eventually she will recognize that her worst fears are not as devastating as she had once thought, and that she can get along quite well with only occasional hand-washing. Desensitization is a specialized technique and should be done only by an experienced mental-health professional.

The therapist can also help put your child's anxieties into perspective ("Tornadoes strike here only once every thirty years or so, and they've never been very powerful; your worries appear to be far out of proportion to what really might happen").

The class of drugs called selective serotonin reuptake inhibitors has been found to be helpful in reducing disabling symptoms. These and other medications are an important part of the current approach to treatment. Like other psychotropic drugs, they should be prescribed only for appropriate symptoms and require close monitoring by a child psychiatrist or pediatrician familiar with these medications and their potentially serious side effects.

27

EATING DISORDERS

American culture places a premium on being physically attractive and having the "perfect" body. This has led to almost a societal obsession with losing weight, being thin, and dieting. Concerns about being overweight begin as early as preschool age, and the drive for thinness intensifies with age. The results can have both physical and psychological repercus-

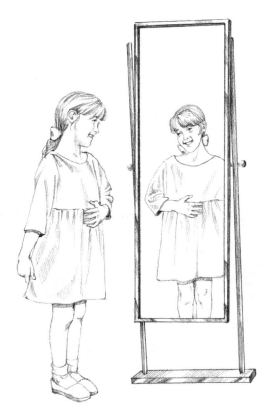

sions, including potentially serious disordered eating.

Disordered eating is an unhealthy preoccupation with food and one's body. It is "emotional" eating and includes compulsive-obsessive eating, anorexia nervosa, bulimia, and most commonly, dieting and restrictive eating. There has been an increased incidence of eating problems during the past two decades. During the middle years, children ages ten to twelve are at greatest risk. More girls and women seem to be affected by eating disorders than males.

In some families, adults use a variety of activities to help them cope with their feelings. They may smoke, use alcohol, work feverishly, exercise intensively, or choose other ways to help them feel better. Many use food and thus become emotional eaters. Most children have ready access to food and so learn to "stuff" their feelings. Whether it is done when they are feeling very high or very low emotionally, it is easy to use food to cope with emotions.

Anorexia nervosa is characterized by self-induced starvation, a troubling degree of weight loss, and a seriously distorted body image fueled by an intense fear of being fat. Anorexia is more common in girls than in boys, but can occur in either sex. The child's body image is so unrealistic and distorted that she complains of looking fat, even when it is obvious to others that she is severely underweight and conspicuously gaunt. Generally, children with anorexia nervosa consume only a few hundred calories each day, while they may engage in rituals of sneaking and hiding food or getting rid of it. They may abuse laxatives and diuretics (drugs that increase urination). They are also preoccupied with exercise to burn off as many calories as possible, by jogging for miles, doing aerobic dancing several times a day, or running up and down stairs constantly in the pursuit of thinness. Girls with anorexia nervosa who have begun menstruating may miss their periods, or stop having periods completely, and pre-adolescent girls who have anorexia nervosa may experience a delay in the onset of menstruation. Anorexia nervosa is relatively rare during the middle years, ages five to twelve.

Bulimia is a different condition but is characterized by some of the same activities. It is often referred to as the binge/purge syndrome. A binge is a period of voracious eating, with an urgency and a need to stuff food, while at the same time having a fear of not being able to stop. Typically the foods that are chosen are high-calorie junk foods, but bingeing can occur with any type of food. Binge eating is out-of-control emotional eating. At times the amount of food eaten is not necessarily excessive; for example, if a girl has been dieting and restricting food intake and then begins to eat, she may binge and feel very out of control, regardless of the actual amount of food she consumes.

Following a binge, purging is common. Girls try to rid their bodies of food, either by self-induced vomiting (sticking a finger or an object like a toothbrush down the throat) or abusing laxatives or diuretics. They may engage in abusive exercise, diet pills, fasting, or dieting, all in an attempt to lose weight. Most girls with bulimia feel quite ashamed of their bingeing and purging, and they become highly skilled at keep-

ing it a secret from friends and family. The strong emotional compulsion to maintain the binge/purge cycle, as well as their success at disguising their problem, makes bulimia difficult to detect and treat. Full-fledged bulimia is also relatively uncommon during the middle years. However, particularly as they enter puberty, children are more commonly engaging in purging without bingeing.

Dieting and restrictive eating are characterized by a disturbing preoccupation with the need to lose weight. These children weigh themselves frequently, engage in fad diets, and are unreasonably restrictive about food intake. This behavior pattern is unrelated to whether the child is over, under, or at a healthy body weight. Being on a diet is the common theme for everyone suffering from disordered eating and can lead to serious problems.

The restrictive-eating child may initially appear only to be a picky eater, cutting out certain foods—maybe refusing to eat any bread—or perhaps becoming a vegetarian. Since these children still have normal appetites, their eating behavior is a way of exerting control in one area of their lives. Because eating is often an important issue in their families, these children find it easy to use their diets to manipulate their parents. Frequently, their disordered eating leads to emotional struggles with their parents. Unfortunately, because of the societal pressure to be thin, parents and other adults sometimes succumb to the controlling eating behavior of their children.

What Causes These Disorders?

As prevalent as these eating problems have become, researchers do not know for certain what causes them. Certainly, society's emphasis on thinness plays a role, as girls strive to look like the models they see in fashion magazines, and boys attempt to emulate TV or sports heroes. If a girl's parents or close friends are overly concerned about thinness and spend much of their energy dieting, or if they even innocently comment that their daughter's jeans are a bit too tight, her concern with thinness can turn into an obsession, particularly if she already has the psychological makeup that puts her at risk for disordered eating.

Beyond this preoccupation with weight and dieting, psychological factors may be involved in these eating disorders. Children with anorexia or bulimia or who chronically diet are frequently depressed, with poor self-esteem, feelings of inadequacy, and stress and trauma in their lives. Young girls with anorexia nervosa tend to be perfectionists and set unrealistically high goals for themselves, both academically and socially. They often have difficulty coping with the anxieties of growing up and maturing sexually, and as their bodies develop, they may use severe dieting to try to postpone these physical changes. These girls also frequently struggle with a grave sense of having lost control of their lives because of family stress, emotional turmoil, or social pressure. Ironically, their self-imposed starvation—however destructive—may be the only part of their lives that they feel they can control.

For girls who binge, the eating is often a way of dealing with stress and boredom. The cakes, cookies, and ice cream that they devour can become "friends," helping to nurture them and ease their anxiety. However, since these girls often feel guilty and ashamed after a bulimic episode, their stress may escalate, making them even more prone to binge and purge again. Girls with disordered eating often have considerable difficulty with intimacy, due to struggles in relationships within their families, and because of their low self-esteem, poor self-concept, and bad self-image (related to embarrassment over their dieting,

vomiting behavior, and the intense effort it takes not to eat).

Eating disorders have complex causes within the child's or adolescent's experiences in her family and the society in which she is raised. There is no certain way to prevent these disorders, but focusing on a child's personal and social strengths rather than on appearance and popularity is a good place to start. (See Chapter 10.)

Prevention and Early Detection

What are the warning signs? Eating disorders may be especially difficult to detect in the middle-years child and younger adolescent. For a ten- to twelve-year-old child, the symptoms of the disorder may be much more subtle than in an older youngster. Failure to gain appropriate weight, rather than more obvious weight loss, may be the only physical sign of a problem. Even if a child is extremely thin, loose clothing may camouflage it in the early stages, and the children become very skilled at hiding their behavior.

Parents of many girls with eating disorders sometimes describe them as model children. Their compulsive tendencies lead them to achieve high grades on their report cards and to keep their rooms exceptionally neat. They may be overly concerned about personal grooming, feeling they always need to look "just right" but never being quite satisfied with their appearance. On the other hand, sometimes these youngsters seem very out of control and have little neatness or apparent structure in their lives.

These girls may never complain about personal problems or express any negative emotions, even though every life has both ups and downs. Not surprisingly, they may talk a lot about their weight and get on the scale frequently. While many girls begin to talk about being fat during these years and sometimes are merely "going along with the crowd," such talk may be a warning that they might begin to take on disordered eating behaviors.

Youngsters with anorexia nervosa spend relatively little time socializing but may devote many of their waking hours to compulsive behavior—rewriting homework assignments until they are perfect or adhering to a fanatical exercise routine. They often perform calisthenics in their bedrooms for literally hours at a time or follow a rigorous program of long-distance running or cycling, constantly pushing themselves to the point of exhaustion. Meanwhile, their personal and social lives may seem empty and devoid of intimacy and depth.

As expected, children with anorexia nervosa may ignore food that is placed in front of them, even if it is just a modest amount. Yet although they eat very little, these youngsters may devote a lot of time to choosing and preparing the food they do consume. They may read calorie charts incessantly, cut their food into small pieces, and prefer to eat slowly by themselves. They often insist on helping with the grocery shopping and cook delicious meals and rich desserts for other family members.

Do not overlook the fact that boys also sometimes develop an eating disorder during late childhood. It is often brought on by the normal increase in weight that accompanies puberty, and by the ever-increasing cultural pressures regarding boys' and men's appearance.

If you suspect a serious eating problem with your child, talk with your pediatrician. *Eating disorders cannot be ignored; they are potentially life-threatening*. Children with anorexia nervosa, if their condition is not brought under control, can quite literally starve themselves to death. Even if the disorder is not fatal, the severe malnutrition can take a terrible toll on the body, causing conditions ranging from heart and kidney damage to a heightened vulnerability to infections. While children with bulimia may not suffer the same type of malnutrition as those with anorexia, the vomiting can seriously injure their esophagus, tooth enamel, gums, and kidneys.

Children who focus on dieting and restrictive eating do not receive the appropriate nutrition to support healthy growth. The use of diet pills, fasting, or other such behavior can lead to severe physical and/or psychological impairment.

Treatment of Eating Disorders

Anorexia nervosa and bulimia are difficult for professionals to treat; for parents, they are virtually impossible to manage successfully alone. Pleading with or punishing your child is not going to change her behavior. Even with the most sophisticated care, cures are difficult and relapses are common. Most children with eating disorders deny having a problem and thus object to treatment. They may be embarrassed by their behavior, and frightened that if they submit to therapy, they are going to gain weight and become "fat."

The earlier the problem is identified and treatment starts, however, the better the chances of success. Once the self-destructive behavior has been well-established, therapy becomes more difficult.

Eating disorders are complex, and the best treatment programs are multidimensional, with medical, psychiatric, and nutritional components. Medications might be prescribed, especially to help the child cope with depression or severe anxiety. Hospitalization or residential treatment may be required, particularly for patients who have lost large amounts of weight or developed serious complications; in extreme cases proper nutrition may be administered with intravenous fluids—or via a tube through the nose and into the stomach—until the child is willing to eat on her own.

Counseling and support are essential components of the treatment program. Therapists will work with the patient to ease her anxieties related to regaining weight, and to help her adopt realistic goals for her own appearance. Because family dynamics play an important role in these disorders, doctors may recommend psychotherapy involving parents and perhaps even siblings. Children need to feel loved but not possessed, pressured, or controlled by their parents.

The entire recovery process, including follow-up care, may take many months and often years. Unfortunately, relapses may occur into the adult years.

28

SOILING (ENCOPRESIS)

Encopresis is one of the more frustrating disorders of middle childhood. It is the passing of stools into the underwear or pajamas, far past the time of normal toilet training. Encopresis affects about 1.5 percent of young schoolchildren and can create tremendous anxiety and embarrassment for children and their families.

Encopresis is not a disease but rather a symptom of a complex relationship between the body and psychological/environmental stresses. Boys with encopresis outnumber girls by a ratio of six to one, although the reasons for this greater prevalence among males is not known. The condition is not related to social class, family size, the child's position in the family, or the age of the parents.

Doctors divide cases of encopresis into two categories: primary and secondary. Children with the primary disorder have had continuous soiling throughout their lives, without any period in which they were successfully toilet trained. By contrast, children with the secondary form may develop this condition after they have been toilet trained, such as upon entering school or encountering other experiences that might be stressful.

Children, parents, grandparents, teachers, and friends alike are often baffled by this problem. Adults sometimes assume that the child is soiling himself on purpose.

While this may not be the case, children can play an active role in managing the processes involved in this disorder.

The Physical Aspects of Encopresis

When encopresis occurs, it begins with stool retention in the colon. Many of these youngsters simply may not respond to the urge to defecate and thus withhold their stools. As the intestinal walls and the nerves within them stretch, nerve sensations in the area diminish. Also, the intestines progressively lose their ability to contract and squeeze the stools out of the body. Therefore, these children find it increasingly difficult to have a normal bowel movement. Most of these children are chronically constipated.

With time, these retained stools become harder, larger, and much more difficult to pass. Bowel movements then can be painful, which further discourages these children from passing the stools.

Eventually, the sphincters (the muscular valves that normally keep stools inside the rectum) are no longer able to hold back all the stool. Large, hard feces may be retained in the colon (large intestine) and rectum, but liquid stool can begin to seep around this impacted mass, passing through the anus and staining the underwear. At other times, semiformed or partial bowel movements may pass into the underwear, and because of the decreased sensation, the child may not be aware of it.

Some of these youngsters are predisposed from birth to *early colonic inertia*—that is, a tendency toward constipation because their intestinal tracts lack full mobility. Early in life these children might have experienced constipation that required dietary and medical management.

Some children develop constipation and encopresis because of unsuccessful toilet training as toddlers. They may have fought the toilet training process, been pushed too fast, or were punished for having accidents. Struggling with their parents for control, they may have voluntarily withheld their stools, straining to hold them as long as they could. Some children may actually have had a fear of the toilet, even thinking that they themselves might be flushed away.

A number of other factors can also contribute to the eventual development of encopresis. Sometimes children may have pain when they have a bowel movement due to an infection or a tear near their rectum. Emotional causes can include limited access to a toilet or shyness over its use (at school, for example), or stressful life events (marital discord between parents, moves to a new neighborhood, family physical or mental illnesses, or new siblings). While most children with encopresis are also constipated, some are not. These children may refuse to use the toilet and simply have normal bowel movements in their underwear or other inappropriate places. In general, these children are demonstrating their attempts to control some difficult aspects of their lives. Professional help is advisable for these children and their families.

Many parents are astonished that their child with encopresis may not even be conscious of the odor emanating from the stool in his pants. When this odor is constant, the smelling centers of the brain may become accustomed to it, and thus the child actually is no longer aware of it. As a result, these youngsters often are surprised when a parent or someone else tells them that they have an odor. While the youngster himself may not be bothered by the smell, the people around him may not be sympathetic to his problem.

The Psychological Aspects of Encopresis

Exasperated parents often place great pressure on their child to change this behavior—something the youngster may be incapable of without help from a pediatrician. While family members may have ideas on how to solve the problem, their efforts generally will fail when they do not understand the physiological mechanisms at work.

Encopresis can lead to a struggle within the family. As parents and siblings become increasingly frustrated and angry, family activities may be curtailed or the child with encopresis may be ostracized from them. By this stage, the problem often has become a family preoccupation.

As the child and family fruitlessly battle over the child's bowel control, the conflict may extend to other areas of the child's life. His schoolwork may suffer; his responsibilities and chores around the home may be ignored. He may also become angry, withdrawn, anxious, and depressed, often as a result of being teased and feeling humiliated.

Management of Encopresis

Encopresis is a chronic, complex—but solvable—problem. However, the longer it exists, the more difficult it is to treat. The child should be taught how the bowel works, and that he can strengthen the muscles and nerves that control bowel function. Parents should not blame the child and make him feel guilty, since that contributes to lower self-esteem and makes him feel less competent to solve the problem.

When encopresis is occurring in a school-age child, a physician experienced in encopresis treatment and interested in working with the child *and* the family should be involved. The treatment goals will probably be fourfold: (1) to establish regular bowel habits in the child; (2) to reduce stool retention; (3) to restore normal physiological control over bowel function; and (4) to defuse conflicts and reduce concerns within the family brought on by the child's symptoms. To accomplish these goals, attention will be focused not only on the physical basis of encopresis but also on its behavioral and psychological components and consequences.

In the initial phase of medical care, the intestinal tract often has to be cleansed with medications. For the first week or two the child may need enemas, strong laxatives, or suppositories to empty the intestinal tract so it can shrink to a more normal size.

The maintenance phase of management involves scheduling regular times to use the toilet in conjunction with daily laxatives like mineral oil or milk of magnesia. Proper diet is important, too, with sufficient fluids and high-fiber foods. These steps will keep the stool soft and prevent constipation. When improperly supervised, these interventions have potential dangers for the health of the child and so should be done only under the supervision of the child's physician. The maintenance phase will usually last two to three months or longer.

Parents often use a behavior modification or reward system that encourages the child's proper toilet habits. He might receive a star or sticker on a chart for each day he goes without soiling and a special small toy, for example, after a week. This approach works best for a child who truly wishes to solve the problem and is fully cooperative in that effort.

Some youngsters have significant behavioral and emotional difficulties that interfere with the treatment program. Psychological counseling for these children helps them deal with issues like peer conflicts, academic difficulties, and low self-esteem, all of which can contribute to encopresis.

Throughout this treatment process, parents should remind the child that there are other youngsters who have the same problem. In fact, children with the same difficulty probably attend his own school.

Children with encopresis may have occasional relapses and failures during and after treatment; these are actually quite normal, particularly in the early phases. Ultimate success may take months or even years.

One of the most important tasks of parents is to seek early treatment for this problem. Many mothers and fathers feel ashamed and unsupported when their child has encopresis. But parents should not just wait for it to go away. They should consult their doctor and make a persistent effort to solve the problem. If the symptoms are allowed to linger, the child's self-esteem and social confidence may be damaged even more.

29

BED-WETTING (ENURESIS)

Bed-wetting is normal and very common among preschoolers, affecting 40 percent of children at age three. It is much less frequent in school-age children, occurring in 20 percent of five-year-olds, 10 percent of six-year-olds, and 3 percent of twelve-year-olds. Thus, during the middle years of childhood, parents may want to seek the assistance of their pediatrician in an effort to reduce or eliminate bed-wetting, or enuresis.

For a child to remain dry at night, her brain must keep a full bladder from emptying. Or a signal from the bladder must be strong enough to awaken the child from sleep and send her to the toilet. It is a complex neurodevelopmental process for the bladder to send the signal, for the brain to receive it, and for the child to respond by awakening and using the toilet.

There are many theories about the causes of bed-wetting. Many parents fear that a disease is causing the difficulty. However, no more than 1 percent of cases actually are related to physical diseases such as kidney or bladder infections, diabetes, or congenital defects of the urinary system. In these instances the child also generally experiences changes in the frequency and volume of daytime urination, or discomfort associated with urination.

In the majority of cases of bed-wetting, however, the cause is simply delayed maturation of bladder control mechanisms, often related to the child's genetic background. These children are physically and psychologically normal.

Emotional problems are an occasional cause of enuresis. For instance, a child who is overwhelmed with stress may develop enuresis, even though she had formerly been dry at night. Children who are being sexually or physically abused may also develop enuresis.

Most school-age children who wet their beds have *primary enuresis*, meaning they have had this condition since birth and have never developed nighttime bladder control. These children often have a family history of this problem, and they seem to have inherited the tendency for developing nighttime bladder control at a later-than-average age. In most cases the child becomes dry at about the same age that her parent(s) did. Interestingly, if one identical twin has a bed-wetting problem, her twin also will; however, fraternal twins (nonidentical twins with different genetic makeups) often do not both have this problem.

Sometimes parents pressure a child to develop nighttime bladder control before her body is ready to do so. These parents may erroneously view bed-wetting as a willful and oppositional act of their child, and thus they may try coercing her to change her behavior. The youngster may become discouraged and depressed when she continues to wet the bed. As hard as she may try, the enuresis is beyond her voluntary control, and she may become frustrated and despondent because of her lack of success.

For the child who wets the bed, parents need to remain supportive and encouraging. They should be sensitive to the child's embarrassment or discomfort over this problem. The youngster may resist spending the night at a friend's house or going to summer camp and may be uncomfortable about her friends' finding out about this condition. Parents can reassure the child that it is not her fault, and the problem *will* get better in time.

Management of Bed-Wetting

Reassure your child that the symptoms of enuresis will pass with age. Until that natural maturation process occurs, however, several techniques might help the situation.

1. *Protecting and changing the bed.* Until your child fully achieves bladder control, encase his bed in a plastic cover to protect it from becoming saturated, thus avoiding a permanent urine smell.

2. *Assuming responsibility.* You may wish to encourage your child to change his own linens when they are wet. This will show that he is taking responsibility for himself, and it will relieve him of the embarrassment of having to alert others in the family when he wets the bed. However, if others in the family don't have similar household tasks, your child may see this as punishment, and in that case it is not recommended.

3. *Try bladder-stretching exercises.* If your child shows an interest in becoming actively involved in decreasing his bed-wetting, he can practice holding his urine as long as possible during the waking hours when he has ready access to a toilet. (Weekends are easier than weekdays.) Whenever he feels the urge to go, he should wait an additional ten minutes or longer until the bladder spasms stop. As he learns to resist and postpone the elimination of urine, he may enhance his bladder capacity and develop greater urine control.

4. *Develop his ability for self-awakening.* Your child can try training himself to wake up in the middle of the night—perhaps initially with the help of an alarm clock—in order to empty his bladder and, if necessary, change his clothes. To avoid wetness, he may have to awaken two to three times during the night. Reward him when he can successfully accomplish this goal. It is not advisable for parents to awaken their youngster before they go to sleep.

5. *Use a bed-wetting alarm device.* When your child reaches age seven or eight and still is having little success at achieving nighttime dryness, you might try an alarm device. It senses the presence of urine and triggers a buzzer that awakens him. This device should be positioned on or close to the child's underwear so it will detect the wetness immediately and sound the alarm; upon awakening, the youngster should go to the bathroom and then reset the alarm before returning to sleep.

These alarms are available at most pharmacies and usually cost from $40 to $50. Although they provide a 60 to 90 percent cure rate, there is a 20 to 45 percent incidence of relapse once youngsters stop using the system. They tend to be most helpful when children are starting to experience occasional dry nights, indicating that they are gradually developing some control on their own.

6. *Eliminate all teasing and negative comments within the family about bedwetting.* In particular, talk with siblings who are teasing a child who has not yet acquired this developmental skill. Parents do best when they ignore completely the occurrence of wet beds, and certainly they should avoid making it a part of regular conversations with the child.

Seeking Additional Help

If your child has primary enuresis, you might wish to discuss the problem with your pediatrician in order to understand it better and simply to be reassured that it is normal.

When a child develops enuresis after having been dry at night in the past, she should be evaluated by her physician. This may be a sign that the condition is disease-related or associated with psychological stress.

In some cases, particularly if your youngster is exhibiting emotional strain because of her enuresis, your pediatrician may perform a physical examination, do a urinalysis, and review your child's entire developmental history. He or she may also suggest one or more of the following treatments.

Medications

The use of drugs to treat bed-wetting is controversial. Since primary enuresis typically resolves itself as the child matures, some doctors worry that reliance on medications may pose more risk (because of side effects) than benefits.

When doctors do prescribe drugs, imipramine is most often their first choice. It is a tricyclic antidepressant taken at bedtime, and about half of children have a good response to it. Others placed on this medication may have no response at all, or may relapse after showing some improvement.

Ask your pediatrician about imipramine's side effects. Some children are drowsy on the medication, have a dry mouth, gain weight, or experience dizziness, difficulty concentrating, or trouble sleeping. In rare cases and in large doses, it can create heart rhythm disturbances.

On occasion, a drug called DDAVP (desmopressin acetate) may be prescribed. It is an antidiuretic hormone, that reduces the amount of urine released by the kidneys. DDAVP is inhaled through the nose at bedtime and seems capable of relieving bed-wetting in some children. It is an expensive treatment best used for special circumstances such as overnights with friends or grandparents or attendance at summer camp.

Psychological Therapy

When enuresis is due to stress or causes emotional distress, psychological intervention may be helpful to resolve the bedwetting. Sometimes hypnosis is useful in giving children more control over nighttime wetting. Proponents of hypnosis as a treatment for bed-wetting have shown a cure rate of 75 to 80 percent. While hypnosis is known to be quite safe and often effective, its mechanism is unknown.

Fortunately, as each year passes, bedwetting will decrease as the child's body matures; most children stop before adolescence.

30

CHILD ABUSE

Nearly all mothers and fathers can point to incidents in which they fell short of their ideal as parents—perhaps a moment of frustration in which they believed they were somehow abusive to their youngsters when, in retrospect, they really hadn't been. Most parents will never actually be child abusers, and most children will never be abused.

By definition, child abuse includes a number of forms of severe maltreatment, including physical abuse, physical neglect, verbal abuse, emotional abuse, and sexual abuse. Some unfortunate children experience multiple types of abuse. For instance, a child who experiences repeated instances of emotional abuse might also be victimized by occasional, deliberate physical violence. Severe physical abuse—even if only a rare outburst by overwhelmed parents with out-of-control anger—can inflict permanent damage on children and, in some cases, death.

Parental neglect—in which a child receives little or no supervision in and around his home, for example—can have tragic consequences if injuries occur. Even when it poses no immediate threat to a child's safety, prolonged or repeated neglect—in which his basic needs for clothing, nutrition, medical care, education, shelter, and nurturance are not met—can have adverse physical, social, developmental, and emotional consequences.

The number of cases of child abuse is on the rise, with reports of abuse to child-protection agencies increasing dramatically in recent years. According to one study there were three reports of child abuse for each one hundred children in the United States in 1985 alone. With societal drug and alcohol problems so severe, and the number of children in poverty growing, the incidence of child abuse is likely to continue to rise.

Most abusers are members of the child's family—if not a parent, then a close relative (such as an uncle or an older brother or sister), or a member of the household. And a number of factors can contribute to their abuse of children. Pressures on the family, both internal and external, can take a toll. When parents are feeling financial strain, job stress, or marital problems, their anger and frustration may make them more prone to strike out at their child. At certain times of the day—perhaps in the early evening after a hard day at work—parents may find it particularly difficult to control their tempers when youngsters misbehave or merely try their patience. Parents who are socially isolated, without adequate sources of emotional support or a helping hand with daily tasks and responsibilities, are more likely to lose control and abuse their children.

Alcohol and other drug use by parents is often a contributor to child abuse. By re-

Signs of Physical Abuse

These indicators may suggest a youngster has been physically abused:

- The child has had repeated injuries that are unexplainable or unusual.

- He appears withdrawn, passive, depressed, and cries a lot.

- Conversely, he is unusually aggressive, disruptive in the classroom, or destructive of his personal property and that of others. He throws toys across the room or becomes violent toward a pet.

- He seems overly tired and mentions that he has trouble sleeping and frequent nightmares.

- The child seems genuinely afraid of a parent or other caretaker.

- He spends a lot of time at the playground and appears hesitant to go home after school, as if he were fearful of something there.

- His parents seem to be isolated from other mothers and fathers in the neighborhood, do not participate in school activities, and may have a drinking or other drug-abuse problem. They appear preoccupied with their own lives at the expense of caring properly for their youngster.

- The parent is unwilling to talk about his child's injuries, or is noticeably anxious when he or she does so.

ducing inhibitions, alcohol consumption often allows anger to explode in a parent who is confronted by his or her child's misbehavior. Some drugs, such as amphetamines, can increase agitation and thus can contribute to an abusive situation in the home. Children who are abused are sometimes those with learning or behavioral problems—conditions that themselves place more stress on and create more conflict within the family.

Physical Abuse

Parents who were physically abused themselves as children, or who were or are intimidated verbally and physically by adults around them, often resort to similar means when they discipline their own youngsters.

The use of force, especially violence toward other people, is a behavior learned from parents and inflicted on children. And when life stresses—from poverty to illness to alcoholism—exist, they increase the risk of abuse. Some abused children live in families replete with domestic violence—where spouses have physical battles and wives are often beaten.

If you suspect that a child you know is being abused—perhaps a niece or a nephew, a child in the neighborhood, or a classmate of your youngster—you have a responsibility to become involved. Teachers are often the first to see the changes in a child's physical appearance, emotional condition, and behavior, changes that suggest she is being hurt or is in trouble. In many states, teachers (as well as physicians, dentists, and other professionals) are legally obligated to report suspected cases of abuse—and for good reason: Every year, children die from abuse, often even after someone became aware that they were being victimized.

Use some common sense in trying to determine whether a child is actually being physically abused. For instance, normal, active children have some bruises and bumps that come from everyday playing. However, these routine bruises tend to occur over bony areas such as knees, elbows, and shins. If you see a child who has injuries on other parts of the body—the stomach, the cheeks, the ears, the buttocks, the mouth, or the thighs—this should raise your suspicions. Black eyes, human bite marks, and burns in the shape of round cigarette butts are *not* symptoms of everyday play.

The adjoining box describes some other signs of possible physical abuse.

In the overwhelming majority of child-abuse cases, parents do not consciously intend to injure their children. Most abusive episodes arise when adults have difficulty coping with life situations and lose control. However, even if their intentions are not malicious, a parent who abuses a child may do it again, especially if his or her underlying stresses are not addressed. As a result, society often has to intervene in order to protect the child and assist the family.

Once a case has been investigated by law enforcement and social agencies, local social service bureaus may institute various forms of services and treatment to help the family. However, the safety and protection of the child are the first priority, and thus children are sometimes removed from their family and placed in a foster home, at least temporarily; at the same time, efforts are made to work with the parents to address underlying problems and teach them coping skills to ensure that episodes of abuse are not repeated. If you have abused your own child or feel that such behavior

may occur, talk with a trusted individual such as a physician or a clergyman. He or she may refer you to a professional or an agency where you can obtain help, including assistance in dealing with your own fears and guilt. Both parents and children may benefit from some guidance and counseling, individually and together, perhaps at shelters for domestic violence that can help break the cycle. You will be guided toward dealing with your emotions without resorting to violence. You will have the opportunity to discuss your own parenting experiences and your current life stresses. You will be shown ways to cope effectively with stresses so that you do not fall into inflicting injuries upon your youngster. You have a responsibility to your child and to yourself to find ways to relate at home that are nonviolent, day after day.

If you feel that you are in the midst of a crisis, call your local chapter of Parents Anonymous or a crisis hotline, which can provide you with some prompt support. Thereafter, the more formal treatment process should begin.

Finally, you might also get involved to help reduce the incidence of child abuse in your community at large. You can become an advocate for a caring and respectful environment for all children. True, some segments of society still condone corporal punishment and even outwardly abusive behavior toward children—but this is wrong. You can work with local schools to eliminate physical punishment and to promote and teach constructive ways to deal with anger and conflict.

Emotional Abuse

Not all abuse is physical. Neglecting your child's needs for emotional support, love, and caring is also a form of abuse. Emotional abuse is one of the most pervasive and damaging forms of child abuse. Belittling, ridiculing, name calling, and being disrespectful and unreasonably critical toward your youngster can have serious emotional consequences and long-term repercussions. Like more violent forms of abuse, emotional abuse can impair your child's self-image and self-esteem and interfere with his ability to function well in society. He may have difficulty making friends and relating to peers. In fact, he may avoid participating in activities with other children, and being in situations in which he's required to give and receive affection. Instead, he may be prone to being aggressive and oppositional. He might also develop learning difficulties or hyperactivity or have problems such as bed-wetting or soiling. Or he might act "pseudomature," becoming a caretaker for adults and others far beyond roles appropriate for his age and development.

When this emotional abuse occurs, especially repeatedly over an extended period of time, it can have a lifelong impact, affecting a youngster's happiness, relationships, and success. He may become somber, unable to enjoy himself, and prone to self-defeating behaviors. At the extreme, he can become self-destructive, engaging in self-mutilation and even attempting suicide.

As with other types of abuse, emotional abuse is often inflicted by parents who themselves were raised in an environment where they experienced emotional mistreatment by their own mothers and fathers. Being made aware of the way they are treating their children is an important first step for these parents in bringing their abusive behavior to a halt. Often they are not conscious that their behavior is damaging; if they knew what they were doing and were more sensitive to their child's pain, they would probably want to do something to stop it.

Visiting a physician or a clergyman is a good way to start looking for help with emotional abuse. You might be referred to a mental-health professional or to community organizations or churches that offer parenting classes aimed specifically at helping you talk to and problem-solve with your child.

On sexual abuse, see "Sexual Abuse," page 50.

PART VI

FAMILY MATTERS

THE IMPORTANCE OF THE FAMILY

Children in their middle years treasure their families and feel they are special and irreplaceable. Families provide children with a sense of belonging and a unique identity. Families are, or should be, a source of emotional support and comfort, warmth and nurturing, protection and security. Family relationships provide children with a critical sense of being valued and with a vital network of historical linkages and social support. Within every healthy family there is a sense of reciprocity—a giving and taking of love and empathy by every family member.

Families are much more than groups of individuals. They have their own goals and aspirations. They also are places where every child and adult should feel that he or she is special and be encouraged to pursue his or her own dreams; a place where everyone's individuality is permitted to flourish. Although every family has conflicts, all the family members should feel as though they can express themselves openly, share their feelings, and have their opinions listened to with understanding. In fact, conflicts and disagreements are a normal part of family life and are important insofar as they permit people to communicate their differences and ventilate their feelings.

The family instructs children and gives guidance about personal values and social behavior. It instills discipline and helps them learn and internalize codes of conduct that will serve them for the rest of their lives. It helps them develop positive interpersonal relationships, and it provides an environment that encourages learning both in the home and at school. It gives children a sense of history and a secure base from which to grow and develop. Yet, as important as these functions are, they do not happen automatically. Every parent knows it takes hard work to keep the family going as an effective, adaptive, and functional unit.

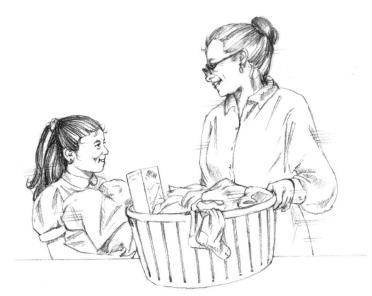

Families come in all shapes and sizes—there is no such thing as a "normal" family.

THE MYTH OF THE PERFECT FAMILY

The American family is a rapidly changing institution. You may have grown up in the stereotypical American family—two parents and one or more children, with a father who worked outside the home and a mother who stayed home and cared for the children and the household. Today, with the entry of so many more women into the workforce, with the increasing divorce rate, and with the growing number of single-parent households, other family structures have become more common.

If your own family is not like the one you grew up in, your situation is certainly not unusual. Currently, 30 percent of American families are now headed by single parents, either divorced, widowed, or never married. Some children live in foster families; others live in step-families or in gay and lesbian families. In more than two thirds of families, both parents work outside the home.

Even if your own family fits the more traditional mold, your children will almost certainly have some friends who live in households with different structures. From time to time you can expect your youngsters to ask questions like "Why do people get divorced?" "How come Jimmy's mother and father don't live together?" "Why does Annette's father live with another lady?" Because families are so important to children, parents need to be able to answer such questions with more than mere slogans or quick replies. By asking these questions, children are trying to understand two things about families: the different structures that families can take and the changes in structure, lifestyles, and relationships that can occur.

Any group of people living together in a household can create and call themselves a family. For example, to share expenses a divorced mother with two children may live with another divorced woman with children; together, they may consider themselves a family. A grandparent who lives with her daughter, son-in-law, and grandchildren may become an integral part of their family. The variations of family structures and definition are almost endless, but they have certain qualities in common: Family members share their lives emotionally and together fulfill the multiple responsibilities of family life.

A VISION OF THE FAMILY

Your child's notion—as well as your own ideas—of the family and how it should work have largely been shaped by personal experiences. If you grew up as an only child, for example, and you have four youngsters of your own who compete for attention, privacy, or possessions, you might feel that there's something wrong with the way your family is functioning and might tend to become overcontrolling. Or if you were one of two girls who grew up in a household where everyone was relatively cooperative, and you have three sons who are rambunctious, you may be concerned about relationships within the family because things are not in sync with your early experiences.

Other factors can help shape your vision of the family and how it actually works. Religious and moral beliefs, for example, help form your ideas of the way things "should" be. Your economic situation and living conditions will influence the functioning of your family, perhaps in ways that run counter to your preconceptions. Today's geographic mobility can put distance between extended families, with hundreds or thousands of miles separating grandpar-

Myths About the Family

Here are some commonly held beliefs about the family, all of which are more fiction than fact.

MYTH: The "nuclear family" is a universal phenomenon.

The nuclear family is generally defined as a family group made up of only a father, mother, and children. Although most people tend to think that this particular family structure has always been the dominant one, that is not the case.

The nuclear family is a relatively recent phenomenon, becoming common only within the last century. Before then, the "traditional" family was multigenerational, with grandparents often living with their children on farms as well as in urban environments, typically with other relatives living nearby. The nuclear family has evolved in response to a number of factors: better health and longer lives, economic development, industrialization, urbanization, geographic mobility, and migration to the suburbs. These changes have resulted in physical separation of extended-family members and in progressive fragmentation of the family.

MYTH: Family harmony is the rule, not the exception.

Although family life is often romanticized, it has always been filled with conflicts and tension. Difficulties between spouses are commonplace, with disagreements arising over issues ranging from how the children should be raised to how the family finances should be budgeted. Husbands and wives also often struggle with their inability to sustain romantic infatuation beyond the first few years of their marriage, thus having to learn to maintain a relationship in which partnership and companionship may become more important than passionate love.

Parent-children conflicts are commonplace too. As parents assert their authority, and children try to assert their autonomy appropriately, strife is inevitable.

While we often expect families to be above the chaos that exists in the rest of society, that outlook places unrealistic expectations upon the family. In the real world, families are not always a haven, since they, too, can be filled with conflict. Although stress and disagreements are common, they can be destructive to families, especially when conflict gets out of hand. Families are under constant stress, being pushed and pulled from many directions, often without the support systems of extended families that may have existed in the past.

MYTH: The stability of a family is a measure of its success.

Change is a part of life. Death, illness, physical separation, financial strains, divorce . . . these are some of the events families have to adjust to. Consequently, stability shouldn't be the only measure of a family's success. Many families function quite well, despite frequent disruptions. In fact, one important measure of a family's success is its ability to adjust to change. Daily life is full of stresses that constantly demand accommodation from family members.

MYTH: Parents control their children's fate.

In reality, parents *cannot* determine how their children will turn out. Inevitably, children assert their autonomy, creating a niche for themselves separate from their parents. At the same time, many factors external to both the child and family can influence the way a child develops.

Even within the same family there can be tremendous individual variations among siblings in intelligence, temperament, mood, and sociability. Yet despite these differences, parents are responsible for imparting to each child a sense of being loved and accepted, for helping each child to succeed at various developmental tasks, and for socializing each child into respecting the rules and accepting the responsibilities society imposes. These are indeed awesome tasks.

Some parents perceive themselves as having total responsibility for their children's fate. This belief places a heavy and unrealistic emotional burden on them as well as their youngsters. If the children are having problems, they often feel a sense of failure; likewise, the children feel as though they have let their family down if they do not live up to their parents' expectations. In essence, parents can influence and shape but cannot control their children's lives.

ents and their grandchildren; if you grew up with your grandparents nearby, the new realities may be uncomfortable for you.

The prevailing cultural values as depicted and transmitted by the media may not coincide with your notion of family. Television, motion pictures, and other media bombard us each day with fantasy images of the family. And if your family doesn't measure up to these depictions—if your family isn't always as happy as those families on the TV commercials, or doesn't settle arguments within a thirty-minute time slot—you might feel you aren't doing as good a job as you should. Some of the media more accurately portray the evolving roles that males and females can play today, with both fathers and mothers having more options in sharing the breadwinning and child-raising responsibilities.

To repeat, there are many variations of "normal," some of which may not conform to your expectations. You might feel something is awry with your own family when nothing is wrong at all. You may just have to rethink your expectations of what a family should be.

THE FAMILY WITH SCHOOL-AGE CHILDREN

During the middle years of your youngster's childhood, many changes will occur within the family. Your child is more independent than before, better able to care for herself, and more capable of contributing to chores and other household responsibilities. Most families discover that routines can be established, and in many ways life seems more settled. However, youngsters still need parental supervision and guidance.

During the middle childhood years, parents have two tasks that are especially important. The first is learning to allow and encourage your child to enter the new world of school and friends alone. The second is learning to be parents at a distance. Once children enter school, parents spend less than half as much time with them as they did before. Parents thus need to be more efficient, more vigilant, and still very much involved in their children's lives in order to monitor, guide, and support them effectively.

During the school years your youngster may develop more self-confidence, overcome fears and self-doubts, test the limits of her autonomy, find role models, and learn and internalize moral and spiritual values. You and the rest of the family should pay particular attention to the following areas, which will become increasingly significant during this time of life:

School

School assumes a central role in your youngster's life when she reaches the age of five or six, drawing much of her attention and energy away from the family unit. Her elementary-school years can become a time of enormous satisfaction and excitement. As she learns to read and master other academic skills, she will develop a love of learning and a pride in her achievements. This can contribute to her self-esteem, not only because of her accomplishments in the classroom but also as she separates successfully from the home environment. In the process her teacher can become a source of support and an important role model in her life.

For some children, however, school may cause frustration and stress. Learning disabilities can interfere with the joy of learning. Poor study habits and/or a lack of motivation can create academic difficulties. Sometimes youngsters may have a poor relationship with their teachers, or they may experience separation anxiety that can interfere with their school attendance.

To make your own child's education as positive and productive as possible, closely monitor her academic progress and social adjustment, and get to know her teacher. Discuss with your child what she is learning in the classroom and how she feels about school. Encourage her to demonstrate her newly learned skills and to practice them with you. Supervise your child's homework (but don't do it for her), and make sure she is preparing herself well for tests. Limit the amount of television she watches and encourage her to read, write, and express herself creatively through hobbies and sports. If she (or her teacher) reports any problem areas, communicate openly with school personnel, and try to figure out how best to help your youngster overcome her difficulties. Consult your pediatrician for suggestions to help solve these problems.

(For more information about your child's education, see Part VII, "Children in School.")

Friendships

As important as your child's family is to her, friends and acquaintances will become increasingly significant during middle childhood. She will spend more time with her peers, both in and out of school. These playmates will provide companionship, and your youngster will probably become preoccupied with being socially accepted by her friends. She will feel a strong need for both conformity (to be just like the others) and recognition (to be seen as unique).

Your family will also have to deal with the stresses associated with your child's peer relationships. From time to time she may have conflicts with friends, which can undermine her self-esteem. Maybe she will be excluded from a circle that she really wants to be a part of, leading to unhappiness and loneliness.

During these years, monitor your child's choice of friends and supervise, but do not interfere with, her play activities. Get to know her friends' parents and share with them your observations about the children's activities. Offer support, understanding, and guidance to your child when problems arise in her peer relationships. When a conflict occurs, try to understand how your

Is My Family Functioning Normally?

"Is my family functioning normally?"

Many parents ask themselves this question, but there is no simple answer, since there can be such broad definitions of the term *normal.*

Still, there are several characteristics that are generally identified with a well-functioning family. Some have been mentioned earlier: support; love and caring for other family members; providing security and a sense of belonging; open communication; making each person within the family feel important, valued, respected, and esteemed.

Here are some other qualities to consider when evaluating how well your own family is functioning.

- Is there ample humor and fun within your family, despite the very real demands of daily life?

- Does your family have rules that have been clearly stated and are evenly applied, yet are flexible and respond to new situations and changes in the family?

- Are the family's expectations of each person reasonable, realistic, mutually agreed upon, and generally fulfilled?

- Do family members achieve most of their individual goals, and are their personal needs being met?

- Do parents and children have genuine respect for one another, demonstrating love, caring, trust, and concern, even when there are disagreements?

- Is your family able to mature and change without everyone getting upset or unhappy?

---

child feels about it, and what she sees as the factors contributing to it. Then discuss how the other child might view the problem, and together work out ways to resolve the conflict. At the same time keep in mind that the family cannot solve every peer-related difficulty—for example, you cannot run to the playground and intervene whenever a conflict arises. Even so, you can offer support and guidance, conveying your own values and expectations.

(For more information, see Chapter 9, "Developing Social Skills.")

Outside Activities

During middle childhood your youngster will develop a number of outside interests, from sports to Scouting, from music lessons to clubs. Many of these activities will require a commitment on the family's part, in terms of time and, in some cases, money. It may also require parental patience and tolerance as children experiment with different programs before finding the ones they prefer.

In general, the family—most particularly the parents—should be willing to support the child with resources, encouragement, supervision, chauffeuring, and, at times, direct participation.

FAMILY LEADERSHIP

Families are not democracies. Each family has its own ways of deciding who has the power and authority within the family unit, and which rights, privileges, obligations, and roles are assigned to each family member.

In most families parents are expected to be the leaders or executives of the family; children are expected to follow the leadership of their parents. As children in the middle years grow older, they will ask for, and certainly should be allowed, more autonomy, and their opinions should be considered when decisions are made; however, parents are the final authorities.

Of course there will always be disagreements among the generations. Your child may want to go to the beach on a family vacation; you may want to go to the mountains. He may think he has too many chores to do; you may think he has just the right amount. Let him speak his mind, but the ultimate decision is yours. Explain why you've made the judgment you have, without becoming defensive or apologetic. You won't always be popular in these decisions, but your youngster is still going to love you.

Although generational hierarchies are the most obvious ones within families, other types of hierarchies exist as well. Sometimes they depend on gender. In patriarchal societies such as ours, men have traditionally had power over women, including within the family. Traditionally, fathers have been the providers and authority figures, but while they may be the final decision-makers, they often have assumed only limited functions beyond that in the family. Mothers have been the caretakers, responsible for the emotional side of the family; they have kept the family together and functioning smoothly. What this means is that mothers and fathers are likely to hold different positions in the family hierarchy, that mothers take primary responsibility and that fathers may have only partial responsibility for day-to-day parental decisions.

Today, however, there are challenges to this traditional gender-based structure. In many families both fathers and mothers are bringing home paychecks. And while women still seem to shoulder the larger share of responsibility for the day-to-day operations of the family, more fathers are assuming greater roles in child-raising and household duties.

It is useful to consider what roles each family member takes within the family, and whether everyone is satisfied with the current arrangement. For example, the oldest children in the family may take on the parental role of caring for their younger siblings. Or grandparents may acquire an important place within the family by assuming a central child-rearing role while parents work.

Think about who is responsible for what within your own family and how the current arrangement is working. Some responsibilities may be open to negotiation, particularly if the family does not seem to be functioning optimally. For example, an older child may be resentful of having too much responsibility for watching over the younger children, while the younger children may also resent the older child playing a parental role. This will result in arguments whenever the oldest child is left in charge. Parents need to review what is going on, discuss how the children are feeling about it, and come up with some alternatives.

FAMILY BOUNDARIES

As families grow up, the so-called boundaries that define how family members relate to one another change. When your child was a newborn, for example, you may have been so closely involved with her that your separateness from each other was virtually nonexistent; you may have been with or near her almost twenty-four hours a day, meeting her every demand for food, cuddling, clean diapers, and other basic needs. As your child matured, the situation changed, and greater emotional distance developed between the two of you. For instance, she may always have shared with you what happened at school, but at age eight or nine she may suddenly stop doing so. She may be trying to assert some independence and trying to negotiate a new boundary that, in essence, says, "This is mine and not always yours to know."

When these situations come up, you need to learn to respect your child's wishes and allow her some privacy. You might inquire why she does not want to talk as much about her school day; but if she is not having problems in the classroom, respect her wishes. Do not pressure her to talk, but still provide opportunities for her to do so. For example:

"What happened today at school, Jennifer?"

"Nothing."

"Don't you feel like talking about your day?"

"There's nothing to talk about."

"Well, if there's anything you'd like to tell me about school, I'd love to hear it. But if you don't want to talk about school, that's okay too."

Bear in mind that at some point early in middle childhood—usually by the second or third grade—children prefer to spend more time playing and talking with their friends than with their parents. This is an example of a child's renegotiating boundaries and relationships.

On the other hand, certain secrets are *not* appropriate to keep. For example, when a child is endangering herself (by experimenting with drugs, perhaps), you need to say, "I have the right to know what is going on!" Or if your child has been approached sexually by an older child, adolescent, or adult, you need to get involved immediately.

These family boundaries, incidentally, are a two-way street. Everyone in the family needs some privacy, including you as a parent. Closed doors and shut dresser drawers must be respected. Teach your child about privacy by respecting her space and belongings.

Also keep in mind that children are not adults. In the middle years of childhood, youngsters are not emotionally and developmentally ready to understand or take on the stresses that adults face. So don't expect a child of this age to serve as your confidante or "best friend," burdening her with your problems and concerns. On the one hand, your child will be sensitive to your moods and will recognize if something is wrong or is troubling you; when this happens, be honest with her, explaining that you are experiencing some difficulties that may take some time to work through. However, a lengthy and complete disclosure of your problems is unwise; particularly if your sharing is intended to elicit emotional support for you, that can become a burden for your child and is not justified.

The best approach is to acknowledge to your child that a problem exists. Discuss how it might affect the family's routines, but voice optimism that in time the difficulty will be resolved and things will be fine. Encourage your youngster to talk about her feelings about what you are going through. But you need to respond in a way to reassure and support her.

If you wish, discuss any concrete actions she can take that would be of help. If you have lost your job, for example, and there will be pressures upon the family finances, perhaps you and your child can together think of ways she could help save a little money—perhaps by taking a sack lunch to school rather than buying it there, or postponing a planned activity or purchase until you become employed again. These actions by your youngster, however, should not become an emotional burden on her, nor should you present them in a way to make her feel responsible for "fixing" the problem.

DEALING WITH FAMILY CONFLICTS

How does your family handle the disagreements that occur in your household? Conflicts are basic to human relationships; they are inevitable and should not be avoided. However, family members should know how to negotiate and resolve these conflicts. To negotiate, parents and children both need to make a genuine attempt to understand the attitudes, feelings, and desires of one another. When disagreements are resolved successfully, family life is enhanced and relationships are strengthened.

Some families cannot seem to settle conflicts. Family members may deny that problems exist. Or they may draw a third person into the conflict, supposedly to mediate the difficulty, but who instead may take a position on one side or the other and thereby make the disagreement worse. Sometimes when they are unable to resolve their conflict, the warring parties may join together to focus attention on another family member as a way to avoid dealing with the real problem.

Within every family, certain alliances, coalitions, and rivalries exist. At times, mother and daughter might form an alliance against father and son. Or the two parents might unite against the children on a particular issue. But within a healthy family these coalitions are not fixed, they change from situation to situation, and they do not disrupt the functioning of the family. If they become rigid and long-lasting, however, they can do damage to the family.

It is natural to be unaware that any alliances exist within your family. But to get a better sense of your family's dynamics, ask yourself questions like: "What family member do I tend to agree (or disagree) with most often? When my children are fighting, whose side do I generally take? With whom in the family do I usually spend my free time? Who in the family most easily angers me?"

FAMILY PROBLEMS

Family problems come in all shapes and sizes; some are short-lived and easily managed, while others are more chronic and difficult to handle. Stress points include events such as illness and injury, changing jobs, changing schools, moving, and financial difficulties.

Each family develops its own ways of coping with these stresses, some of which work better than others. Unsuccessful coping can be recognized by a number of characteristics, including the following:

Poor Communication

Family members either avoid talking with one another, or have not learned how to listen well to what others are trying to say through their words, expressions, or actions.

Inability to Resolve
Conflicts and Disagreements

This usually occurs because family members avoid discussing problems or even avoid admitting that problems exist. This allows the conflicts to continue—which, while causing some discomfort and unhappiness, allows the family to avoid what they see as the greater discomfort of facing the problem. Some families just have not learned the skills of negotiating or, for some other reason, cannot let go of bad or hurt feelings. Children are likely to pattern their behavior after their parents' behavior and may learn to refuse to talk about feelings and problems.

Poor Problem-Solving

Family members have trouble deciding what problems really exist, who is responsible, the options for solving them, and how the family can agree upon an option and act upon it. There may not be agreement on what the priorities are within the family.

Poor Division of Responsibilities

Families often have not decided how family responsibilities will be divided among family members. When that happens, family life can become chaotic, and many things do not get accomplished. At the other extreme, some families are not flexible at all, and family members do not help one another out or fairly reassign responsibilities as family circumstances change.

Insufficient Emotional Support

Families are, especially for children, the most important source of emotional support. During the middle years, children find it hard to obtain this emotional support outside the family. Children do not perform or develop well without this support.

Maintaining a Healthy Family

In order to provide a supportive, emotionally healthy family environment, you need to devote some thought and energy to the following questions:

- *Do you treat each child as an individual?* Each child has his own temperament, his own way of viewing and interacting with the world around him. Parents may love their children equally, but naturally will have different sorts of relationships with each of them. Individualize your relationship with each of your children, reinforcing their strengths and talents and avoiding making unflattering comparisons with their siblings or friends.

- *Does your family have regular routines?* Children and parents benefit from having some predictable day-to-day routines. Morning schedules, mealtimes, and bedtimes are easier for everyone when they follow a pattern. Children also appreciate family rituals and traditions around birthdays, holidays, and vacations.

- *Is your family an active participant in your extended family and the community?* Families work better when they feel connected and supported by friends and relatives. Usually such relationships require that parents make an active effort to get together with others socially or for civic projects.

Intolerance of Differences

Families function best when the individuality of each family member is acknowledged and appreciated. At the least, even if someone else's personal traits or characteristics are not highly valued, each family member needs to tolerate these traits and respect that individual. When family members withhold love from one another because of personal differences, children are likely to have a difficult time developing a healthy self-image, and they will have low self-esteem and poor social skills.

- *Are your expectations of yourself and other family members realistic?* Your child's self-awareness, knowledge, and skills are constantly changing. Observe, read, and talk to others to learn what can reasonably be expected of your child at each stage of development. Parents, too, have limitations on what they can accomplish, given their resources and the time available. There are no "superparents," just individuals doing their best.

- *Does the time you spend with your family members contribute to good relationships among you?* Most of the time you and your child and your spouse spend together should be fun, relaxed, meaningful, and relatively conflict-free.

- *As a parent, singly or as a couple, are you taking care of your own needs?* You should be leading a healthy personal life (including proper diet, exercise, and sleep habits). Set aside time, however brief, for things you enjoy. Your children will thrive when your own emotional needs are being met. They do best when they are reared by parents who are in a harmonious relationship with each other.

- *Do you take moral and social responsibility for your own life?* You are the most important role model for your child. Demonstrate your value system through actions as well as words.

Overdependency on Others

Children need to succeed in order to feel capable of successfully managing life's stresses and challenges. If they are taught or encouraged to depend on others (within the family or outside it) to solve their problems, they will have low self-esteem and limited initiative and will have trouble succeeding in the world.

Chronic Crises

Families who have some of the above characteristics are likely to have trouble coping with life's inevitable crises. In these families even relatively simple problems are not resolved but take on the appearance and feel of major dilemmas. Thus, by their lack of successful coping skills, these families create additional problems for themselves and go from crisis to crisis, with little relief and little pleasure from life or from one another.

Although we all strive for perfection, there is no perfect family. Each family has its own strengths and weaknesses, assets and liabilities, challenges and problems. If your family seems overwhelmed with problems, or if there is a breakdown in relationships within your family, it is probably time for outside help.

As a parent, your task is to meet the multiple demands of family life with energy and creativity. By doing so, you will enable your children to grow and develop in positive, healthy ways and to experience satisfaction and success.

STRENGTHENING
YOUR FAMILY

F amily life is filled with positive and negative experiences, calm times and hectic ones. Getting the kids off to school in the morning . . . sharing the day's experiences at the dinner table . . . dealing with arguments and conflicts . . . managing financial pressures; all are parts of everyday life for families.

This chapter discusses some of the experiences shared by virtually every family, as well as offering practical guidelines for helping the family function as efficiently as possible.

FAMILY ROUTINES

Every family needs routines. They help to organize life and keep it from becoming too chaotic.

Children in the middle years do best when routines are regular, predictable, and consistent. Even so, one of a family's greatest challenges is to establish comfortable, effective routines, which should achieve a happy compromise between the disorder and confusion that can occur without them and the rigidity and boredom that can come with too much structure and regimentation, where children are given no choice and little flexibility. As a parent, review the routines in your household to ensure that they accomplish what you want.

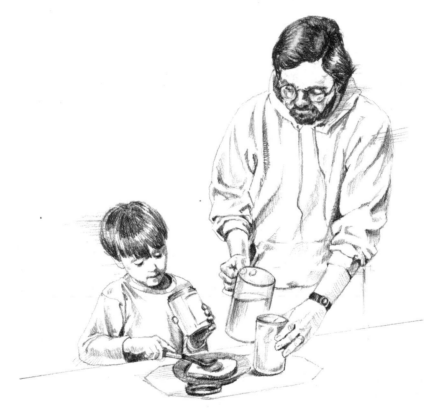

Children should participate in meal preparation—it increases the importance of family mealtime.

Weekdays

Mornings. Most households are stressful places on weekday mornings. The children are preparing for school. Mother and father are trying to get the youngsters out the door while making sure that they themselves get to work on time.

To make the household function well in the morning, everyone needs to know what has to be done to get ready for the day. Many parents get a head start on the morning by putting as many things in order as possible the night before. Prior to going to sleep, they have their children pack up their books and papers for the next day. They also make lunches and lay out their youngsters' clothes.

Of course, there are probably dozens of obstacles that can interfere with a smooth-running morning. For example, your child may disagree with your choice of clothes for her. Try to resolve these squabbles with a minimum of discussion or arguing. Sometimes children can be pacified by giving them some choice in the matter; for instance: "It's going to be chilly today, so you have to wear a sweater. Would you like to wear the blue one or the red one?" Or, "If you really don't like this raincoat, we'll talk about getting you another one soon; but at least for this week, you have to wear this one to keep you from getting wet."

Keep the wake-up routine cheerful and positive. Until your child is able to use an alarm clock, you should awaken her each morning. Gently but firmly rouse her and remain nearby until she is fully awake and out of bed. If she has trouble waking up, you might need to be more forceful, like pulling the covers back. Persistent difficulty in awakening may indicate that she is getting to sleep too late or is suffering from a sleep disturbance.

As a general guideline, limit your child's bathing or washing to ten minutes. Be sure she eats breakfast too; even if she is not hungry in the morning, have her get *some* food in her system to start the day. Some children regularly use the toilet after breakfast; allow these children adequate time so they do not feel rushed and omit this part of their routine.

Some children dawdle in the morning: If you set aside thirty minutes for them to take care of all the morning's tasks, they will take forty minutes; if you increase the time allotment to forty minutes, they will take fifty minutes. To keep your youngster moving at a steady pace, try offering her gentle encouragement and reinforcement. For example, some parents say, "If you want to watch fifteen minutes of television before you leave for school, be ready to go by seven forty-five and you will earn the right to turn on the TV." (See "Procrastinating and Dawdling" on page 380.)

If your child is one of those who simply has trouble remembering what to do next, check with her every five minutes to make sure she has moved from washing her face to dressing herself, and so on, and give her some positive feedback when she's doing well ("I'm glad to see you're brushing your teeth. Keep up the good work").

Also, try doing a little homework of your own, timing how long it takes your child to get ready in the morning without your nagging or pushing her along. Determine the amount of time she needs to get dressed, wash herself, eat breakfast, brush her teeth, and get things ready for school. Some parents discover that they are expecting their children to get everything done much faster than the youngsters are actually capable of; for example, they may be giving their children only twenty-five minutes to accomplish tasks that actually take thirty-five. If necessary, schedule your child's wake-up time a little earlier so the morning will proceed more smoothly.

In order to remind children of their responsibilities, many parents make a list of the tasks involved in getting ready in the morning. Charts and drawings about the morning routine can be fun to make as a family and can offer youngsters a chance to discuss how they view the process and where they might be stuck. This strategy helps to pinpoint where problems are likely to arise and how to reshape the routines to reduce the chaos and confusion that can accompany morning time.

If you and/or your children just aren't "morning people," all of you need a little extra affection and gentle fun time before getting going. It might be nice to spend a few moments fooling around or talking about something pleasant before starting the morning routine.

If mornings are generally hassled and full of stress, you should monitor your own behavior to see if it might be contributing to the problem. Yelling, scolding, criticizing, and engaging in fruitless arguments will undermine your authority and diminish your child's respect for the rules. Even if things aren't going as planned, keep your emotional reactions under control, and handle any conflicts or mishaps with a certain amount of good humor.

Finally, round out each morning by saying goodbye to your youngster. A simple hug and a wave as she heads out the front door or slides out of the car are extremely important. They will give her a positive feeling with which to begin the day's activities.

After School. During middle childhood, children need adult supervision. After school the presence of an adult will provide them with safety, structure, support, and a sense of well-being. While some parents have their children return each afternoon to an empty home, these "latchkey" kids are more susceptible to misbehavior, risk-taking, and anxiety. (For a further discussion of latchkey children, see Chapter 41.)

For this age group, the American Academy of Pediatrics recommends that a child come home to a parent, other adult, or a responsible adolescent.

Particularly for younger children in the middle years, an after-school schedule is also useful, although every minute does not need to be planned. The routine should include a snack, exercise, relaxation, and study, in whatever order works best for your child. In general, after six to eight hours of school, children need time for active play, both to invigorate themselves so they are better able to complete the tasks before them and to help them stay fit. Watching television or playing computer games is not a good substitute for this active play.

Nonetheless, some youngsters try to complete as much of their homework as possible *before* dinner; TV watching and other pleasurable activities wait until later. Most children, however, go outside for some play and exercise after coming home, saving the homework until later, perhaps after sunset when playing outdoors is impractical.

As an alternative to coming home after classes end, a variety of after-school programs and child-care settings are available in most communities. Many are offered through the public schools, city agencies, or community organizations (YMCA, Boys and Girls Club) and are reasonably priced.

Of course, before enrolling your child in one of these after-school programs, visit the site while youngsters are there. The staff should relate to children in a sensitive way, and the child-to-adult ratio ideally should not exceed ten- or twelve-to-one, and the size of the group should be no more than twenty-four. The facilities should be clean, safe, functional, and have convenient outdoor play areas. (See "Finding Good Childcare," page 411.)

Evenings. Dinner should be an important time for your family. As often as possible, all family members should eat together at the dinner table, without the distraction of television or radio. In many families, in fact, this is the only time of day when the whole family is together.

During dinner the family can share the day's activities and participate in enjoyable conversation. Everyone should be encouraged to take part, and negative comments and criticism should be discouraged.

It is important for children to participate in the preparation and clean-up of dinner. In middle childhood, they are capable of taking on a regular chore such as preparing part of the meal, setting the table, helping to serve, clearing the table, or rinsing the dishes. When they help in this way, it will increase their awareness of the importance of dinnertime and raise their level of investment in making dinner a good family experience.

If the entire family is unable to eat dinner at the same time—perhaps because Dad or Mom gets home late from work—try to schedule another time during the evening when the family can congregate for even twenty or thirty minutes of discussion, reading aloud, or playing games. Many parents have discovered that this is a wise investment of time during the middle years of childhood. Not only is this a period to enjoy your children—while they are still young—but if you have a strong history of sharing good times with your youngsters, you will probably find it easier to make a difference in their lives during adolescence, when problems might arise and need resolving. At that time your relationship will already have become strong and important to both of you, and that strength can help carry you through tough experiences.

During the evening your children will need to finish their dinner-related tasks, perform their other chores (such as emptying the garbage or putting things away), and complete their homework assignments. Once these are done, they can relax by reading, having a conversation, playing games, or watching television. These should be seen as earned privileges and rewards

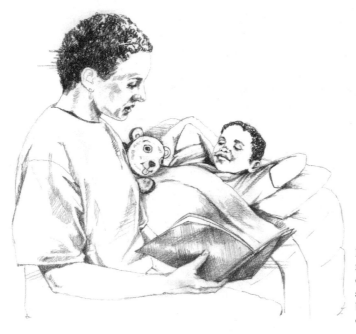

Nighttime rituals, such as reading, can help ease a child to sleep and strengthen the relationship between parents and children.

rather than inalienable rights. If a child fails to finish her chores, she should forfeit some of her free-time leisure activities.

Bedtime. After leisure time, most youngsters are expected to take a bath and get ready for bed. On school nights children need a regular time to go to sleep. Lights can go out at different times for different children in the family, depending on how much sleep each youngster needs; some children in the middle years need ten hours a night, while others function fine the next day on just eight hours. When deciding what time your child needs to go to bed, pay attention to how she functions the next day; if she is groggy and struggles through the morning and afternoon, then she needs an earlier bedtime.

Nighttime rituals can help ease a youngster to sleep, as well as promote intimacy between parents and children. These rituals can include storytelling, reading aloud, conversation, and songs. Try to avoid exciting play and activities before bedtime. Your child might enjoy reading in bed for thirty minutes before the lights are turned off. Or she might like to listen to the radio for a few minutes in bed just before falling asleep.

A few minutes of conversation at bedtime affords a good opportunity to resolve any persisting conflicts, putting them to rest so the child has a peaceful night and the conflicts don't continue into the following day. For instance, if you had an argument earlier in the evening, or there were some hassles related to homework, neither of you should take these conflicts to sleep. Say something like, "I know we had an argument. Let's put it to rest and start tomorrow fresh. I was unhappy with your behavior, but it's over now. I love you very much."

Before you turn out the lights, kiss your child good-night. This will reinforce her sense of being loved.

Weekends

Weekends are good times for family togetherness. After a long week of work and school, the entire family can spend extended periods of time together on Saturday and Sunday. You might go shopping as a family, visit museums and zoos, do chores that everyone participates in, go on hikes or bike rides, or attend religious services.

In the middle years of childhood, since peers are becoming more important in your youngster's life, she may want to spend part of her weekends playing with friends too. Since knowing your child's friends is important, you might invite them to join your family in some activity. Find a balance between family time and your child's other priorities, while also allotting time for yourself for your own personal interests. Your child may have homework, too, as well as obligations to a sports team or other activities.

Many families carefully plan the weekend to avoid conflicts over time allocation. If one of your children is interested in tennis lessons and the other is determined to take ballet, work out a practical schedule for getting them to and from these activities. Morning routines will usually have to be altered so as to get the children ready in time, and car-pooling arrangements may need to be made.

When one of the youngsters has a special school assignment due, the weekend may be the best time for her to work on it. She should have all the materials she needs for the project, and thus trips to the library and stationery store may need to be done the previous week. Keep some time open in which you'll be available to help her if the need arises.

On weekends children in the middle years can usually be allowed a later bedtime than during the week. However, keep in mind that there may be some consequences to her staying up later: She may feel tired the next day, or if she sleeps later the following morning, she will have a shortened weekend day.

One additional thought about the weekends: Although family time is essential, it is equally important for parents to set aside some time just for themselves. Too often, as mothers and fathers work hard at parenting, they neglect their own relationship. But when parents go out on a Saturday night, at least once a month but preferably more often, it sends a positive message to the children—namely, that even though they are loved, they are not the center of the universe, and their parents have their own relationship and don't need to have the children around every minute. At the same time, the children may be able to spend time with a babysitter they like, watching a movie on the VCR, cooking some popcorn, or telling scary stories.

(For more information, see Chapter 36, "Babysitters and Other Caretakers.")

YOUR FAMILY RITUALS

Every family should have activities that they enjoy together and that become a regular, predictable, and integral part of their lives. Some can be serious pursuits, like attending community functions or religious services as a family; others can be more lighthearted, like going fishing. Whatever they are, they can help bond a family together.

These are some rituals that many families have made parts of their lives:

Important Conversations. Communication between parents and children should be a top priority in your family. Set aside time to talk, discussing the day's and the week's activities, sharing feelings and really listening to one another.

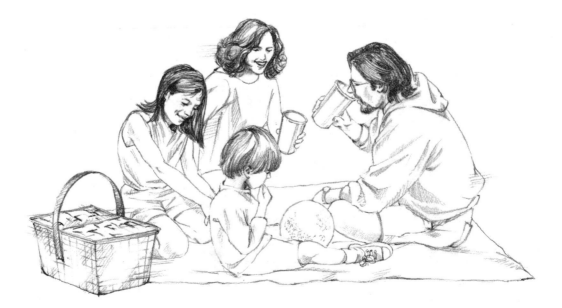

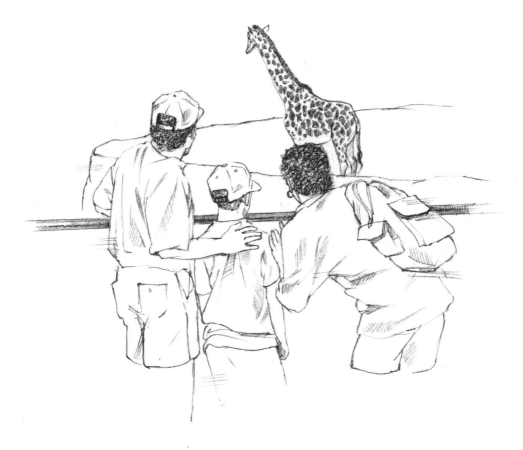

Respect the privacy of each of your youngsters as they begin to assert their independence during these middle years; they may have certain problems and difficulties they may not want to divulge to their brothers and sisters. You should be able to have a one-on-one conversation with each child without all the other children listening to it. If you honor his wishes for confidentiality, this can build trust between you.

Some families establish a weekly time for a family meeting. When everyone is present, family issues, relationships, plans, and experiences are discussed, and everyone from the youngest to the oldest gets a chance to be heard and to participate.

Recreation and Cultural Activities. Family recreation is an important way to strengthen the family. Sports (participation and spectator), games, movies, and walks in the park are good ways to increase cohesiveness and reduce stress.

Cultural activities can be valuable too. Visits to museums, libraries, plays, musicals, and concerts can expand the family's horizons and deepen appreciation for the arts.

Shopping. Shopping trips can provide regular opportunities for parents and children to spend time together. Whether you are grocery shopping or buying birthday gifts, these excursions can be fun and exciting for youngsters in middle childhood. Let your children make lists, find items in the store, carry the bags to the car, and unpack them once you return home. Allowing your child some choices and assigning some meaningful responsibilities can help build his self-confidence.

Reading and Singing Aloud. Reading and singing aloud as a family promotes feelings of closeness and an appreciation for music and books. Parents should

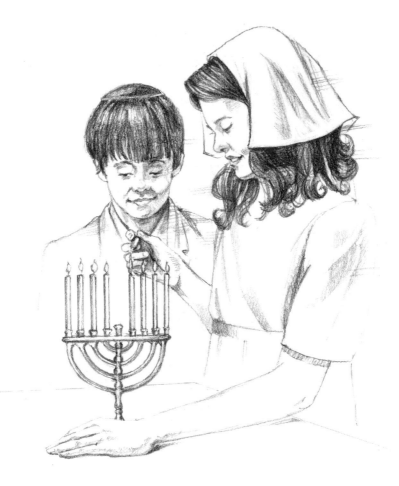

find out what stories their children like to read, and what music they like to listen to. It is lots of fun to take turns reading aloud, and to let the children hear the stories and songs you enjoyed when you were growing up.

Holiday Traditions. These are another source of fun family activities. By learning about the history, significance, and rituals of a particular holiday, children will feel a greater sense of involvement in the holiday preparations and celebrations.

Spiritual Pursuits. For many families, religion plays an important role in providing a moral tradition, a set of values, and a network of friends and neighbors who can provide support. Attending services is something family members can do together.

You do not necessarily need to go to a church, synagogue, or other place of worship regularly, however, to share moral values with your children and help them develop a sense of their history and the continuity of the family. Many families develop a strong spiritual life without the formal structure of organized religion.

FAMILY DISRUPTIONS

No matter how harmonious you may want your family life to be, some disruptions and disturbances are inevitable. When they occur, they can be stressful for every member of the family. Here are some of the most common events and circumstances that can interfere with the normal course of family life.

Illness and Injury

Whether it is a parent or a child who becomes ill or injured, the entire family is affected. While even a short-term illness like the flu can disrupt the normal activities of a family, a chronic disease (from cancer to epilepsy) can create lengthy and even permanent disturbances in the way a family functions.

For a youngster in middle childhood, reactions to illness depend on a number of factors, including the nature of the illness (its severity, course, and treatments), her previous experiences with medical problems, her overall ability to cope, and the support she receives from the family.

You may need to do some adjusting to the illness as well. With a short-term disease you might feel stress and annoyance until the condition disappears. With a chronic illness your reactions may be more severe. You might experience guilt, fear, anger, helplessness, and hopelessness. You may need to set aside time for treatments as well as conferences with physicians and other

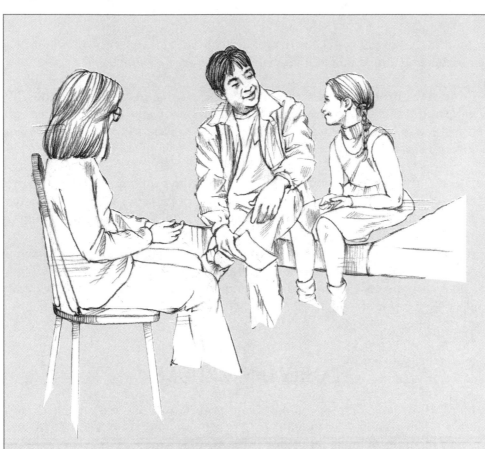

How to Have a Family Meeting

Weekly family meetings are an effective and pleasant way to bring the family together, to improve communication, to set weekly goals, to recognize and reward progress, and to determine each member's needs and feelings.

health-care professionals. You will need to learn as much as possible about the illness and its care.

Also, with a chronic or long-lasting disease, you need to comfort your child. Explain the condition as honestly and fully as possible, and what she can expect by way of treatment and cure. Be realistic; do not make promises that can't be kept. Encourage your youngster to express her feelings, too; not only

1. The meetings should occur at a regular, pleasant time—for instance, after dinner, with dessert.

2. Parents can serve as discussion leaders and make sure that any ground rules are clearly explained and understood.

3. The meetings should emphasize both individual and family needs, goals, and accomplishments and discuss positive events and efforts. During the meeting parents can give allowances and praise and reward behavior progress and changes. They can also share other relevant family information, such as an upcoming family vacation or school event to prepare for.

4. Each family member should be allowed to speak without criticism or interruption, to share his or her thoughts, feelings, achievements, and hopes.

5. The meeting is not a time or place to scold, punish, recall past mistakes, blow off steam, or single out a particular person. Those issues should be taken up separately and individually.

6. The meetings should last no more than twenty or thirty minutes unless the family wants to continue.

7. Everyone should understand and accept that parents have the final word in difficult decisions.

8. A record should be kept of the main points, rewards, progress toward goals, new goals and agreements.

9. Before the meeting ends, anyone who wants to should have a chance to say how he or she thinks the meeting went, and what might be done to make the next meeting better.

should she feel free to talk with you about anything on her mind, but she should be able to trust her doctor. Discuss how to communicate about the illness with friends, classmates, and teachers. If it appears that your child is having strong emotional reactions or troubling behavior, she might also benefit from some counseling.

(For additional information, see Part VIII, "Chronic Health Problems.")

Parental Mental or Substance-Abuse Problems

If you or your spouse are depressed or have another mental or emotional illness, your child is growing up differently than her peers. Depression in a parent affects all family members and colors their relationships with one another and with people outside of the home. Depressed parents tend to create a less positive emotional tone in the way their family interacts. They do not respond as quickly or as appropriately to the emotional needs of their children. They are also more likely to be controlling and coercive in relating to their youngsters, rather than discussing and negotiating issues.

Many children of depressed parents feel rejected and develop low self-esteem. They may have problems relating to their peers and thus are less likely to become involved in social activities. These children can often benefit from close relationships with adults outside the family and from professional counseling to help them develop ways of coping with the stresses within their families.

The children of alcoholics and other drug abusers may have similar problems. Although family experiences vary, these youngsters often grow up with more negative life experiences, and a decreased sense of togetherness and open communication. Drinking is also tied to a greater incidence of parental depression, family violence, and marital problems. Active participation in school and extracurricular activities can go a long way toward helping these children achieve success and happiness. In the meantime, affected parents need to seek professional help for their drinking and drug-abuse problems.

Arguments and Conflicts

Disputes between you and your children are inevitable in family life. If your family never has arguments, it probably means that issues are being avoided. To become productive adults, children need to be able to voice their opinions—even if they disagree with yours—and feel they are being taken seriously.

Even so, you can and should keep the negative impact of arguments to a minimum by adhering to the following guidelines:

- Be selective about the issues you fight over. When a potential problem arises, decide if it is really worth the battle; some issues probably are not. For example, if your child wants to wear an old pair of sneakers to school rather than the newer pair you recently bought her, or if she wants to wear her hair a little longer than you would prefer, you might decide to let her have her way, choosing to take a stand on more important matters instead. Pick your battles carefully.

- As long as arguments stay within certain boundaries, they are an acceptable and productive form of communication. They can continue as long as they are under control, respectful, and are moving toward a solution. But discontinue them if they degenerate into name-calling, if calm voices are replaced by shouting, or if you and your child are going around in circles without progressing toward a resolution. Never laugh at your child, no matter how ludicrous her arguments sound to you; by laughing you are essentially ridiculing her and what she is saying.

  If you are unhappy with the essay your child wrote about the Civil War for school, for example, the two of you can discuss what you perceive to be its shortcomings. But remember, it is *her* school assignment and *her* responsibility. Her teacher is the ultimate judge. If the dialogue between you and your child starts to get personal ("You don't know what you're talking about!"), then it's time for a break. Tell your child: "This discussion isn't going anywhere. We need to stop, cool down, and come back to it later." Resume the dialogue later in the day, when one or both of you might have a new approach to the problem.

  Some families actually schedule these follow-up discussions. A parent might say, "Come back with five points to support your argument, and I'll have five to support mine." Families can even create a format for these dialogues: The child speaks uninterrupted for five minutes, and then the parent responds during the next five minutes; after another round of five minutes each, you might find areas where you can agree or compromise.

- Let your child win sometimes. When you and your youngster argue, you need to do more than listen to her point of view; when she presents a persuasive case, be willing to say, "You convinced me. We'll do it your way." Let your youngster know that you value her point of view, and that through communication, conflicts can be resolved—and that sometimes she can win.

- If conflicts about particular issues recur again and again, take a look at the root causes. Think deeply about why you and your child are arguing about these matters, and try taking some preventive action. For example, if your youngster rebels against going to bed each night, she may be using her outbursts as a way to stay up a little longer, or to get more attention. Or if she repeatedly argues about doing her homework, try to put an end to these conflicts by actually writing up a contract stipulating the expectations, responsibilities, rewards, and punishments for doing and not doing homework. Remember that the homework assignment is made by the teacher and is your child's responsibility. She may not do it your way, but if she is satisfying the school's requirements, you should not turn it into an issue at home. Both you and your child should sign the contract, agree to abide by it, and (hopefully) end the disagreements about the subject.

Do not forget that children learn how to handle disagreements by watching their parents' example. How readily do you and your partner have "good" arguments, which end in successful reconciliation? Or do you stay angry, or avoid fights altogether? Your children model themselves on you.

Departures and Returns

Do you or your spouse frequently travel on business? These can be disruptive times for your child and for the family as a whole. To minimize problems, prepare your youngster for these out-of-town trips. Spend as much time as it takes to explain where you are going and why.

Your child may be sad, anxious, angry, or all of these before and during your travels. You need to acknowledge and accept her feelings: "I know you're going to miss me. I understand that you feel this way. I'm going to miss you too." In addition to missing you, your child may also feel inconvenienced, insecure, unsafe, or worried about how you and she will fare during your absence.

Remind your youngster that you will be back soon. And while you are away,

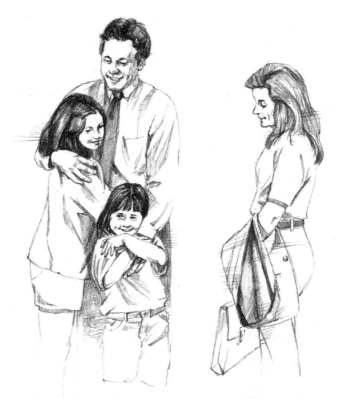

Parents' travel can be disruptive for their children.

maintain contact with phone calls (each day if possible), as well as postcards or letters. Once you come home, make your return special; spend some extra time with your child and do something together that she enjoys.

Unexpected Setbacks

What happens when you lose your job? Or when the family has financial problems? These disruptions can be very unsettling for your child, particularly if you are not honest and do not help her deal with the situation directly.

If the family is having financial difficulties, for instance, your youngster does not need to know all the specifics; however, she deserves an explanation of why she may not be able to return to the same summer camp she attended last year, or why you may not be able to buy her the exact pair of sneakers she wants. Children need to know: "Mom lost her job, so we're going to have to reduce our spending until she finds a new one."

Children can be just as concerned about disruptions in the extended family—for example, the news that her uncle and aunt are getting a divorce. Don't be surprised if she asks what exactly is happening and how it might affect her relationship with her cousins. She also might ask you: "Are you and Dad going to get a divorce too?"

It is unwise to protect your child from these kinds of family problems. Keep in mind that if she sees you becoming anxious, without an obvious reason, she may misinterpret it ("Oh, no, is Mom upset with *me*?"). Keep the channels of communication open, encourage your child to express her own feelings, and explain how you and your spouse are trying to get the situation back on track. And reaffirm the importance and the stability of your family: "Even though Dad has lost his job, we are all going to stay together as a family and we are all going to be okay."

SPECIAL EVENTS IN THE FAMILY

Birthdays, anniversaries, holidays, weddings, and summer vacations—these are special times in a family's life and can create lasting memories.

However, as treasured and important as these events are, some families try to make too much of them. Parents may try to turn each birthday party into the best one ever. Or they feel they have to fulfill every wish on their children's gift lists. Inevitably, that kind of attitude creates anxiety and disappointment, since few events turn out perfectly.

Tell your child to draw up a list of things he wants so that you and others who plan to give him gifts have something to choose from. Have him underline

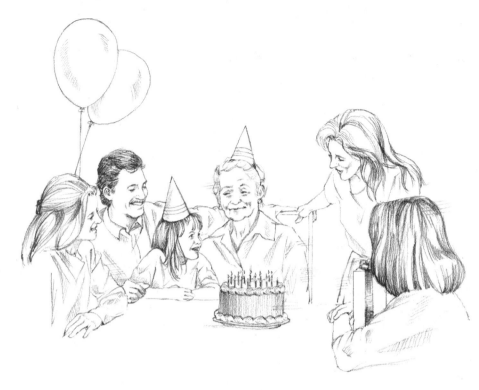

Celebrating special events, like birthdays, are important times for a family.

or indicate his top preferences in some other manner. This way, he will understand from the beginning that he won't get everything on the list, and he won't be disappointed. And if you can, try to surprise him with something *not* on his list.

If your family budget does not allow you to buy your child most of what he wants, do not feel guilty; instead, buy one or two gifts that will mean the most, rather than a dozen that don't. Even if you can provide for your child's every wish, some selectivity can teach him to set priorities and to learn values.

More important, spend time with and show your love for your child; this is much more significant and lasting than material items. Remember that special events—from family gatherings to attendance at school recitals—are times to demonstrate the specialness of the people you care about.

A summer vacation needs careful planning, not only taking the children's input into account, but also paying attention to how the adults want to spend it. Planning vacations is a good opportunity for families to sit down and talk together. A family vacation needs to be *everyone's* vacation, and that may mean not going to the place that the children have put at the top of their list. ("Dad and I have decided that we're not going to Disney World again; this summer, we're going to a national park for some camping.") As long as your destination has something there for your children, you do not necessarily have to go where they want to every year.

In making decisions about vacations, think back to the summers of your own childhood. What did you like most about your family vacations? What do you wish you had done more often? The answers to these questions will help guide you toward what may be important to your own child. More than anything, children remember that their vacations took them to locations other than their home, that the family got to spend time together, and that there were long days and memorable experiences they did not get to enjoy the rest of the year.

Finally, when planning your vacation, be realistic. Too often, parents try to squeeze too much into the vacation, and the family ends up finding their time together stressful, not relaxing.

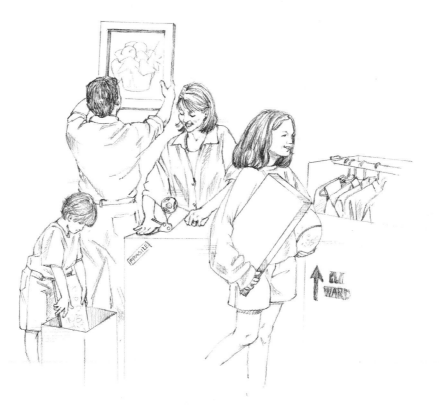

FAMILY MOVES

In today's shrinking world, job loss, promotions, and transfers are forcing some families to move frequently, across town, across the country, and even around the world. These moves can be quite difficult for the whole family but particularly for the children.

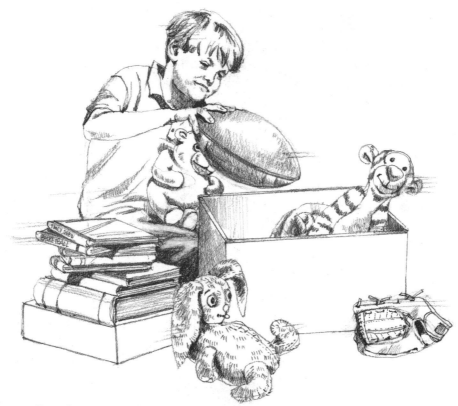

To make a move easier on your children, include them in the planning process.

Most people think that, in general, moving is harder on an older child—high school students, for instance, who are asserting their identities, forming meaningful friendships, and becoming achievement-oriented. Older children do benefit from permanence and stability. Nevertheless, youngsters in middle childhood have some major adjustments to make, too, even if they seem more flexible. Children, of course, are different, and no two will handle a move quite the same. Stresses such as moving will tend to accentuate different aspects of your child's personality.

Positive and Negative Aspects

Children tend to think about the negative side when a family moves. There is the loss of friends and, along with it, loss of a sense of belonging. In the new community the children will be newcomers, strangers, and may need to learn some different social rules. In changing schools they might have to leave behind extracurricular activities—a sports team, a school drama program—that were important to them. Upon arriving at their new school, they may find themselves either academically ahead of or behind their new classmates, depending on the curriculum in the previous school.

In helping your child prepare for a move, place as much emphasis as possible on the positive aspects of what awaits her. This is an opportunity for her to live in and learn about a new city, perhaps even a new country, and its people. She may be exposed to new cultural traditions and interesting and different ways of life. It also is a chance to meet new people and make new friends. Explain how the family will benefit from the move.

For some children, particularly those who may have experienced academic failure or been rejected by classmates at their old school, the opportunity for a new beginning is an exciting prospect. It gives them a chance to be accepted in a new setting and to make friends free of their former reputations and self-images. If this is the case, talk about and plan what you and your child will do differently in your new community. Be cautious, however, of unreasonable expectations that a move will make things wonderful. Children take their likes and dislikes and personal strengths and weaknesses with them.

Making the Transition Easier

There are a number of ways in which you can make the move easier on your children. Keep these suggestions in mind during the planning stages and as you are adjusting to the new neighborhood:

Let Your Child Express Her Feelings. Give your child adequate notice to get used to the idea of moving—even a year in advance may be appropriate. Acknowledge her sadness about leaving behind friends and familiar places. Let her know you are sympathetic and that you understand that she might feel nervous about what awaits her, whether it is the new people, the new school, or the new bus ride. At the same time, tell her you will try to make the move as easy as possible for the entire family, and emphasize some of the positive aspects listed earlier.

If you are also experiencing stress about the move, be open with these feelings. At the same time, keep in mind that your own anxiety might rub off on your child. For that reason, try maintaining and communicating an optimistic attitude about what lies ahead. The stress of moving is greatest about two weeks before and after the move. Be sure to take some breaks to relax and play.

Emphasize the Excitement of Moving. Remind your child that while the move may be making everyone a bit uneasy, it will also be adventurous and interesting. Use the example of the pioneers or the immigrants who overcame their own fears and traveled to new lands, where they encountered new and stimulating experiences. Give her some age-appropriate books that describe families moving from one city to another. Encourage your child to make plans for the move. Have her make lists of tasks and projects to do.

Take Your Child to the Community Where You Will Be Moving. She will probably discover that the new city is really not that different from the one she is leaving. Drive by her new school, and even visit it for a few minutes so she can get a sense of what awaits her. Much of her fear of the unknown should dissipate with this trip.

Look for new things your child might enjoy. For example, if the family is moving to a larger house, maybe your child will get a room of her own for the first time. Perhaps the new city has a zoo or a science museum that she might find interesting. If you are moving to a different climate, there may be opportunities for new activities (skiing, sledding, ice skating; or, in warmer climates, the chance to play outdoors year-round). Plan in advance to enroll your child in sports, clubs, lessons, and the like so she has something to look forward to and so she doesn't lose out on opportunities.

Give your child the chance to participate in decisions that directly affect her. For instance, what kind of wallpaper would she like for her room? If the new house permits the family to get a new pet, what kind would she prefer?

Become Involved in the New Community Yourself. As you meet new people through local schools, groups, or organizations, you can be opening some doors for your child to make new friends. Reach out to people who have children the same age as your own child. Invite them over to make it easier for your youngster to meet other children. Investigate community sports activities, YMCAs, and Boys' and Girls' Clubs. As your child sees you finding your place in the new neighborhood, she will feel more comfortable and secure doing the same. If you are successful in finding a new friend for your youngster before school starts, your child will have the security of knowing someone on the first day of school.

Maintain Contact with the Old Community. If your child wants to keep her old friendships intact, help her do so. Host a farewell party with her friends, and take photographs as keepsakes. Encourage her to write letters and make phone calls. If possible, visit the old neighborhood from time to time, and invite some of her old friends to spend weekends and vacations with you. Let her know that even though you have moved, she does not have to break the ties that have been so important to her.

Make the Move a Family Event. If you plan the move as a family, and support one another as you adjust to the new community, it can bring your family closer together. Let your child know that you will be available to help her deal with any problems and concerns that arise.

YOUR DEVELOPMENT AS A PARENT

P arents develop along with their children, responding to the different challenges that growing children present and changing their style of parenting as their family matures.

In this chapter you will find a discussion of some of the factors that influence parents, and have an opportunity to look at specific issues with which your family may already be dealing. The questions and ideas that follow may provoke some thinking, help you understand the parenting decisions you make, and give you suggestions that may make your family function more effectively.

No single approach to parenting works for all families. Parenting is hard work and an extremely personal experience. Each family—and within that family, each parent-child relationship—is different.

There are many theories and recommended practices about family life and child-rearing. You need to find out what works best for you and your own youngsters. Keeping your family functioning well will often be a matter of trial and error. Even so, a better understanding of your own parenting style and why you are drawn to the decisions you make and the expectations you have will help you become the type of parent you wish to be.

PARENTING INFLUENCES

Many of the factors that influence the way you act within your family had their origins long before you became a mother or a father.

Your Childhood Experiences

When most parents set their standards and expectations for parenting, they take into account their recollections of their own youth. As a first step toward understanding your own approach to parenting, and to use that information in a positive way, examine it through the prism of your own childhood. To begin, answer the following questions:

1. What do you remember about the family you grew up in, particularly your relationships with your mother and father? What do you appreciate most about their way of raising you?

2. What did you most enjoy doing with each of your parents? The answer to this question might give you a clue to the activities your own child might enjoy doing with you.

3. What were the greatest difficulties you had with your parents? This information might help you avoid problem areas with your own youngster, while understanding why you respond to certain parental situations the way you do. For instance, if you felt your parents were too strict, you might become too permissive with your own child; or if you believe your mother and father were too withdrawn and quiet, you might insist upon talking with your child a lot.

4. What do you feel were their greatest shortcomings as parents? If your own father became abusive when he got angry, for example, you might feel anxious whenever tempers flare in your own household, and you might try to avoid angry confrontations.

Even though you may consciously try to avoid the actions of your parents that you thought were wrong, do not be surprised or upset if you find not only your parents' words but also their tone of voice coming out of your mouth. Pay attention to this experience and remember that children learn from what they see and hear.

You can also learn a lot from childhood relationships with your brothers and sisters. Ask yourself questions like: What were the best aspects of your relationship with your siblings? What did you enjoy doing most with them? What problems and conflicts did you have with them? How do you feel your parents handled these conflicts?

If you were an only child, you might have difficulty adjusting to the way your own youngsters relate to one another; you may find their fighting quite disturbing, although if you had grown up with siblings, you would understand better that sibling bickering is quite normal. Or if you were the oldest (or the youngest) child in your family, you might unconsciously identify more with your own oldest (or youngest) child.

As you reflect back on your childhood, think about the significant events that took place. What do you remember about moves to a new city? Starting school? Illnesses or injuries? Losses (the death of a pet, a friend moving away, a stolen bicycle)? These childhood memories can affect how you relate to your own youngsters today. If you had a tough time moving to a new neighborhood when you were young, you might find it hard to put your own child through the same experience. If the first day at a new school was always difficult for you, you might feel especially anxious when your child changes schools.

Also, examine your own memories of teachers and classmates, your academic performance, what you liked and disliked about school, and important school events (tests, oral reports, class trips, science fairs). Think back upon your childhood friendships, too: best friends, adversaries, activities with other children, and how you adjusted to changes in friendships.

As you reflect upon these childhood experiences, you might recognize how they have influenced your responses to your own child's interactions with others—and not always in a positive way. For instance, your youngster may prefer coming home after school, playing a musical instrument, doing homework, and not spending much time in social activities. However, if you yearned to be more popular when you were young, you might push your son to participate more in sports, 4-H, or Scouting activities, although he might have no interest in them. These are issues you need to become more sensitive to.

As part of this self-examination, talk with your youngster about your own childhood recollections. He will love to hear stories about what life was like for you when you were his age. It will give him a sense of history and belonging. It will also help him through difficult times once he finds out that you, too, might not have been invited to a party you really wanted to go to, or that, like him, you had fears about giving an oral report in front of the class.

Your Personality Traits

You cannot change your personality. But by understanding your personal characteristics, you will get a better sense of how you approach others (including the members of your family) and what your strengths and weaknesses as a parent might be.

Take a few minutes to list your personality traits. Are you shy or outgoing? Are you intellectual or intuitive? Open-minded or opinionated? Self-accepting or self-critical? Self-assured or insecure? Moody and temperamental, or stable and even-keeled? Disorganized or obsessive-compulsive? Rarely is anyone always one way or another, but we all have tendencies we should recognize as we approach childrearing.

Although children are born with uniquely individual temperaments, certain personality traits develop through life experiences. For example, if your child has a tendency to be verbally expressive of his feelings, or if he is an affectionate child, he probably acquired these characteristics growing up in the family environment. Or if you or your spouse complains a lot, he may tend to whine. Generally, children identify more with one parent than the other and unconsciously assume more of that parent's traits.

If your own personality characteristics fit with or match those of your child, you may find living with him much easier than if your personalities conflict. (See "Temperament," page 123.) Also, the more accepting you are of your own traits, the more you can relax and be a better spouse and parent.

Keep in mind, however, that certain personal characteristics can have a negative impact on the family—for example, judgmental people tend to be critical of themselves as well as of others, which can interfere with the way they relate to their children; the offspring of judgmental parents often grow up feeling inferior or rejected. At the other extreme, however, some parents may accept *anything* their child does, even if he has adopted bad habits or negative values. You need to find a balance between these two extremes and communicate and try to model those personal traits you value.

Your Early Parenting Experiences

There is a whole history to your parent-child relationship that began at the moment your youngster was born. To help you better understand the present, try to gain some insights into where you have been as a family. Think back on your experiences with your child when he was a baby, a toddler, and a preschooler. Ask yourself:

- How active a parent were you in those early years? Did you play a major child-raising role in the family, or were there other demands (such as long hours at work) that kept you from being as involved as you would have liked?

- What were your most enjoyable parenting and family experiences during those years?

Since those first years of your child's life, your parenting techniques may have changed. Perhaps you were quite anxious as a new parent but gained confidence as the months and years passed. Ask yourself questions like:

- What have you learned as a parent? What were the hardest skills to learn?

- What were your best traits as a parent of a young child? What were the areas in which you had the most problems? For example, did you find it difficult to relate to your child before he started to talk? Was it difficult for you to set limits when he entered toddlerhood? How did he respond to you in your parenting role?

- What did you want to change about yourself as a parent as your child grew? How successful have you been in making those changes? Keep in mind that as your child grows, you and the entire family need to change too. In essence, you are proceeding through your own development as a parent.

Even if you made mistakes during those early years, you can amend them now. If you missed out on certain family experiences because you were working too hard, you still have many years to enjoy your spouse and children. In general, children are understanding and forgive their parents for shortcomings and faults. And if you weren't there when your child took his first steps or rode his tricycle for the first time, you can be there for other special events to come, like your child's school play and his soccer games.

Your Current Parenting Experiences

Spend some time thinking about how you are doing as a parent during these middle years of your youngster's childhood. This is a challenging time, in which your child is seeking more independence and is questioning the family's rules. And, from time to time, you may have to help him with school-related problems. He will be developing more peer relationships, too, and his interactions with siblings may change.

How well are you parenting your child during this time in his life? In what areas are you doing well? Where do you think you need more help?

Your Child's Developmental Needs and Personality Traits

Your youngster, like all children, is unique, and thus there are differences in parenting each child. Some children are easier to manage than others. Some are more troubled than others. Each child's own characteristics will affect your approach to parenting and the way your family functions. (See "Why They Are Similar and Different," page 360.)

As your middle-years child moves through particular stages of development, your own personality can influence just how well you adapt to these phases. For example, if you tend to be a parent who values routines and sets a lot of rules, you may have particular difficulty with a rebellious and controlling child. In the same way, if you are an energetic and sometimes impatient person, you might have trouble with a low-key and slow-moving youngster. Mothers may feel closer to their daughters, may play with and relate to them more easily than to their sons. These are the types of issues to reflect upon in order to better understand your relationship with your family.

Stages of Parenting

As you may have surmised from the previous discussion, parents go through stages as their children grow and develop. You had certain responses to your child when he was an infant and preschooler and are now experiencing new stresses as he enters school and negotiates new relationships outside the family. Children's entry into school and growing independence give parents an opportunity to review their images of parenthood, to ask themselves how successful and realistic they have been, and to consider what changes they would like to make in their relationships with their children. These years have been called a time of interpretation—interpreting yourself to your child and interpreting your child's developing personality. During these years separation becomes an issue for many parents: The child who once relied on them for almost everything has now become more independent. The trade-off is that the child may be more capable of new forms of companionship with his mother and father.

As children approach adolescence, parents must learn again, as they did during their child's preschool years, to cope with challenges to parental authority.

It is important for parents to consider how they have experienced these different stages and whether they are feeling secure with the nature of their parenting. Above all, parenting means being open to change.

Your Current Life Issues

For many men and women, the stress in their lives interferes with their ability to parent. If they are unhappy on the job, for instance, they might return home preoccupied and tense at the end of the day and be unable to handle the tasks of running a family as effectively.

Take a moment to assess how you feel about these and other important aspects of your life.

- Your career and occupation

- Your relationships at work

- Your living conditions, including your home and neighborhood

- Your lifestyle, including time for yourself and leisure activities

- Aging: growing older, slowing down, and experiencing changes in your body

- Your relationship with your spouse or partner

- Your relationship with your parents and siblings

- Your friendships

Evaluate problems in these areas, and how they might be influencing your family life. Whenever possible, find ways to deal with these difficulties in your life more effectively, so they will not interfere with your parent-child relationships.

For example, if you are like many parents, your day is so filled with job and family responsibilities that you have absolutely no "down time," when *you* become a priority. Keep in mind, however, that most parents are happier people (and thus better parents) when they make time for things they find pleasurable. As your children move through their school years, they will develop interests and responsibilities (from friends to homework) that can provide you with more time for those activities that you find enriching. You do *not* need to devote every free moment to playing checkers or baseball with your children; in fact, as long as you are also setting aside some time for your youngsters, they will probably feel good knowing that you are pursuing interests that you really enjoy.

Your Relationship with Your Child's Other Parent

To some degree, your own parenting style is affected by your adult relationships, most particularly the one with your youngster's other parent, whether you are married to that person, separated, or divorced. Think about how the two of you have divided up the tasks of parenting—from making sure your child gets up in the morning on time, to tucking him in at night, and everything in between. How well is this arrangement working? Do either of you feel any resentment about this division of labor? If so, how is this expressed?

Ideally, both parents should work as a team, providing nurturance for their children and family, showing consistency and providing support for each other on issues like discipline. The two of you should communicate regularly about what is happening with your children. If there are particular issues that you regularly disagree on, you need to discuss and try to resolve them.

Here are some other topics to contemplate:

- Do you trust the other parent of your child—that is, how comfortable do you feel with his or her style of parenting? If you go away for an evening or a few days, leaving your child in the care of the other parent, are you confident that he or she will care for your youngster responsibly? What are his or her strengths and weaknesses? How do you respond to his or her difficulties with your child?

- Do you and the other parent have similar values and priorities regarding the family? Do you have similar expectations of your child's behavior?

- What kind of role models are the two of you providing for your child? Do you and the other parent apply the same standards of behavior for yourselves that you do for your children—that is, do the two of you expect your child to behave in a way that you yourself live up to?

As well as doing some self-evaluation on the issues described on the preceding pages, compare notes on these topics with your child's other parent. Use this information as a springboard to deal directly with any family difficulties that exist.

PROBLEMS AND SOLUTIONS OF CO-PARENTING

As you and your spouse (or ex-spouse) share the responsibilities of parenting and managing the family's day-to-day activities, problems will arise. Here are a few of the most common difficulties that today's parents encounter:

Inconsistency

Often parents differ in their rules and expectations for their child. Mom might say, "You can't watch TV until your homework is finished"; but when she's away, Dad may say, "Go ahead and watch TV if you want to." Dad might insist that the child's bedtime is 8:30; Mom may say that stretching it until 9:00 is fine.

Similar conflicts can develop over issues like approaches to discipline, or a child's choice of friends. When these inconsistencies occur, one parent inevitably undermines the authority of the other.

To begin to resolve this problem, you and your spouse need to be explicit with each other about what your rules and expectations are. If necessary, write them down, review them, and be sure they are workable. In areas in which you differ, find a compromise that you both can live with—and stick by it.

Noncommunication

If you and your spouse do not talk about the issues the family faces, one of you may be left out of important matters you should be informed about.

To avoid this situation, you and your spouse need to commit yourselves to communicate about every significant issue in your family life. At least once a day the two of you need to check in with each other and discuss what happened that day that was important. At the same time, talk about long-term issues that may be confronting the family.

Confusion

Uncertainty about what stands to take and what rules to impose can create turmoil within the family. Too often, parents are perplexed about issues like the degree of supervision required for their children and the amount of freedom to give them. Parents frequently do not make decisions at all, and that can leave their children puzzled and dismayed over what is expected of them.

You and your spouse need to resolve your own ambivalence on important family matters and agree on a position on these issues. Then you must clearly inform the entire family about your decisions and how their own lives will be affected by them.

Competition

Sometimes rivalry can develop between parents over their children's attention and love. If Dad wants his daughter to spend Saturday afternoon fishing with him but Mom wants her to go shopping with her, they may struggle to get their

The Impact of Marital Problems

Interpersonal relationships do not exist in a vacuum. If you and your spouse are having marital difficulties, they are likely to disrupt the entire family. When your marriage is not going well, your parenting skills and your children will suffer.

The adults in the most successful families do not neglect marital problems. They commit themselves to spending time together as a couple and working together to resolve any misunderstandings, jealousies, or conflicts. They make a commitment to communicate, praise, and forgive each other; they try to understand each other; and they routinely examine their relationship and how it can be improved.

Sometimes children are a convenient excuse for not dealing with serious marital difficulties. Parents may think, "The kids require so much of our attention now; once they're grown, we'll have a lot of time to talk about the problems we have in our own relationship." But that is a prescription for marital and parenting disaster. Problems tend only to become worse with time, and once your children are grown, you may not have much of a foundation to build on—if you are still together at all. So don't be complacent and let problems persist without attempting to solve them.

way, putting the child in an unenviable position, right in the middle of the conflict.

The two of you need to find ways to cooperate, not compete, with each other. That doesn't mean you have to agree on everything; but it does mean that you are committed to working together toward a more harmonious relationship and family life, and you are not going to let differences undermine your common goals. Each of you needs to demonstrate some flexibility.

As you form ground rules for the family, identify the areas in which each parent excels. That parent should then exert leadership in the areas of his or her strength, so the decision-making responsibilities are divided within the family.

Overt Conflict

Too often, parents argue and openly challenge each other on family-related matters. Perhaps their child has gotten into trouble at school, and the parents disagree about how to handle it; the mother may think the child should be grounded, while the father believes it wasn't her fault. They start to argue—sometimes for hours or even over a period of days—and eventually, rather than resolving the problem amicably, one parent wins out because the other ultimately gives in, at least for the moment. Nevertheless, the parental power struggle often begins all over again at a later time with a different issue, with some of the same anger from the previous conflict resurfacing. The wounds never fully heal and the animosity builds.

Clearly, this is not a healthy situation. Parents need to learn the skills of conflict resolution. These include:

- Listening

- Clarifying points of difference

- Taking each other's feelings seriously

- Generating alternative solutions together

- Negotiating

Remember, the way you handle conflict in your family is how your child learns to manage disagreement. Many community colleges offer seminars and courses on conflict resolution.

PARENTING PRINCIPLES

Parenting is one of life's biggest challenges. It requires loving, respecting, and empathizing with your children. It involves protecting, guiding, communicating, teaching, showing patience, setting limits, and resolving conflicts. If you feel you fall short in some of these areas, bear in mind that they are acquired skills. They can be learned and improved upon at any time.

Successful parenting begins with understanding and valuing yourself and your children. Without self-respect, you may have difficulty tolerating the inevitable trials of family life.

Too often, parents strive for perfection, but there is no such thing as the perfect family and the perfect parent. Every member of the family unit needs to work toward accepting the humanness of every other member, including faults and limitations. Rather than striving to be perfect, everyone should work toward being "as good as I possibly can."

A second key to successful parenting is understanding your child—reading his cues correctly, engaging in dialogue and listening carefully, and appreciating these things that make your child unique.

When family difficulties arise, trust your gut and listen to your heart as well as your head. You may have better parenting instincts than you think. Because there are few definitively "right" answers, use your experience as a guide. Also, both inside and outside the family, have people you can talk to, share feelings with, and turn to for support and guidance. Do not allow parenting to become a lonely experience, or you risk having frustration and fatigue get the best of you.

BROTHERS
AND SISTERS

As their children grow up, parents are often surprised to discover how different each child is from the others, even though they have grown up in the same family. Of course, differences among siblings are the rule, not the exception. One challenge for parents is to deal with these differences without seeming to favor one child over another.

Except for twins, the most obvious differences among siblings are in age and sex. Differences are also evident in temperament, interests, confidence, resilience, vulnerability, social style, sense of security, achievement in a variety of domains, physical and mental health, rate of physical and sexual maturation, and physical appearance. And while diversity and differences may be a source of pride for parents, they may also be a source of confusion and frustration, as well as uneven attention, praise, and other displays of affection.

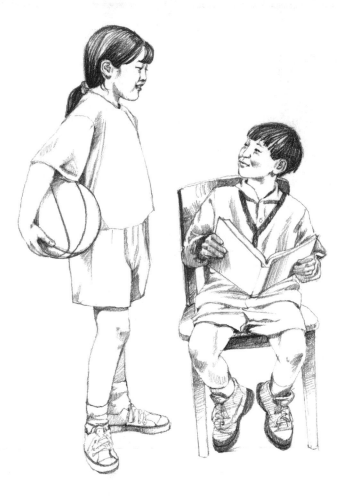

WHY THEY ARE
SIMILAR AND DIFFERENT

What are the factors that influence your child's personality and other attributes? Two major influences are at work: *nature* (genetic factors, heredity) and *nurture* (experience). These interact with each other in ways that are particular to each child. To better understand the similarities and differences among siblings, let's look at both of these factors more closely.

Nature

Because of heredity—the biological or genetic influences of the same two parents on each child—parents might expect their children to be alike. But overall, children have only about a fifty-fifty chance of developing any particular inherited trait (physical appearance, personality, intelligence, aptitudes, health), and even when these traits are present, they can vary.

For instance, researchers have found that siblings tend to be more similar in their physical characteristics than in their likelihood of developing the same diseases. Also, while siblings may resemble one another in their intellectual aptitude and other psychological characteristics early in life, these similarities generally diminish by adulthood, while differences become more pronounced. Even in childhood, siblings with similar levels of intelligence may differ in their school achievement, since academic success can be strongly affected by the different life experiences of each child.

Nurture

Nurture (or experience) refers to the *non*hereditary influences on your child's development. They include social factors such as relationships with siblings, peers, parents, and other adults, as well as environmental influences like illnesses, accidents, nutrition, and cultural experiences. Other forces come into play as well, including your child's perceptions of herself and others, past experiences, self-expectations, and the expectations others have of her.

Siblings share some experiences but have many others that are not shared. While shared experiences generally contribute toward similarities, even a shared experience may affect each child differently. And since most experiences are unshared, they contribute to differences between children too.

In the early school years, for instance, qualities such as intelligence and academic achievement are largely determined by heredity and shared experience. However, as children grow, they have more unshared experiences, which gradually help differentiate one sibling from another. Siblings even perceive and interpret shared events differently, and these different perceptions can be important in shaping a child's development and self-image.

INFLUENCE OF PARENTS AND SIBLINGS

Do you treat all your children alike? Probably not. You should relate to and treat each youngster differently. Treating each child as an individual is part of what makes that child a unique person and is a way of appreciating his special characteristics.

A husband and wife become and learn how to be parents with their first child, who for a while is their only child. As a result, their relationship with that first child will be different from their relationships with subsequent children. Since parents develop and learn along with their children, parents' actions, conversational style, and displays of emotion will change with each new youngster.

Not only do parents change their style as they gain experience raising children, but each youngster has his or her own style and needs, initially because of birth order and inborn traits, and later because of experiences. Older children need to be treated differently from younger ones. High-strung children need different approaches than do easygoing ones. On every issue—rules, expectations, chores, responsibilities, rewards, and punishment—parents must individualize their parenting while trying to remain fair to all. This last goal is nearly impossible to achieve. Even if parents interact with their youngsters in a comparable manner, each child may perceive these actions differently.

Your behavior toward your children is determined in part by the age and developmental stage of each youngster. For example, you probably have tended to treat all your children in a somewhat similar way at the same age or level of development. A mother may be physically affectionate to her two children in their respective toddler years but less visibly affectionate when they reach school age. In a situation like this, the older child may perceive that the younger sibling is receiving more affection. Parents *should* treat children differently at different ages; problems occur when parents are not able to act appropriately for their child's developmental age and needs.

Birth order and family size also influence your children's development. The experience of an only child is different from that of a child in a larger family. An older child's experience is different from a younger one's: The older child has a younger sibling, while the younger child has an older sibling. A third child has two older siblings, and so on. Because of birth order and family size, no two children experience the same family the same way.

The birth order of your children also will affect the way you relate to them, the way they respond, the experiences they have, and thus the way they develop as individuals. For instance, firstborn children may feel neglected or unloved after the arrival of a new sibling. Though their parents may expect or at least hope for them to be more responsible and self-sufficient, firstborns may act younger or more babylike in order to attract parental attention. In turn, the parents may express frustration or anger with them because of their babyish behavior.

The temperaments of each parent and each child influence the way each interacts with the other. A parent whose temperament fares best with order and predictability could find raising a disorganized, spontaneous, impulsive child a daily challenge. On the other hand, easygoing parents and children can readily make allowances for one another.

Each pair of family members has a unique relationship. A child relates in different ways to his father and to his mother. His sibling relates to each parent in his or her own way. Each sibling relates to each brother or sister in a particular way. Children are quite sensitive to these differences within family relationships; they monitor them, respond to them, and relate to one another in a manner based upon the nature of their experiences and how they perceive them.

Therefore, some of the differences among siblings reflect how they perceive their roles and relationships within their families—how they have been loved, appreciated, respected, and understood. These factors can influence their self-confidence, sense of trust, and ability to cope with challenges and disappointments.

Over the years the relationships among siblings can contribute to increasing differences. Siblings compete for the affection and attention of their parents; they may compare themselves with one another, become aware of one another's strengths and weaknesses, and try to find the most comfortable and rewarding role for themselves within the family unit. In this dynamic interaction, differences develop and can become more pronounced with time, affecting everything from self-esteem and behavioral style to life goals and career choices.

BIOLOGICAL DIFFERENCES

Age and sex are the most readily apparent differences and similarities among siblings. Older children expect certain privileges, in part due to the greater level of responsibility they are expected to assume in the household. Younger children expect special consideration because they are less independent.

Sometimes parents have difficulty treating children of similar ages differently, even though they realize that each child could benefit if they did. Boys and girls are treated differently in our society, and some of that difference may be seen as unfair by a child.

Some children are different because of a problem in physical, psychological, or social functioning. For example, a child with a learning disability may need extra time being read to or helped with homework. The special attention these children require can be a source of jealousy and conflict unless it is handled well. Sometimes, however, children who seem different from their siblings because of an evident handicap have learned to handle that problem well and actually differ more in some less obvious way, such as in their personalities.

Parents face a difficult juggling act in meeting the varying needs and expectations of their children without falling into the trap of being accused of favoritism. If you learn how to listen to and observe your children, you will be more aware of their different perceptions and needs and thus can respond more successfully to each of your particular children and to the whole family.

INFLUENCES OUTSIDE THE FAMILY

The new people and experiences encountered by children in school, play, and other everyday events all contribute to sibling differences. Each encounter provides a unique opportunity for the child to test her innate personality and learned skills and wisdom with different people and new social situations. These interactions continually shape a youngster's perceptions, attitudes, beliefs, understanding, and behavior.

For instance, a child often has a particular relationship with friends. When a friend of one child is in the house, other siblings may join in their playing, but each will have a different way of relating to the visitor. These peer experiences can contribute significantly to the way a child views herself, and they magnify the differences between her and her siblings.

At the same time, keep in mind that the way a child interacts with other people is strongly influenced by her relationships within her own family. Thus, family experiences not only shape the personalities of individual children but also establish the patterns of interactions that will occur outside the family.

WHAT DIFFERENCES MEAN FOR PARENTS

Siblings are destined to be more different than alike. But as you watch your children grow up, remember that their similarities or differences are not as important as their overall development toward becoming positive, productive, healthy, and kind human beings.

In order for your youngsters to reach those goals, they need to feel loved, trusted, competent, and respected for who they are, not for who they are in comparison with their siblings. Children who are raised in this way will develop resiliency, self-confidence, the capacity for risk-taking, the ability to set and achieve goals, and a sensitivity and respect for others.

Of course, you should be monitoring your children's relationships with one another to help them learn to avoid and resolve conflicts. At the same time, make an effort to accept, appreciate, and respect the basic uniqueness of each of your children. Honestly appraise each youngster's strengths and weaknesses, and encourage his or her growth and development based on that appraisal. As you nurture each youngster's individuality, he or she will develop into a special person of whom you will be proud.

35

SIBLING RIVALRY

Nearly every parent with more than one child has experienced the frustration of sibling rivalry. Despite the best attempts at keeping harmony in the family, brothers and sisters will fight over toys, tattle on one another, argue, tease, criticize, or become physically abusive, leading mothers and fathers to ask themselves: "What have I done wrong? Why can't our household be peaceful?"

As annoying and upsetting as this rivalry can be, it is quite normal. Some jealousy and friction between siblings is a part of growing up, although it is worse in some families than in others.

Why does rivalry among your children occur? In part, it is a competition for your attention and love. You are very important in their lives, and they would rather not share you with anyone, particularly a brother or sister. That in itself is enough to cause dissension. Other factors contribute to this rivalry as well, including the personalities of your youngsters, their mutual or differing interests, their ages, the amount of time they spend with one another and with you, and even the favoritism you may show toward one child, however unintentional. With so many factors at play, some squabbling is inevitable. (See Chapter 34 for a discussion of sibling differences and similarities.)

THE POSITIVE AND NEGATIVE
SIDES OF SIBLINGS

Brothers and sisters do more than compete with one another. They also play very positive roles in each other's lives. They provide companionship and serve as ready playmates and confidants. They help one another learn to relate to the outside world. At times, they may find themselves protecting each other, perhaps from a neighborhood ruffian. As they grow, they have many of the same experiences and will share similar memories of family gatherings, holidays, vacations, even family crises. They may have little secrets they share only with one another. These kinds of experiences can bond them for a lifetime.

Even the minor bickering is not all negative. Some squabbling is part of childhood and human nature. Children will try to dominate one another, to assert their authority, and to test different aspects of human relationships. Provoking responses from a brother or sister, pleasant or conflicted, is part of children's normal and necessary learning. Through these interactions, siblings learn to be assertive, say what they are feeling, defend themselves, and find solutions to their disputes. Also, as they compete with one another, they can push themselves to excel.

However, when the rivalry becomes mean-spirited and creates constant stress and tension within the family, consuming a lot of your time in breaking up and resolving arguments, then it has gone beyond the bounds of normal sibling competitiveness. If one of your children is aggressive or violent toward another, it has gone too far.

WHAT TO EXPECT

Although sibling rivalry can be present at any age, it tends to become more intense as children grow older, often peaking in the eight- to twelve-year-old range. Youngsters of the same sex are usually more competitive, as are siblings close in age or those who have similar interests.

In many cases, the oldest child in the family feels a greater sense of rivalry than the younger ones. The younger children may look up to and idolize the older brother or sister; by contrast, the oldest youngster may see his siblings as intrusions upon his privacy or the family unit and a threat to the special attention and status he is used to getting from his mother and father.

At its worst, sibling rivalry can take a serious emotional toll upon one or more children in the family. A youngster's self-esteem can suffer if he is being constantly harassed, belittled, or bullied by a brother or sister. This contentiousness can leave him feeling slighted, undervalued, and unloved, particularly if he believes that his parents favor his sibling. If he is often punched by a sibling, his physical well-being may be in jeopardy too.

STEPSIBLINGS

Stepfamilies are creating another variation of sibling rivalry. With current high divorce and remarriage rates, the number of stepsiblings is growing, creating new situations and conflicts. When two families become one, children who barely know each other may be sharing bedrooms and bathrooms, fighting over toys, and battling over which programs to watch on TV. At the same time, they are trying to adapt to a new marriage, new stepparents, and maybe a new house. It is a difficult adjustment.

Stepfamilies may produce other situations that can create antagonism among children. The twelve-year-old daughter of one spouse may feel real anger if she is frequently burdened with the responsibility of babysitting for the three-year-old child of the other marriage partner. Also, when there are conflicts within the new family—for instance, disagreements over whom to visit during holidays—youngsters often band together with their own parent, forming camps and aggravating any rivalries that may already exist. (See Chapter 44, "Stepfamilies.")

WHAT PARENTS CAN DO

Sibling rivalry can change the dynamics of the entire family. Fortunately, however, there are ways to prevent or at least minimize problems.

Preparing for the Birth of a Sibling

Prior to the birth of a new baby, you can prepare your child for the addition to the family. A youngster beyond the age of five is usually not as threatened by a newborn as a younger child is, particularly if the middle-years youngster has

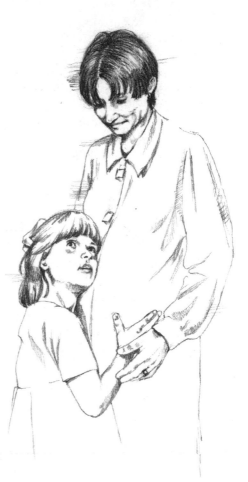

To prepare your child for the birth of a sibling, be honest and truthful about what is about to happen, using language she can understand.

good self-esteem and feels loved and valued. Nevertheless, resentments are likely to surface because of the attention the infant receives.

To prepare your child, be honest and truthful about what is about to happen, using language he can understand. Explain the impending arrival of his new brother or sister, noting the changes that may affect him—both the good and the not-so-good. Have him help get the house ready for the arrival of his new sibling, fixing up the baby's bedroom, picking out a new crib, buying diapers. If your child is going to be moved to a different bedroom, make the move at least several weeks before the new baby is born, thereby spreading out the changes in his life over a longer period. However, children can be impatient, so don't focus on preparing for the baby too far in advance.

Mothers and new babies are being discharged from hospitals very soon after birth. However, if there is time soon after the delivery, have your older child come to the hospital so that he feels part of the expanding family. Then, when you bring the baby home, make the newborn's sibling feel that he has a role to play in caring for the baby. Tell him he can hold the infant whenever he wants, although he must ask you first. Compliment him when he is gentle and loving toward the baby. When friends and relatives visit, ask them to give some attention to your older child too.

During the first few busy weeks, do not neglect the needs and activities of your older youngster. Give him permission to talk about any negative feelings he is having about the new sibling. Tell him: "A new baby means a lot more work for me, but if you ever feel that I'm not spending enough time with you, let me know so I can give you plenty of extra love." Make an effort to spend some time alone with him each day; use that as an opportunity to make him feel like the most important person in your life.

Rivalry of Older Children

As children grow and mature, sibling rivalry can worsen. You can minimize that possibility by treating your youngsters as individuals. Every child should be recognized for his or her distinct achievements and strengths. Make sure you listen to each child, demonstrate your concern for his interests and needs, and if possible, enjoy time alone with him. Show all your children that they are loved and valued.

To cut down on conflicts, clearly explain that there are different rules for each child based on age. Although you will do your best to be fair, things will not always be *equal* for the siblings. While a twelve-year-old may stay up till 9:30 at night, an eight-year-old's bedtime might be 8:30. While an eleven-year-old may be able to go to the movies with a friend without an adult accompanying them, a six-year-old isn't yet ready for that. (At the same time, do not force your middle-years child to assume too much responsibility for the care of his younger sibling, always having to take his little brother or sister with him when he goes to the movies.) Explain to your younger child that he will enjoy the same privileges when he becomes a little older. Don't push your younger child prematurely into situations and experiences for which he isn't yet ready.

Teach your youngsters that each one has his own "space" and belongings. Your middle-years child might have to learn to ask his older sibling for permission to play with a board game that doesn't belong to him. He also should learn to respect the privacy of his brother or sister.

When it comes to chores in the family, make certain they are divided fairly. If there is a particular household job that none of the children enjoys—perhaps helping with the dinner dishes or carrying out the trash—be sure that everyone takes a turn with this responsibility.

Cooperation and compassion are other important values to teach. As you spend time together as a family, children can learn the importance of supporting and caring for one another. They should be sensitive to any emotional distress that others in the family may feel from time to time, thinking beyond themselves and their own individual needs.

Children learn a lot about relating to others by observing how their parents interact. Be conscious that the way you and your partner treat each other, respect each other, and resolve your differences is a model that your children are likely to follow.

Avoid making comparisons between the children. For instance, one child may be an academic high-achiever, while another struggles to get C's; or one child may be a star athlete on the Little League team, while another can barely swing a bat. Or one child may have a particular talent that is not appreciated by other family members, and thus he may feel neglected or resentful and act out his feelings. Differences can be acknowledged in a positive way without negative judgments and comparisons being made. However, insensitive discussion of these differences can be very hurtful and may escalate hostility and anger between siblings.

Rather than making comparisons, look for the strengths in each of your children and encourage their individuality. You might have to search out new interests and activities, nurturing them in each child. Also, find an activity each of your youngsters can do just with you, so they know you see them as special individuals.

Children who might feel they are being outshone by a sibling—who sense they are living in the shadow of a smarter or more talented brother or sister—may feel anger toward that sibling unless parents take the trouble to make them feel special too. A child's own personal activities, however, can help him experience success and find a niche where he is not in competition with his sibling.

Resolving Problems

As much as possible, siblings have a responsibility to solve their own conflicts reasonably and appropriately. Parents should set parameters of how siblings may resolve their disagreements—for example, through discussion and perhaps even yelling, but not through physical violence. Act as an impartial arbiter, and help the children themselves negotiate their differences and solve their mutual problems. Arrange regularly scheduled family meetings in which each child voices his concerns and desires. Additional meetings can be convened quickly for unforeseen incidents and issues that should be aired. In these discussions, allow each youngster to express his grievances toward the other, without interruption, name-calling, or other abusive language. Let them know that while these disagreements among siblings are normal, hurtful language and physical aggression are not permissible. After all sides are heard, restate the opposing viewpoints. Ask the children themselves to propose solutions to the conflict, and help them reach a middle ground. Initially, they will

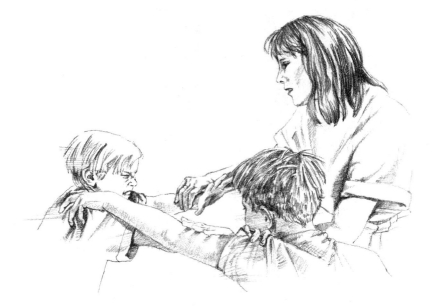

Parents should encourage siblings to solve their own disagreements, but they may need to intervene when things get out of control.

need help, reminders, practice, and rule enforcement from you. Eventually, they should be able to do this on their own.

Do not let these sibling squabbles get out of control. You need to intervene when the children have overstepped the guidelines, particularly when physical or emotional abuse is taking place.

Find out the reason for your children's anger toward one another. It might be as simple as an argument over the choice of a TV program. However, it can go much deeper, perhaps with one child taking out on a sibling the hostility he feels toward *you*. (After all, it is much safer to lash out at a brother or sister than to shout or swing at a parent.) Intense rivalry may reflect family tension or problems that are expressed through the children, but don't originate between them.

As you teach and discipline, be careful not to label one child as being the cause for all sibling conflicts, making him the scapegoat in the family. In some families, a timeout for both children works well, letting tempers cool down before a solution is sought. (See page 213.)

At times, once the facts are on the table, it is clear that one child is at fault. In those instances you may need to intervene with some punishment and/or guidelines to prevent the situation from recurring. Be fair and firm with your decision, making a statement like: "Bobby, when your brother is doing his homework in his room, you can't walk in and begin playing with his toys. He needs it to be quiet. Knock on his door, but if he asks you not to come in, you have to obey."

Guidelines for Parental Management of Sibling Rivalry

- Be fair.

- Avoid making comparisons between your children.

- Encourage the children to work out their own differences.

- Avoid taking sides on sibling conflicts. Be impartial, and do not show a preference for one child or another.

- Set guidelines on how children can disagree and resolve conflicts.

- Discourage tattling.

- When it is necessary to punish or reprimand, do it with the child alone in a quiet, private place.

- Use regular family meetings for all family members to express their thoughts and feelings, as well as to plan the week's events and to give positive recognition and rewards (allowance, special privileges).

As children grow older, sibling rivalries sometimes decrease in intensity. An eleven- or twelve-year-old may develop more interests outside the home—perhaps youth sports or Scouting activities—and that can ease sibling conflicts. However, in some families there is no decrease in rivalry. As older children become increasingly opinionated and physically stronger, they may become more aggressive in asserting their place in the family.

If you are persistent, however, your efforts toward encouraging cooperation will be worthwhile. By adulthood, if not before, your offspring will tend to become closer. In most cases they will grow into lifelong friends.

36

BABYSITTERS AND OTHER CARETAKERS

One of the most telling aspects of middle-years development is that at the beginning of this time of life, children require nearly continuous supervision, while at the end, they are much more autonomous. During the early years of middle childhood, they need babysitters, but as they approach adolescence, they may start to take on some limited childcare responsibilities themselves.

Finding good babysitters for your school-age children can be a daunting task. If you do not choose them wisely, serious disruptions in family life can occur. While it would be nice to find the perfect sitter simply by placing an advertisement in the newspaper, the reality is that the process of recruiting and selecting caretakers is often quite difficult.

The first step is to determine what type of help you are looking for. Are you interested in someone who can watch the children on Saturday nights while you go out to a movie, or do you need a person to help out on a daily basis? Are you considering hiring someone to live in your home and to assume other duties such as housekeeping? How much can you afford to spend? What are your children like, and what kind of person do you think would be best suited to watch them? These questions need to be kept in mind when selecting childcare.

Choosing Childcare

If you are looking for an occasional babysitter, you might decide to employ responsible adolescents from the neighborhood, typically teenagers who are looking to make extra spending money. There is an advantage to having young people as babysitters, since they are generally energetic, playful, fun-loving, and entertaining for your children. The disadvantage is that they may be less strict than you are with discipline, and they may not be experienced in handling problem situations. If your child is close to twelve years old, you will need someone considerably older to babysit. A teenager only one or two years older is not likely to have much authority. Be sure to speak with the parents of any teenager you are considering hiring, to get a sense of how he or she handles responsibility. It is also a good idea to check with other families who have used the teenager for babysitting.

The best strategy is to develop a list of three or four sitters who know your child and can be called upon if your regular sitter is busy or ill. Make sure they all understand the rules that apply to sitting at your home regarding TV watching, visitors, smoking or drinking, telephone use, and taking your child outside.

If you need a sitter on a more regular basis, you may need to employ an older person. Newspaper advertisements, agencies, and word of mouth are the most common means of recruiting people. Sometimes local colleges have rosters of students interested in babysitting. And what qualities should you be looking for in this babysitter? In general, he or she needs to be mature, reliable, friendly, and pleasant with children. He or she should be someone with whom your child enjoys spending time. In fact, as your youngster gets older, she should have some say in your selection of caretakers.

Interview applicants thoroughly to get a sense of their reliability and competence. Ask them about other positions they have held, the ages of children they have cared for, and what their responsibilities included. Inquire about how they would handle various situations (such as your child not wanting to do homework). Ask about activities they enjoy doing with children. If you think reading or singing to your child is important, look for a babysitter who enjoys these activities. Explain fully your expectations—for example, will the childcare involve housecleaning? Ask for and carefully check references.

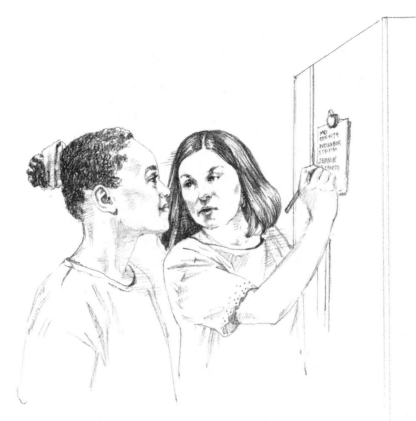

Babysitters should always be provided with a list of emergency phone numbers.

If one person stands out among those you've interviewed, have him or her come for a "visit" while you are home. Introduce him or her to your child, and pay him or her for an hour of childcare while you are there to watch. Evaluate this first encounter in helping you make a final decision. Later, ask your child about the sitter, and be sensitive to her comments. Trust your intuition about whether the sitter will work out, and follow that feeling.

The hourly rate for babysitting varies from community to community. In general, pay should increase with responsibility and with the competence of the babysitter. Caring for multiple children or adding household chores to childcare merits a higher hourly rate.

Some families prefer to hire an "au pair." Typically, this is a college-age person from another country who agrees to live and work in the United States for a specified period of time (usually one year). While an au pair can be expensive, he or she can bring cultural richness into your family. Recognize, however, that many of these individuals also need to be given support and assistance in adjusting to the United States. To find an au pair, use an agency that specializes in these placements.

When Your Child Wants to Babysit

In the middle years, many children learn babysitting skills by being taken care of by an older sister or brother, or by helping their parents care for younger siblings. At some point, they may express an interest in becoming a sitter, and by the age of thirteen, they may be ready to do so.

Schools and organizations (YMCA, local hospitals) often provide courses in babysitting. However, nothing can compare to experience, preferably under the observation of an adult. Preteenagers, boys and girls, can seek some "on-the-job" training by working as a mother's helper, assisting in the care of young children when a parent is present in the home. This is particularly valuable if the family has expressed some interest in hiring your child as a babysitter in the near future. She can observe how the parents interact with their children, while getting to know the youngsters before taking full responsibility for them. She will also discover the tasks involved in babysitting, and how each child must be approached somewhat differently.

If your child has shown interest in becoming a sitter, emphasize to her the responsibility of taking care of someone else's children. When she is asked to sit, help her plan her schedule so other tasks (such as homework) do not conflict with the hours she has committed to childcare. Also, assist her in formulating questions to ask the parents who are hiring her, such as what is expected of her and what she will be paid. Be willing to help her think of some activities she might be able to do with the children.

Some families develop cooperative arrangements with neighbors or family friends who also have children. Families take turns providing childcare for one another. Even in these cases, be sure you are clear about the rules you expect to be applied to your children. It is also helpful to keep track of how much childcare each family is providing, so no family feels that the exchange of service is out of balance.

No matter what kind of sitter you select, make sure that the person with whom you leave your child has a list of all emergency phone numbers, including where you can be reached, and the names and numbers of trusted neighbors, relatives, and your child's pediatrician. The emergency hotline number (such as 911) in your locale, and the number of the poison control center, should be displayed on or near the phone.

In the weeks and months ahead, monitor your sitter and how he or she gets along with your child. Work with the sitter to improve his or her understanding of your youngster. Give advice and suggestions, but also reinforce his or her positive qualities.

What should you do if your child challenges the babysitter's authority? First, find out exactly what happened, talking to both the child and the babysitter. Then, except under extraordinary circumstances, stand behind the sitter. If you don't, your youngster will lose respect for the sitter and make it even more difficult the next time you leave home. However, if your child expresses a dislike for a sitter or protests when hearing who is going to sit, take their opinions and concerns seriously. Explore what the problem is, and remember that with regard to childcare, your child's safety and well-being get top priority.

Finally, be considerate of your sitter's time. Schedule and (if necessary) cancel well in advance. Respect the sitter's wishes to be with his or her family and friends on holidays and other special occasions. Remember, a good sitter is a valuable resource.

37

RESPONSIBILITIES AND CHORES

As children enter and move through their school years, they become increasingly able to manage matters like homework and school projects on their own. Consequently, each year they should take on more responsibilities in the classroom and at home. During the middle years of childhood most youngsters can help clean their rooms, make their beds, pick up their toys, and help out in the kitchen or the yard. Some feed and care for pets. These daily chores and responsibilities are an important part of learning that life requires work, not just play.

Normally, of course, children are still preoccupied with their desire to have fun. While they may pitch in, particularly if helping out gives them time with their parents, children are not likely to ask for household tasks, and parents often need to assign responsibilities as part of belonging to the family. At this age, many children find it difficult to follow through and complete their chores, at least ini-

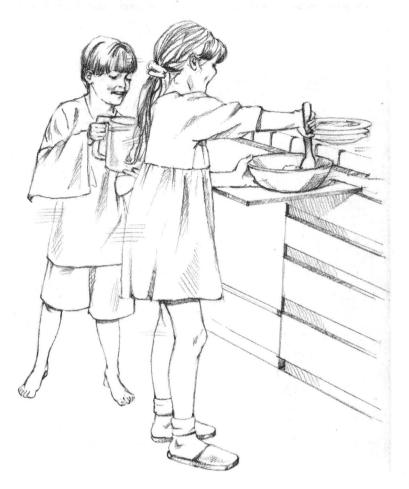

tially. Responsibility and initiative are learned through a gradual process of guidance and reward.

PROCRASTINATING AND DAWDLING

As your own child takes on more responsibilities, he will probably have periods of acting *ir*responsibly, procrastinating and dawdling. Most children do. During these times you need to step in and, with encouragement and gentle guidance, point him in the right direction.

Sometimes parents may demand too much of their children, or may see a problem in everything their children do. They may burden them with too many responsibilities—an unfair number of chores, excess hours of taking

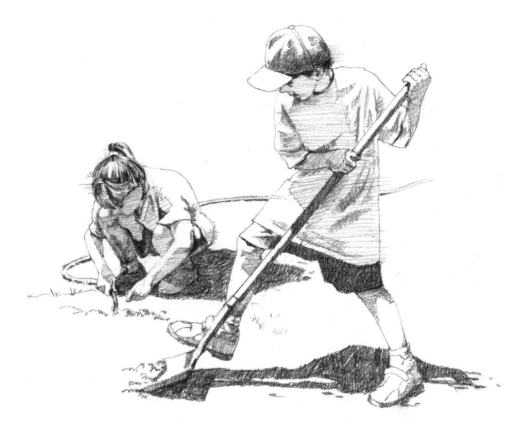

care of younger siblings, or a too rigorous schedule of after-school activities. When that happens, children may feel overwhelmed and resist taking on any responsibilities at all. Parents need to guard against this kind of overloading, while still making sure that their youngsters are assuming an appropriate level of responsibility. Children, of course, differ in the personal traits and temperament they bring to tasks. Some are simply not very persistent and drift away in the middle of chores. Others have difficulty getting organized. Still others have trouble shifting from one activity to another. You should have a good sense of your child's style, and shape your expectations accordingly.

Children need to have some obligations and duties within the family, or they will not learn to accept responsibility. In unstructured home environments, or in families who are very permissive and where little is expected of children, youngsters are losing out on some valuable learning experiences, and their development of a sense of responsibility and initiative may not happen until later in life, if ever. As a result, whenever demands are placed upon these children, they appear to procrastinate or dawdle, never having learned to get started meeting their responsibilities and completing them.

WHAT PARENTS CAN DO

If your own child procrastinates and dawdles, especially around responsibilities and chores, here are some simple management techniques that are often helpful:

1. Carefully spell out the tasks your child must perform. Make sure she understands what is expected of her on a daily and a weekly basis. Star charts or chore lists posted in your youngster's room or on the refrigerator should clearly show what your expectations are. With a school-age child, particularly one who has not taken on responsibilities before, you should introduce one new task at a time; if you spring a long list on her, she will probably fail and rebel.

2. Honest praise from you can be the most effective way of motivating your child and guaranteeing her success. As your youngster completes a regular task, praise her and the job she did. Initiating tasks on her own without a reminder, completing a special task, or doing an unusually good job with a regular one might merit a reward of some sort. You may also want to consider tangible rewards like allowances and stickers tied to completed chores.

3. Your child may be greatly helped in remembering to do chores if your family life has a structure and routines. Encourage her to do her chores at the same time each day. Routines of other activities—including meals, homework, play, and bedtime—also can teach organization and help her develop responsibility.

4. Schedule weekly family meetings to review your child's progress. Ask her to discuss her ideas about chores and other responsibilities. Create new or modified "contracts" of the chores that are expected of her. Most important, supervise and support your child, which is the best way to ensure that she is being responsible.

5. When your youngster does not complete her chores and other responsibilities, it may be necessary to discipline her. For example, you might decide to revoke certain privileges or special activities that mean a lot to her. Although some parents may feel that badgering or scolding a child to

Allowances for the Middle-Years Child

For children in this age group, an allowance serves two purposes:

- An allowance motivates children to assume responsibilities around the home. These tasks should contribute to the family's (and not just the child's) well-being. Yes, children need to learn to care for themselves (clean up their room), but they also need to contribute to the family.

- An allowance introduces children to the value of money—to saving, budgeting, and planning. These are life skills that are important to acquire. School-age children are not ready to assume the responsibility for purchasing necessary items, from clothing to school supplies, but their allowance can be used for discretionary purchases. For that reason, it should be only a modest amount. However, since discretionary purchases tend to increase with age, so should a child's allowance.

Make sure your child clearly understands the purpose of an allowance. If you use it as a reward or payment for chores, then the rules should be clear about what your youngster needs to do to earn that money, and you need to abide by the agreement that you make. If the allowance is provided for discretionary spending and to teach money management, then a different set of rules apply. Spell out the amount, purpose, and expectations for the money in advance, and monitor the spending to teach important decision-making lessons.

the point of starting an argument will get her to accept more responsibility, this approach is rarely effective. Rewarding successes and providing encouragement is always much more effective.

In some cases a procrastinating youngster may be helped by professional intervention. Review your concerns with your own pediatrician, who may be able to reassure you that your child is behaving normally. On the other hand, the pediatrician may consider a referral to a child psychiatrist or psychologist for an evaluation, not only if your child *consistently* fails to complete everyday home responsibilities but also if irresponsibility is evident at school.

This evaluation might also help determine if other problems are present that may only appear to be procrastination. For example, a youngster with an attention difficulty may have trouble concentrating on her homework; for this child, procrastination is not the problem. Treatment in this situation should be aimed at managing the attention deficit itself.

Early efforts to help children who consistently avoid responsibility are important for their future success.

TELEVISION AND OTHER MEDIA

Every day children are inundated by endless messages intended to educate, entertain, or influence their behavior. Many of these sounds and images appear in media with the explicit intention of selling a product. Others, such as movies, computer games, and music, are the product. Children in the middle years are frequent users of these products and important targets of advertisements. It takes commitment and effort on the part of parents to monitor and help interpret these external influences on children.

Television is the most pervasive medium and occupies a central place in the lives of millions of children. For these youngsters TV is a loyal companion that entertains and informs them day after day.

Almost every American household has a TV set, and in about half of these homes there are two or more sets. Although viewer habits vary, the average child in the middle years views two to four hours of TV each day. Many children watch TV for more hours than they devote to any other waking activity. Over the course of a year they spend more time with the television set than they do at school, playing sports, or with family and friends. By their high school graduation day they will have watched 15,000 to 18,000 hours of television, compared with 11,000 hours devoted to classroom instruction. Not surprisingly, during the formative school years TV affects children's lifestyles, values, health, eating habits, family interactions, sleeping habits, and selection of role models. Despite ongoing debate about whether TV viewing is harmful, one thing is certain—when a child is watching TV, he is not doing something else that could be more positive.

FAMILIES AND TV

Families lose important opportunities when TV viewing replaces time parents and children can spend together, and children lose out when TV substitutes for household responsibilities or is used as an alternative for healthy after-school activities.

Due to television, many families function differently than they did a generation ago. TV viewing has encroached upon many family activities—even on shared mealtimes. In some households family discussions are almost nonexistent. In many families there has even been an end to constructive disagreement, which can be a form of learning and a stimulus to problem-solving and character formation.

Thus, in too many homes, everything seems to revolve around television. Youngsters often say things like "I'll do my chores, Dad, after this show is over," or "I can't go out to dinner with the family now; my favorite program is coming on."

Ironically, some children are busier than ever, with many scheduled activities—soccer, Scouting, music lessons—and less free time. Yet TV, not the family, dominates whatever time remains. The TV set also draws youngsters away from their homework, often creating conflict and tension within the family. As a rule, homework and TV don't mix; if your child needs to study, the television set should be off.

PHYSICAL HEALTH AND TV

Do not overlook the effect that TV can have on physical health. Glued to the television set, children spend less time outdoors, cutting back on their exercise, and their fitness suffers.

Studies show that children who watch a lot of television are likely to be overweight, compared with their more physically active peers. While viewing TV, children often snack on calorie-rich salty or sugary junk foods. These

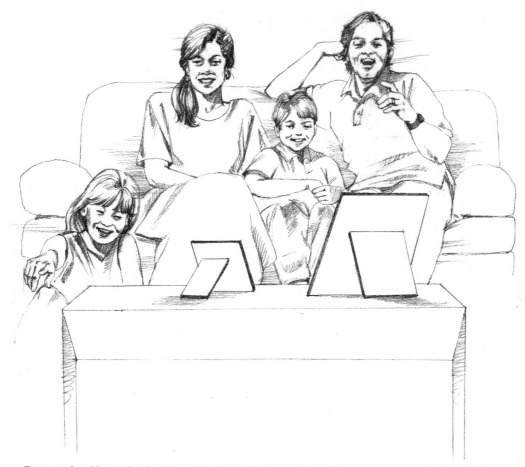

Parents should watch television with their children and use TV programs as springboards for family discussions.

snacks further serve to reduce their appetite for regular, healthy family meals. To counteract this problem, keep some healthy foods—perhaps carrot sticks and other low-calorie snacks—near the TV set. Even better, get your child outside for some physical activity.

LEARNING AND TV

There is a lot about television that concerns pediatricians, especially the passive nature of TV viewing. The next time your child watches TV, look at her instead of the screen and ask yourself, "What is she doing?" or perhaps more appropriately, "What is she *not* doing?" Sitting in front of the television set, children are giving up opportunities for more active intellectual, emotional, artistic, and physical growth. Instead of playing outdoors, reading a book, conversing, exercising, or doing homework, they spend hours sitting, entranced by what is on TV. Children learn best in the context of relationships and meaningful interaction with people they respect. In most cases, even in a group, television viewing is a passive, solitary activity.

Children who have learned critical viewing skills and who belong to families that actively select high-quality programs can learn from television viewing. For some children, especially young ones, TV can be a source of rote language. However, these circumstances are the exception. In general, while watching television, your child is probably not doing any of the following:

- Asking questions

- Solving problems

- Being creative

- Exercising initiative

- Practicing eye-hand coordination

- Scanning (useful in reading)

- Practicing motor skills

- Thinking critically, logically, and analytically

- Practicing communication skills

- Playing interactive games with other children or adults (helpful for developing patience, self-control, cooperation, sportsmanship)

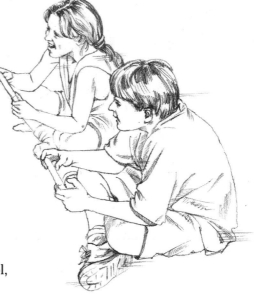

While parents often worry about television's negative influence, it can play a positive role in children's lives. If the programs a child watches are carefully selected, TV can provide her with good entertainment, exposure to other cultures, and positive social values. News programs can inform her about current events. Through special programs she can learn about the wonders of nature and the fascination of history. When the family watches together, TV can provide an opportunity for them to share time with one another.

Although there is some worthwhile television programming, you will have to look for it actively. Too much of prime-time television is dominated by programs that depict violence and aggression or promote family-role stereotypes that may not reinforce the values you hold. Many shows portray criminal activity or sexual promiscuity, with little or no attention to moral implications or dangerous outcomes. Some cartoons are designed to make it difficult for children to distinguish between fantasy and reality. Media glamorize harmful and dangerous behavior, especially the use of alcohol, tobacco, and other drugs. Music videos contain frequent references to or graphic displays of sexual behavior, drug and alcohol abuse, and suicide. Commercials and other advertising expose children to products that parents often do not approve of and cannot afford. They normalize and promote the adoption of unhealthy behaviors by children and adolescents.

Greater than any other single concern for many parents is television violence and its effects on their children. Studies suggest that TV, music video, and motion picture violence can cause antisocial behavior in youngsters and

WHERE WE STAND

Media, which include television, movies, magazines, advertisements, the Internet and computers, video games, and music, have an important influence on child development and behavior in our society. It can affect what children learn, how they view their world and how they interact with others. Research has shown that some media can be a public health risk factor to children and adolescents, leading to risk-taking behaviors, aggression, or negative attitudes about nutrition, sexuality, and self-image. Parents must realize the influence media can have and monitor children's exposure in terms of both quantity and quality.

Pediatricians, parents, and teachers should help children develop critical thinking and viewing skills about what and how things are portrayed in the media. When children understand that media are constructed to elicit a specific opinion or response, they become more critical of the messages they see and hear. Children who are "media educated" are less likely to be influenced by media messages and more likely to withstand potentially harmful effects.

Children are exposed to violence in television, movies, video games, and music. Media glamorize the use of guns and wrongly teach youngsters that it's all right to use violence to resolve problems. Children need to know that violence on TV and in the movies is not real. By watching television with their children, and discussing the content, parents can address objectionable content and use the medium as a springboard for family discussion.

Quality programming can both entertain and educate children, but too much TV viewing detracts from time spent reading or using other active learning skills. It also has been associated with obesity. The AAP recommends that TV viewing by children be limited to one to two quality hours per day.

make children more likely to hurt others, behave more aggressively on the playground, and display callousness toward other people's pain. It can also create fear and suspicion in young viewers. You need to be an involved parent, making a conscientious effort to minimize or eliminate your youngster's viewing of violence on television. (See the suggestions in the box on page 389.)

MEDIA EDUCATION: WHAT PARENTS CAN DO

You do not need to relinquish your control of the TV set to your child. Here are some suggestions to help you keep your youngster's viewing in balance:

- Set firm limits on the amount of TV your child watches. Keep his viewing to a preplanned hour or two daily. Ordinarily, homework assignments and household chores should be completed prior to TV viewing, but TV should not be used as a reward. Providing alternatives to TV—such as after-school sports, hobbies, chores, and family activities—can make the transition easier.

- Encourage and help your child to plan his TV viewing in advance. With your guidance he should organize his time and choose programs from the TV listings at the beginning of each week. Keep copies of the family viewing schedule posted in visible locations (by the TV or on the refrigerator) to serve as a reminder.

- Screen the television shows that your child watches. Sit down and watch TV with him, and when any depictions of sex, alcohol or drug abuse, violence, or negative stereotypes should appear, use them as springboards for family discussions, helping your child put them in context. Use TV to promote dialogue that can reinforce family values. Also, guide your children toward becoming more critical viewers by discussing the behavior and attitudes of characters, as well as the sales pitches in commercials: Children may want the toys and junk foods advertised on TV, but you can explain how commercials are aimed at persuading people to buy items they may not need or which may not be good for them.

- When good programs air at inconvenient times—perhaps educational programs telecast during school hours, or programs that conflict with family activities—videotape them (if you have access to the equipment) so your child can watch them at a later date. This will demonstrate your respect for his viewing rights and your willingness to honor the contract or agreement you have about his TV watching.

- Keep books and magazines in the TV room, as well as board games. Make regular trips to the library with your child and help him select books to read.

- Set an example of behavior you wish to instill. Parents are powerful role models. If you want your child to read more, that is what you should do. If you would like him to go outdoors for some physical activity, invite him to do so as part of an enjoyable family exercise program.

- Do not permit TV watching during dinner. The evening meal is often the only time that families are able to be together for any sustained period. If the TV set is on at the same time, it will interfere with or terminate conversation.

- Do not allow your child to have a TV set in his bedroom. Not only will he tend to watch more TV indiscriminately if there is a set in his room—with little if any parental monitoring of his program choices—but he will probably isolate himself there, thus reducing time with the family. When a youngster watches TV in his own bedroom, his viewing may also cut down on his sleep, causing problems with fatigue the following day at school.

- Pressure your local television stations to schedule programming aimed at children and to get rid of commercials you find offensive. Let the station managers know not only what you do not like, but also what you enjoy. Good programs often have poor ratings, but letters of praise can help keep them on the air. Organizations like Action for Children's Television (46 Austin Street, Newtonville, ID 02160) have taken an assertive role in trying to improve TV programming for children.

- If TV becomes a source of tension and conflict, simply unplug it for a while. Some families institute TV-free days or weeks. Children become very creative and are certainly more available when TV is not dominating their attention and time.

WHERE WE STAND

The primary goal of commercial children's television is to sell products—from toys to junk food—to youngsters. Young children in particular cannot distinguish between programs and their commercials, nor do they fully understand that commercials are designed to sell them (and their parents) something.

Television is also guilty of distorting reality on matters such as drugs, alcohol, tobacco, sexuality, family relations, and sex roles.

The American Academy of Pediatrics strongly supports legislative efforts to improve the quality of children's programming. The AAP also advocates for content-based TV ratings systems.

PETS

Whether they are dogs or cats, hamsters, fish, or parakeets, pets are found in millions of American households. Most families at least consider acquiring a pet, and for children an animal to love and care for can provide one of their most memorable experiences. The attachment to animals developed in childhood can last a lifetime.

By the middle years most youngsters are capable of having their own pet. Not only can they fully enjoy the animal, but they are old enough to assume some or all of the responsibility for its care. At the same time, the presence of a pet can teach important lessons about showing love, respect, sensitivity, and gentleness toward another living creature.

A youngster's self-esteem can also be improved by having a pet, largely as she recognizes that she is capable of handling the caretaking duties. She might also feel particularly good about herself if she becomes an "expert" on the type of pet she has and perhaps competes for awards in pet shows or 4-H programs. Pets can help children gain status or acceptance among their peers too.

Despite the benefits, you and your child should not take lightly the decision to adopt a pet. Make sure you and your youngster understand that the responsibilities associated with a pet are continuous—and if she commits herself to bathing the dog or cleaning the litter box, it is a long-term obligation, one that will probably last for years.

Also, while having a pet can be very rewarding, an improperly handled animal can be provoked to bite. Be sure that your youngster appreciates that keeping a live animal as a pet is a serious undertaking.

CHOOSING A PET

When selecting a pet, keep your child's developmental stage in mind. If this is going to be *his* pet—and thus he agrees to care for it—choose an animal whose needs can be met by your child. Some pets—like dogs or cats—require daily attention; they must be fed, groomed, cleaned up after, and exercised. Others—like fish, turtles, birds, guinea pigs, and hamsters—demand minimal care and may be a good choice for a younger child who needs to learn about what

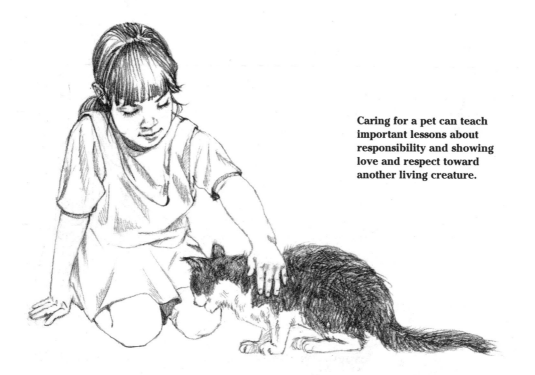

Caring for a pet can teach important lessons about responsibility and showing love and respect toward another living creature.

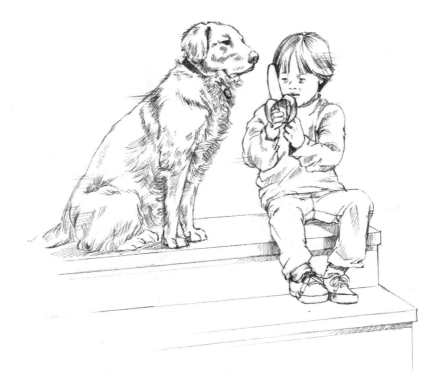

is involved in having a pet. A goldfish, for example, requires feeding only every two to three days, with its water changed only periodically; by contrast, a dog cannot be neglected for even a single day.

Also, some pets have easygoing temperaments conducive to being around children. For instance, dogs such as retrievers and beagles tend to be gentle with kids, while other breeds, such as boxers, German shepherds, pit bulls, Doberman pinschers, and miniature French poodles, may be more unpredictable. Keep the animal's characteristics in mind when selecting a pet.

The dander (shed skin cells, hairs, and feathers) of some animals can evoke allergic symptoms in certain children. If your child has allergies (eczema, hay fever, asthma) or your family has a strong history of allergic disorders, bringing a pet into the house may not be a good idea. Ask your pediatrician or a local veterinarian for advice.

Almost every type of pet is a potential source of disease that can infect your child. All reptiles, for example, can carry and transmit salmonella bacteria that can cause serious diarrhea. However, as long as your child practices reasonable hygiene, especially handwashing after playing with a pet and before eating, they should be safe. Children whose immune systems are suppressed, however, need to be especially careful, and generally should avoid most pets. Buy pets only from reputable breeders and shelters. Otherwise you increase the risk of purchasing an ill or diseased animal and endangering your child and yourself.

Before bringing the pet home, discuss with your child the needs of the animal and everything that is involved in caring for it. Books on pet care from the library or the pet store can help him understand what is expected of him. So can a visit to a friend who has a pet, where your youngster can see firsthand what care of a pet involves.

How should you react if your child loses interest in caring for the pet several weeks or months after the family adopts it? If he has made a commitment to be the primary caretaker but does not live up to that agreement, perhaps someone else in the family would be willing to take over the responsibility. If not, let your child know that you are unwilling to jeopardize the well-being of the pet because of his neglect, and unless his interest in the animal changes, you are going to find another home for it.

During this discussion do not accuse your child of any personal inadequacy ("You are too selfish to care for a pet"). Instead, be as logical as possible, saying something like "The dog needs a dependable caretaker, and you haven't followed through on your promise. We need to find another family who can care for him."

SAFETY AROUND A PET

Although most animals are friendly, some can be dangerous. More than any other age group, children between the ages of five and nine are the victims of animal bites; about 5 percent of youngsters of this age are bitten each year. Children nine to fourteen are next in line as the most frequent victims of bites.

When a new pet comes into the home—or if your child is sometimes exposed to dogs or cats in the neighborhood—make sure he knows how to minimize his chances of being bitten or scratched. Most often, a child is at risk if he teases, hurts, or plays too roughly with an animal. A dog might lash out to defend itself or to protect what it considers its territory or food. Incidents are rare in which a dog aggressively attacks when unprovoked. The box on page 397 offers some guidelines on how to reduce the chance of bites.

If your child is bitten by a pet or other animal, do not ignore the wound. Infections can occur—more often from cat bites than dog bites—and on rare occasions a particularly vicious attack by a dog can even be fatal. (For care of these wounds, see "Animal Bites," page 608.) Be sure any dogs or cats you own are fully immunized to protect both your pet and your family.

The bites of wild animals such as raccoons and bats pose a special risk of rabies, particularly in some locales. Bites by wild animals should be examined promptly by your pediatrician, and public health recommendations about treatment to prevent rabies should be followed. Often the psychological harm associated with an animal bite is at least as serious as the physical wound it-

Avoiding Problems with Animals

How can your child protect himself from attacks from his own or other pets? Here are some suggestions to talk over with your youngster.

- Do not pet or otherwise disturb a dog or cat that is sleeping or eating.

- Do not tease or abuse an animal.

- Never pet an unfamiliar dog or cat. Also, be cautious about touching puppies or kittens within view of their mother.

- When a child is approached by an unfamiliar dog, he should not run; that can often make the dog aggressive. Instead, he should refrain from making direct eye contact, slowly back away, and avoid sudden movements while still keeping the dog within view.

- If your child is riding his bike and is being chased by a dog, he should not try to pedal quickly away from it. Rather, he should stop the bike and dismount from it so that the bike is between him and the dog. Before long, the animal may lose interest in a nonmoving "target."

self. Once bitten—or even snapped at or growled at by a dog—a child may develop a lifetime fear of all dogs and other animals. If your child becomes afraid of your own dog because it has bitten her, point out that your pet is normally good-natured but can sometimes become angry if it is teased, threatened, or abused. Ask what happened that might have provoked your pet to bite. In the immediate aftermath of the biting incident, consider a cooling-off period for a few days, in which you keep the dog in the back yard or a separate part of the house to give your child a chance to calm down. After that, your child may have to adjust the way she behaves with the animal.

Teasing or maltreating animals is not only dangerous, it may be a symptom that your child is having some emotional problems. Purposeful maltreatment of an animal is a cause for concern and should be discussed with your child's pediatrician. If your child continues to tease animals after you have talked about it with her and made it clear to her that this is unkind as well as dangerous, your child may benefit from the counseling of your pediatrician or a mental-health professional. (See Chapter 16, "Seeking Professional Help.")

A PET'S AFFECTION

A pet's love is unconditional, and the bond that develops between child and animal can become important to both of them. Even when children are rejected by friends and are feeling lonely, they can still depend on their pet for acceptance.

Latchkey children—who come home from school to an empty house because of working parents—often rely on a pet for companionship and sometimes protection. Dogs, especially big ones, can be excellent guards. Be sure you choose the breed of dog carefully—a large, overly aggressive dog can cause great harm.

Pets are also often recommended for children with chronic illnesses and handicaps, serving as good companions for these youngsters. Some psychotherapists use animals as part of their treatment of disturbed children, employing dogs or cats as a way to teach love, friendship, and responsibility.

WHEN A PET DIES

The loss of a pet—either through death or because it has run away—can be emotionally traumatic for a child. If your family loses a pet, spend some time with your youngster, helping him understand his feelings and deal with his sadness. Do not make light of the loss or of his hurt. Share with him any sorrow over the pet that you may be experiencing. This is a good chance for you to teach him something about life and death.

Occasionally a child will feel guilty over the traumatic death of a pet, perhaps because the dog was not properly tied up. In cases like this be especially sensitive to what your child is undergoing. Do not punish him for his lack of responsibility; the consequences of his behavior are lesson enough.

Sometimes acquiring a new pet can help the child get over the loss of the old one. Explain to your youngster that while another animal cannot replace the pet that has died, it can become a new companion and something he can love. Let him help decide if and when the family should get a new pet, and let him participate in the choice.

CHOOSING A
SUMMER CAMP

Camp experience can be an important part of growing up. It offers a time for children to learn about themselves, other people, and about aspects of the world to which they might not normally be exposed. They meet and interact with new children, often from different parts of the city and state, and with different backgrounds. An overnight camp may also be a child's first experience being away from her family for more than just an overnight visit with a friend or a grandparent. Camp can be pure recreation, and it can be educational and a place to learn new skills and proficiencies. Some camps are designed to offer special and therapeutic experiences for children, helping them mature and learn to be more responsible for themselves.

Camp should be a time to learn cooperation and consideration for others. However, for some children it can be a stressful and unpleasant experience. Individual differences which have been unapparent or unimportant at school may become of concern to the

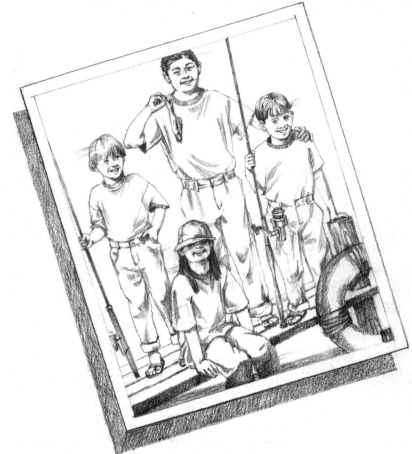

Camp provides opportunities to meet and interact with children from different places and with different backgrounds.

child and focused upon by other children and adults. Away from the security of their family and familiar surroundings, fears and insecurities can be magnified, and the camp experience may be unpleasant and sometimes traumatic.

Although middle childhood is the time when most children have their first camp experience, you need to determine whether and when your child is ready. She needs to have the physical and emotional maturity to live away from home for a week or two. Perhaps the key indicator of readiness is whether she is excited and enthusiastic about attending camp. Some camps are designed especially for younger children (ages six through nine) and thus are accustomed to giving some extra support to youngsters who may have some fears about being away from home for the first time.

Before your child decides to attend an overnight or resident camp, see how she does at a day camp first. If that turns out to be a positive experience, then you can start thinking seriously about an overnight camp.

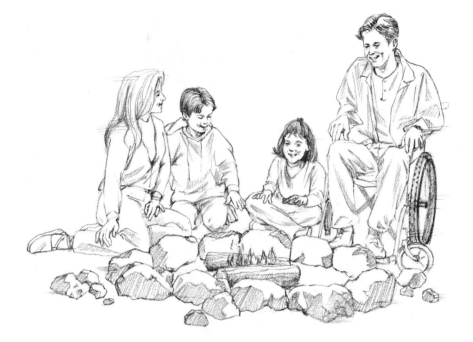

MATCHING YOUR CHILD TO A CAMP

There are probably dozens of summer camps in your area. Cost, of course, is an important consideration, and more expensive does not necessarily mean better. Your family budget will of course influence your choice of camps. Some very fine camping experiences are available at a reasonable price through the YMCA, the Scouts, and church groups. Send for brochures of the camps in which you are interested, and look at them with your child. If he has a particular interest—for example, if you think that he would have a special attraction to a camp specializing in sports or music—be sure to look into these facilities. Or if he has certain health problems—perhaps diabetes or a disability that keeps him confined to a wheelchair—there are camps devoted exclusively to these children, and which have medical personnel and facilities on-site to ensure that the needs of the youngsters are met. Your pediatrician can help you identify such specialized programs. Keep in mind that some camps "mainstream" children with health problems, mixing them with other children. Youngsters do very well in these settings; this approach provides valuable learning experiences for all campers, whether they have health problems or not.

As a parent, you are probably the best judge of where your child will be happiest and have the most valuable experience. Ideally, visit the camp and meet the camp director and counselors, and observe the activities that are available. Ask the camp director for the names of parents of past campers whom you can contact to get their impressions and advice.

There are other factors to take into consideration. For example, do the children attending the camp represent a mix of social classes and cultures? How structured is the schedule of daily activities, and how much freedom in choosing activities is best for your child? Also ask whether the camp is accredited by the American Camping Association (ACA), indicating that it has met or exceeded a set of standards that include staff qualifications, first-aid and other health care facilities, and transportation. Inquire about the staff's background and training, and the staff-to-camper ratio. The ACA ratio requirements vary according to the age and health of the children; for instance, for campers with severe mental disabilities, the ratio should be one staff member for each camper. For overnight camp, the recommended ratio is one staff member for every six campers in the seven-to-eight-year-old range; and a one-to-eight ratio for ages nine to fourteen. For day camp, the recommended ratio is one staff member for every eight campers in the six-to-eight-year-old range, and one-to-ten for ages nine to fourteen.

When investigating costs, be sure to inquire as to whether the camp fees are all-inclusive, or whether there are additional charges for laundry, accident insurance, special lessons, and so on.

GETTING READY FOR CAMP

Once the choice of a camp has been made, then it is time to prepare your child for her camping experience. The director of the camp you've selected should tell you well in advance what your child should bring with her, and what you will need to take care of in advance—for instance, a physical examination, an updating of immunizations, and health insurance.

As the time for camp gets closer, encourage your child to talk about what she expects camp to be like, and what she will miss being away from home. Let her air her anxieties, and reassure her that the camp's staff is there to make her comfortable and create an "at home" feeling. Remind her of the fun she will have, and tell her that because of your love for her, you want her to have this enjoyable experience. Also, promise to write her frequently while she's away, and let her know that you want to receive letters from her too.

Among the things to discuss with your child before she leaves for camp is your confidence in her judgment about people and new situations. Although she is there to learn and have more experiences, encourage her to trust her feelings and to resist joining in activities with other campers and counselors with whom she feels uncomfortable. If the opportunity is available prior to camp, or at the time you take your child to camp, take a while to get to know the people who will be caring for your child. As a parent, you should feel involved in your child's away-from-home experience.

Once your child has left for camp, be sure to stay in touch. In fact, it is a good idea to send your first letter to her *before* she leaves for camp, so she receives it on the first day or two that she is there. Tell her you are looking forward to hearing about all of her experiences.

If you are feeling a little guilty about sending her away for a week or two, keep in mind that homesickness is usually short-lived. Once she makes her first new friend and becomes involved in camp activities, her time away from home will probably pass very quickly. Most children adjust rapidly to their new surroundings and enjoy their camping experience immensely.

HOME AGAIN

It is important for you and useful to your child to talk about his camp experience. Encourage your child to tell you about his experiences, what a typical day was like, who his friends were, and how he got along with the staff. Find out what experiences were new, which were most rewarding, and which were difficult for him. Were there especially good moments? Were there bad ones? In particular, unpleasant experiences need to be understood from your child's point of view. Do not dismiss or minimize them. Acknowledge the importance of your child's feelings about them, and be supportive. Speak with the camp personnel if it seems appropriate.

WHEN BOTH PARENTS WORK

Not too many years ago in the typical American family, only the father worked outside the home. Usually the mother was the homemaker and was there to greet the children when they returned home from school each day. But there have been dramatic changes in that picture. Today, the mothers of nearly 76 percent of children over the age of five are in the workforce, and during workdays no parent is at home or readily available. During school hours most children essentially are being looked after by a teacher, and after school, before their parents come home, they may be cared for by another adult—in many cases a relative, a neighbor, or a commercial childcare facility. About 7 percent of middle-years children return from school to an empty house and care for themselves until their mother or father arrives. With most of their waking hours spent away from their parents, the quality of children's everyday experiences is difficult to predict and control.

Millions of families find that they need two wage-earners in order to buy a home, pay the rent, afford vacations, or simply to maintain the family budget. In most communities two-working-parent families are no longer exceptional.

THE IMPACT OF WORKING

When both parents are occupied with their jobs for eight or more hours per day, there are obvious effects on the family. On the positive side, the family has an increased income and thus fewer financial stresses. Also, when both parents work, there is a potential for greater equality in the roles of husband and wife. Depending on the nature of the parents' work, as well as the family's values, fathers may assume more responsibility for childcare and housework than has traditionally been the case. With their wives out in the workplace, men find it easier to define a greater role for themselves in child-raising. This is particularly evident when parents have staggered work schedules—for instance, if the father works daytime hours and is home after school and in the evening, while the mother works a shift such as 4:00 P.M. to midnight. Dad may then be in charge of preparing dinner, cleaning up the kitchen, and helping the children with their homework.

The Risks of Shift Work

Many families are feeling the stress of overcommitted and overscheduled lives. But few families feel it more than those in which parents work at different times of the day. When parents work different shifts and are not home together very often, a strain is put on their relationship and the family. Even more difficult are jobs that have rotating shifts—firefighting and nursing, for instance—forcing parents to work different hours each week; those schedules can prevent families from establishing routines and rhythms and can seriously disrupt family stability.

In these families, husbands and wives often have little or no time together. If they are lucky they have a day or two during the week when they are both off, but their sleep schedules may be so different that they still spend very little time with each other. These people essentially pass messages to each other, and their parenting may be hampered by a minimum of teamwork.

When parents work different shifts, children often sense that a problem exists. They rarely see their parents together, and they sometimes yearn for a "normal" family life. Parents in these situations have to work especially hard at giving their children the feeling that their family really is a unit, despite the difficult schedules. They need to make the most of weekends and vacations and support each other in areas like household responsibilities and discipline.

For some families, shift work is a solution to providing good childcare and supervision for children who would otherwise be left in the care of another adult or on their own. Such arrangements may provide a financial benefit to the family and a sense of comfort to the child.

CHANGING FAMILY ROLES

In two-income families, do men assume an equal share of the everyday responsibilities at home?

Surveys have shown that while many men are willing to help with the grocery shopping and cleaning up in the kitchen after dinner, they still perceive certain tasks as "woman's work," including cooking and doing the laundry. Thus, in these households, there are still some gender-based divisions of chores and responsibilities.

One study found that working mothers average eighteen hours per week of housework, plus ten to fifteen hours per week of childcare, while fathers average three hours of housework and two hours of childcare per week.

Even so, women who work outside the home report significant benefits associated with their jobs. They describe having higher self-esteem and a greater sense of autonomy. When a mother enjoys her work and gains a sense of satisfaction from it, her children can benefit, perhaps more than if she stays home but is unhappy. When women are bringing home a paycheck they often have more leverage in the family, encouraging greater participation by their husbands in keeping the household running ("I have a job too; let's share more of the responsibilities"). With their own source of income, women may not have to ask their husbands for spending money for their own needs and desires; the result may be a greater sense of independence in the relationship.

The husbands of working wives report that they have more respect for their spouses. And because there are two paychecks instead of one, men say they feel that providing the income for the family is less of a burden. With this decrease in financial pressure, many couples describe improvements in their marital relationship.

Nevertheless, families have adjustments to make when both parents work. Their dinners may become simpler than before. Children may eat less often with one or both parents, they may eat more quickly, and their diet may not be as nutritious or well-balanced. Some parents complain that dinnertimes seem more like meals in a restaurant than with a family at home.

Working parents also often sleep less than they once did, since they need to catch up on household duties in the late evening; women average six to six and a half hours of sleep per night, compared with seven and a half hours in the past. That can cause fatigue the following day, which in turn can affect their productivity and temperament both at work and at home.

Working parents may have less time for each other during the week too. If they do not consciously schedule time for each other and for their individual pursuits, these activities may get lost in the hectic pace of family life. As a result, marriage and family life may not seem as fulfilling. Relationships become more stressed, family members do not feel as close and as involved with one another, and family living can become less enjoyable.

When mothers are in the workplace, they sometimes feel guilty that someone else is assuming the daytime child-raising responsibilities, although that guilt tends to be less when their children are of school age, rather than infants or toddlers. Nevertheless, women are often torn between their careers and spending more time with their youngsters. And when they come home tired at the end of the workday, they may have less energy to give to their family, which can create even more maternal guilt. A University of Maryland study found that in 1985, American parents spent an average of only seventeen hours a week with their youngsters.

Even so, working parents—both men and women—frequently say they appreciate their children more than if they were home all day. Particularly if they enjoy their jobs, they say they look forward to spending time with their youngsters in the evenings and on weekends, even if they are fatigued.

One of the realities of a working parent's life is that he or she will inevitably spend less time with the children. Consequently, those few hours a day that everyone is together become extremely important. As much as possible, make them count.

HOW DO THE KIDS FARE?

When both parents work, some children feel neglected. No matter how hectic your life becomes, you need to set aside time each day for your youngsters. Let them know just how important they are to you, not only through words or gifts but through a commitment of time. Two-parent working families may have more money, but material things and access to costly activities are no substitute for a parent's time.

Encourage your children to talk with you about how your job is affecting your relationship with them; if they are upset that you are spending less time with them than in the past, you need to make an extra effort, perhaps by developing a ritual of having them call you at work each day at a certain time. Let them know you really want to hear from them each afternoon.

It's important to keep in mind that stress at work can find its way home. When parents feel overworked or unappreciated at their job, they may vent their frustration and anger at their children or at each other. And the way parents are supervised at work frequently becomes how they "supervise" their

---

Parenting Alert

When both spouses work, there are two particular aspects of parenting that often suffer:

Some parents become less nurturing or less emotionally available. Caught up in the hectic pace of their lives, parents may give their children a little less attention and loving care than they need. Set aside time each evening to show your children some affection. Bedtime is often a good time for that.

Some parents are afraid to set limits. Setting limits is an important component of gaining the respect of your youngsters. For children to grow into happy and secure adults, they need to be sensitive to your feelings and values and listen to what you say. If you see that they follow the rules you set, they will adopt many of your values.

---

children at home. If you have to abide by many rules and rigid policies at work, you may find yourself running a very structured household with lots of rules. Finally, parents tend to encourage their children to develop skills similar to those they use in their work. For example, parents whose jobs involve autonomy and creative problem-solving are likely to guide their children toward those same types of behaviors, while parents whose work rewards organizing information or materials may value those skills at home.

Some parents awaken their families a few minutes earlier each morning so that everyone can eat breakfast together and thus share a few minutes with one another as the day begins. In the evenings they turn off the television set and replace it with family activities like games, sports, music, and conversation.

A family with two wage earners can be a positive influence on children. Everyone—both children and adults—will enjoy some of the benefits. Boys and girls will tend to see the world as a less threatening place, knowing that both Mom and Dad are succeeding in the workplace; girls in particular perceive themselves as having greater career options if they have a mother who works. Children also tend to feel proud that their parents have careers. Depending on their after-school childcare setting, middle-years children also have greater exposure to other youngsters and new social experiences, which can contribute to their development.

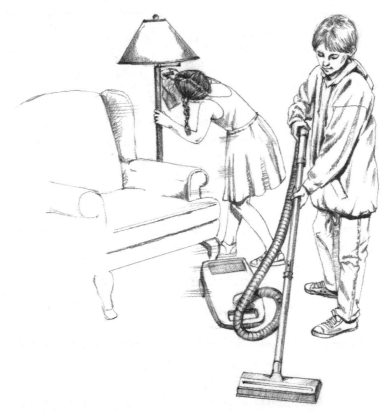

When both parents work, it is often necessary for all family members to assist with household chores.

AVOIDING BURNOUT

Some parents feel terrible strain and fatigue as they try to juggle their responsibilities at home and at work. If you are starting to feel burned out, here are some ideas to help you ease the pressure.

- Throughout your workday, fit some relaxing moments into your routine. Close your office door for ten minutes, shut your eyes, and perform a relaxation exercise. Or during your coffee breaks, forgo coffee and doughnuts and take a short walk instead. Diversions like these can reduce stress, improve efficiency on the job, and make you feel more vitalized when you return home in the evening, thus creating a more amicable family life.

- If you regularly come home tired, try to develop rituals that improve your frame of mind when you arrive home. This may mean spending some time by yourself in order to put a distance between you and the day's stresses. Coming home is an important moment that should be taken seriously.

Your children are eager to be with you and to share their day's experiences.

- Assess how you are spending your time during the day. Look for areas in which you can reduce stress. For instance, can you bring in dinner two or three nights a week? Can you hire a high school or college student to help for an hour or two in the evenings, perhaps doing the laundry or cleaning up the kitchen? If you can save a couple of hours a night this way, you will have more time to spend with your children and/or to relax or sleep.

- Involve the entire family in the evening responsibilities that are such a drain on your time and energy. For example, the family can work together to clean up the kitchen after dinner; with everyone's help it will get done much quicker and free up some time for you in the evening. Do the same on the weekends too: If the house needs cleaning, have everyone pitch in on Saturday morning; this will help build family cohesiveness while finishing the job faster, thus leaving more time for enjoyable family activities.

- Keep your expectations realistic. On certain evenings you might have to choose between going to the market and doing the laundry. Some tasks just may have to wait until the weekend.

- On the weekends, schedule some relaxation time for yourself. Go for a walk or go to the gym. Do some recreational reading. While family time is important and certain chores need to be done, time to unwind and recharge your own batteries is essential too.

FINDING GOOD CHILDCARE

During middle childhood, youngsters need supervision. A responsible adult should be available to get them ready and off to school in the morning and watch over them after school until you return home from work. Even children approaching adolescence—the eleven- and twelve-year-olds—should not come home to an empty house in the afternoon unless they show unusual maturity for their age.

Maturity is the key here and is a much more important criterion than age. Some fourteen-year-olds still require supervision; some twelve-year-olds can be trusted to come home, do their homework, and care for themselves responsibly.

When deciding whether your child can return home to an empty house after school, keep the following in mind: Studies show that preteenagers and teenagers who come home to an unsupervised house—so-called latchkey kids—are more likely to use alcohol and other illegal drugs. One study of five thousand eighth-graders (twelve- and thirteen-year-olds from a range of economic and ethnic backgrounds) concluded that children who care for themselves for eleven or more hours per week were twice as likely to consume alcohol, smoke cigarettes, and use marijuana as children who were supervised.

Although being physically present is the best way to supervise a child, sometimes that is not possible. If alternative adult supervision is not available, parents should make special efforts to supervise their children from a distance. Children should have a set time when they are expected to arrive at home and should check in with a neighbor or with a parent by telephone. Parents and children should agree upon a regular routine for the child that is written down and posted in a conspicuous place alongside emergency telephone numbers. Such a schedule might consist of having a snack, doing homework, feeding a pet, and setting the dinner table. On some days the child may have an after-school activity or go to a friend's house to play. Parents should always know where their unsupervised children are and what they are doing.

When evaluating childcare options, determine whether other family members can handle these responsibilities. For example, does a grandparent or other relative live nearby, and is he or she available and willing to help? Is there a responsible teenager—perhaps an older sibling—who can supervise your child for a couple of hours in the afternoon until you arrive home?

If you choose a commercial after-school program, inquire about the training of the staff. There should be a high child-to-staff ratio, and the rooms and the playground should be safe.

Also talk to personnel at your child's school and at the local YMCA about after-school programs, which are growing in number in many parts of the country. These programs tend to be structured, offer a variety of activities, and include time for homework. Many are reasonably priced.

If cost is an important factor, consider pooling resources with neighbors and hiring one mother to watch the children of a number of families. Or set up a co-op of several families in which each parent shares after-school childcare on a rotating basis.

Some companies now offer their employees flexible time schedules—perhaps allowing mothers and fathers to start work early so they can be home at three o'clock when the kids return from school. Some employees take work home with them, spending their last two job hours at their desks at home. Twelve-hour shifts, with four off-days each week, and part-time employment are other alternative patterns of work that some parents are finding suitable. These options can be effective solutions to the childcare problem for school-age children. Each family has its own needs and each must look for its own best circumstances.

MANAGING SCHOOL HOLIDAYS AND VACATIONS

Not surprisingly, some single and working parents have grown to dread school vacations, legal holidays (like Martin Luther King Jr. Day and Washington's Birthday), and "teacher in-service days." These are days when the child is out of school but parents usually have to be at work. To make matters worse, caregivers whom you might rely on at other times of the year often ask for time off during holidays, and community activities like art classes and Scouting often are cancelled too.

The good side of these situations is that you know they are coming and can plan for them. To help in that process, get copies of your child's school schedule as early as possible so you are aware of vacations several months in advance. Children's vacation schedules often dictate family vacation plans. With sufficient advance notice, you may be able to block out your own vacation time to coincide with that of your youngster.

Few parents have as much vacation time available as do their children, so arrangements have to be made for childcare and supervision within the framework of the demands of the parents' jobs. If your spouse has some flexibility in his or her work schedule, divide the home responsibilities so one of you takes time off during different parts of the children's vacation. Some couples are able to work out a plan where Mom is home in the morning, and Dad replaces her in the afternoon; perhaps one or both can work flexible schedules (6 A.M. to 2 P.M.; 2:30 P.M. to 10:30 P.M.) so that at least one parent is home at all times.

Fortunately, businesses are becoming more sensitive to the family needs of their employees. The federal Medical and Family Leave Act of 1993 is helpful to parents upon the birth or adoption of a child, or when a child is ill, but it does not have any provisions covering school holidays and vacations.

Sometimes neither you nor your spouse will be able to get off work. Or you will need a backup or alternative strategy for unexpected job demands or the sudden loss of a caretaker, both of which require some last-minute juggling of schedules. It is important that school-age children are always supervised, directly if possible and indirectly if not. Indirect supervision means providing a safe environment and a structured schedule of activities, including regular times to check in, even by phone, with a responsible adult. This latter option should be considered only for mature preteenagers and is never the preferred alternative.

When you can't break away from the office, another option is to call upon extended family members to help. Some parents are able to work out a timetable with several families, where each assumes the caretaking responsibilities for all the children one day a week, or they trade hours of babysitting with each other. Some high school and college students, or after-school child-care employees, are willing to work on holidays, perhaps coming to your home to assume the care of the children from several families. (Many high schools and colleges have job-placement offices to find employment for students on vacation; ask for and check references before hiring these young adults for childcare.) You may also inquire about special holiday programs and camps that might be planned by local YMCAs, Boys and Girls Clubs, and other community organizations. If none exist, gather some parents together and, as a group, urge local organizations or city leaders to provide holiday activities for children.

For some parents of school-age children, the best long-term solution is to work at home *all* the time, often in a small home-based business of their own. However, while this can be an ideal option, it is not available to everyone, and working at home poses problems of its own.

Making the Most of Vacations

Before your child's school vacations, do some planning to make them as enjoyable and productive as possible—for both of you. Here are some general strategies that can keep these holidays running smoothly:

1. Teach your child the magic of anticipation, looking ahead at what the next few hours or days hold for the two of you. Help him think positively about the upcoming school vacation time, without worries and doubts. If he has been disappointed with past holidays, he may feel unenthusiastic about what awaits him; but work to make things better this time, while instilling realistic expectations of what he can anticipate. Plan your vacation to be interesting for your child. Build on previous interests and offer some opportunities to learn something new.

2. Be playful at your child's level and interests. Let him make many or most of the decisions about what you will do together.

3. Make ordinary activities fun. Keep things relaxed, without allowing critical or analytical remarks to get in the way. Stay away from "hurriedness" and trying to do too much in too little time. Everyone enjoys some "down time" together, just taking walks or watching some special programs on TV with one another.

4. Don't feel the need to plan elaborate, expensive, or exhausting events and trips. Some parents, often envious of friends who may go on fancy vacations, feel obligated to overspend and overschedule. However, the most valuable gift you can give your child is time together, whether you are bike-riding, enjoying an ice-cream cone on a park bench, or putting to-

gether a photo album and telling stories about when he or she was younger. Your child wants attention from you, and even one fun activity a day together can be very satisfying for both of you.

5. A short, easy, and inexpensive "vacation" can be just a day and a night away. For example, if you feel the need to get away from familiar surroundings, try an overnight stay at a nearby hotel, where the pool, room service, in-room movies, or a nearby miniature golf course can make it into a special vacation. Enjoy the moment rather than comparing your activities with what other families are doing. Sometimes divorced parents try to outdo each other, often with the weekend parent feeling obligated to really do something special and expensive; this usually puts a strain on everyone.

6. Some families find that vacationing together and doing the same things each year become a valued ritual. Knowing what to expect allows more time for enjoying each other rather than fighting about how to solve new problems each day.

SEPARATION, DIVORCE, AND THE SCHOOL-AGE CHILD

W hen parents decide to separate, whether temporarily or permanently, there is an inevitable emotional and psychological impact on their children. Youngsters may mourn for the loss of the familiar family unit. They may be angry at their parents— or even at themselves, if they somehow feel they are to blame for their parents' problems. They might be so distracted by the family disruptions that their schoolwork suffers, or they may withdraw from friends. Children respond to divorce differently, depending on their age, sex, temperament, development, and experience, but in virtually all cases it has some consequences.

By some estimates 50 percent of all marriages will end in divorce, more than half in the first ten years of marriage. When children are involved (which occurs in about 60 percent of divorces), they tend to be young, often no older than their elementary-school years. Although 80 percent of divorced persons eventually remarry, these second (or third) marriages are more likely than first marriages to end in divorce as well. Thus, some children experience divorce in their families more than once.

Currently, about 20 million American children have experienced a divorce of their parents. In addition to formal divorces, some couples separate, then get back together, only to separate again when they are unable to resolve their differences. Just when the child gets her hopes up that the family situation is stabilizing, another split occurs and she has another adjustment to make. This pattern of repeated separations is quite difficult for children.

THE SIGNIFICANCE OF DIVORCE

Although separation and divorce are common, they are not a "normal" experience for anyone, particularly for children. No matter how amicable the divorce, children still view it as a loss when their families are torn apart. On rare occasions—for example, when one parent is physically or emotionally abusive toward the other parent and/or toward the children themselves—youngsters may welcome the divorce. But in the majority of cases children do not want their parents to separate.

Most child-health professionals believe that divorce is preferable to an embittered, conflict-ridden marriage, which can take a terrible toll upon children. On the other hand, few children will experience their parents' relationship as one of continuing bliss, and children develop normally in a household where they feel loved and where parents are at least respectful of one another. Regardless of the circumstances that lead to the decision of parents to divorce, it is a major disruption in the lives of children. Their initial emotional responses may vary: Younger children often describe sadness as their main reaction; older children say they are angry. Almost all have experienced a breach of faith and have a fear of what the future will hold.

For most children, the quality of their parents' marital relationship and the experience of their divorce colors their view of relationships and family for years to come. When they become young adults, some of these youngsters experience problems with relationships that they relate to their early life experience within the family of their childhood.

There are, however, actions that divorcing and divorced parents can take to minimize the trauma their children experience, assist them in adapting to their new circumstances, and help them achieve happy and satisfying relationships throughout their lives. If you are divorced, despite the difficulties you and your ex-spouse are going through, remember that though you no longer share a marriage, you continue to share parenthood. If the two of you, alone or with professional help, can put aside your marital conflicts and get on with your lives, your children will probably fare all right over the long term. The most important predictor of a child's long-term adjustment to divorce is the way his

Talking with Your Child About Divorce

When you and your spouse tell your child about your divorce, she will have many questions. More than anything she will want to know "Am I going to be okay? Do Mom and Dad still love me? Will they be able to take care of me?"

Here are some of the specific questions you might expect from your youngster or that you can bring up yourself.

- "Why are you getting divorced?"

- "Will we ever be a whole family again like before?"

- "Do you still love me?"

- "Was it my fault?"

- "Where am I going to live?"

- "Will I have to change schools?"

- "Will I still spend time with both of you?"

- "Will I be able to see my friends as before?"

- "Will I still be able to see both sets of grandparents?"

- "Will the family still have the same amount of money?"

- "Why can't things be just the same?"

parents adapt to their separation—specifically that the divorce ends the discord the child was experiencing.

WHAT SHOULD YOU TELL THE CHILDREN?

Children have a right to know about impending change in the family, particularly how it is going to affect them. But this kind of information should be saved until you and your spouse have made some final decisions and are able to provide the children with a structured plan and answers to most of their questions. Your youngsters should not be subjected to statements like "Your father and I are thinking about getting a divorce; we'll let you know what we decide."

If you and your spouse make the decision to separate or divorce, explain the situation honestly to your children. Ideally, both you and your spouse should talk with the children about the divorce at the same time. Discuss the situation in language they can understand. For example, if you have a child in the younger years of middle childhood, explain the situation simply and directly:

"Mommy and I have decided that we are going to stop living together. We don't know yet whether it's going to be forever or for a little while. We're getting what's called 'separated.' That means that Daddy will live in one place and Mommy will live in another. We've decided that we just can't live together right now. You are going to live most of the time with Mommy and some of the time with Daddy. But we both still love you just as much as we always have."

As you talk to your child, explain that despite the changes that lie ahead, everyone hopes that life will be better under the new family arrangement. For instance, if your child has been exposed to constant arguments in the home, she will not have to be subjected to them anymore. And as you and your spouse get a new start on life, the two of you will become better, happier parents in many ways.

Allow your child to respond with whatever she is feeling. She may be upset. She may cry. While some parents try to convince their children that they should not feel sad, this is unwise and is often an attempt to ease their own guilt about the impending family disruptions.

Here are statements to children that some parents have found useful:

- "Hearing about the divorce probably makes you angry."

- "Our divorce seems to make you sad."

- "You probably have a lot of strong feelings about Mom and Dad right now."

These "active listening" statements from parents may give a child who is experiencing divorce an opportunity to express herself with thoughts and emotions. When such statements are followed by a brief period of silence, the school-age child is more likely to respond.

You might find that your child is not surprised by the impending separation or divorce at all. By the middle years of childhood, most youngsters are sensitive enough to family dynamics to realize that problems exist in the marriage, and they are probably familiar with divorces in the families of relatives or friends. Your own child may have heard you or your spouse make threats about divorce in the past. She may even have already verbalized her fears about divorce ("You and Dad are going to get divorced, aren't you?").

When choosing the best time to have this discussion—whether at the time of the separation or several days or weeks beforehand—take into account your youngster's maturity level. A five-, six-, or seven-year-old has a frame of reference that extends no further than a week or two into the future, and she may become confused if you are talking about a separation that won't take place for a month or longer. You can give an older child a little more advance notice, allowing her a chance to think about and adjust to the changes ahead and to ask questions. Expect the questions to continue. Most children cannot quite comprehend and adapt to the issues the first or second time they hear them. Additional questions will occur to the child as she grows older and reconsiders what has happened.

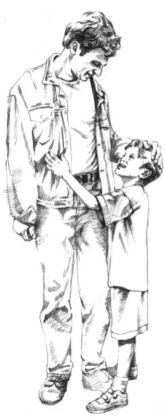

Children cope better with divorce when they have an ongoing relationship with both parents.

ADJUSTING TO THE CHANGES

When a divorce occurs, the family generally moves through a series of stages: In the *predivorce* period, as spouses argue and the distance between them grows, children may be caught up in the marital conflict, either directly or indirectly, and may exhibit acting-out behavior like fighting, disobeying, talking back, and crying for no reason. Then, during the *separation* phase, as one of the spouses leaves the household, children in the middle years may feel quite insecure with the disruptions in their daily routines, with one parent no longer around to pick them up from school, help them with their homework, or tuck them in at night.

As the initial turmoil subsides, the *adjustment* period begins, and children start to cope with their new life circumstances, including new routines, visiting schedules, living arrangements (two homes instead of one), and perhaps a mother who has gone back to work. Frequently, the income and financial resources of the custodial parent (usually the mother) decrease during this time. This economic hardship can make the child's emotional adjustment to divorce even more difficult, particularly if his parents argue a lot about financial matters (and about other issues too). Failure to pay child support is an all-too-common occurrence that can place stress on the entire family and prolong the adjustment process.

Sometimes parents are so caught up in grieving over the loss of their marriage and what it represented for them that they are paralyzed into inaction. Professional help may be necessary to get the family's adjustment and recovery back on track.

Next, during the *reorganization* period, both children and parents reach a new equilibrium and the youngsters feel more stable. Finally, *remarriage* may force new adjustments, with children feeling insecure until they sense that their parent is still emotionally available to them.

Through these stages, youngsters will experience many emotions, including anger, sadness, loneliness, embarrassment, disappointment, fear, and a sense of betrayal. Each of these emotions needs to be recognized, accepted as real, and discussed between parent and child. Youngsters need to feel free to express these feelings within the family.

All children have fantasies about their parents' reconciling. This wish may last for years, representing their desire for the family to be whole again. It is a sign of their loyalty to both parents. Accept this wish without ridiculing it ("Oh, that's so silly!"). It is a normal part of the process of coming to terms with the divorce.

An older child in the middle years may ask, "Did you and Mom ever love each other?" You can respond by explaining that people's feelings change over time. "When you were born, things were better between Daddy and me. But things have gotten more difficult, and we couldn't make them better."

Children may pose questions like "Why didn't you work it out?" or "Why did you let him leave?" They may blame one parent or the other for the divorce. If this happens, acknowledge your child's hurt and anger, and tell him: "That may be the way you see things, but there are other ways to look at it. Sometime when you are not so angry, let's talk more about it." You do not need to become defensive or to go into the details of why your marriage did not work.

On occasion, children blame themselves for what is happening. The five- or six-year-old may feel that he somehow caused his parents' divorce ("They're getting divorced because I was bad"). The child who is a little older may understand that he was not the cause of the divorce but may blame himself for being unable to make things better ("I failed in trying to keep Mom and Dad together").

While you may already have tried to reassure your child that the divorce is not his fault, do not demand that he stop blaming himself. Instead, say something like "I believe you did your best to keep us together." Or "I know you are disappointed, but there is nothing you could have done." Let him know that the divorce was beyond his control.

In the weeks and months ahead, keep the lines of communication open. But while you should invite your child to talk, do not force the conversation if he is not ready. Youngsters in middle childhood are doing a lot of analyzing and intellectualizing of their own and may not always be ready to share what they're thinking. They need to go through the grieving process as they experience and learn to accept the loss of their original family structure. Sometimes a hug is more important than words. In general, older school-age children are more verbal than younger ones, but if your child has always tended to be withdrawn and quiet, he will probably continue to be that way through the divorce. In times of stress, children's usual ways of interacting may be accentuated. In any case, always make yourself available for discussion ("I know you're upset; would you like to discuss it?").

Some parents feel so guilty about the divorce that they will impose less discipline upon their youngsters during this time. However, if your youngster is angry and acting out, you need to set limits and not give in ("I know you're angry, but that doesn't mean you can break your toys or throw things at your sister").

If he is younger, your child may have periods when he seems to be regressing, when sadness and anger that he hasn't exhibited in months resurface, or when he becomes afraid of the dark or asks for help in tasks he has already mastered such as brushing his teeth or doing his homework. Tolerate this behavior for a while, and reassure your youngster that you are still there to care for him.

Sometimes a child's birthday, a special holiday, or a vacation may trigger emotions related to the divorce that he hasn't felt in a while. The necessity to change schools may do the same. In general, children take about six months to a year to move through the postdivorce adjustment process, although a variety of emotions may resurface from time to time thereafter.

Whenever problems occur, try to deal directly with the specific causes. For example, if he's concerned that you and he are not going to have as much money to live on, explain that you're still going to be able to afford what is necessary to live a comfortable life, even if he sometimes might have to do without the most stylish T-shirt or tennis shoes.

Some factors will help your child cope better with your separation or divorce. If he has a sibling he can share the experience with, this can help. Sibling relationships can provide considerable support, because brothers and sisters can understand one another's feelings and reactions on a level that others may not. Research shows that siblings tend to become closer as their parents go through a divorce. However, if siblings fight more during and/or after the divorce, and this problem does not subside on its own, it may be a signal that professional help is warranted.

Relationships with grandparents, aunts, or uncles also can be stabilizing for middle-years children. Give your child access to these relatives, and do not make him feel guilty if he wants to see your former in-laws, for example. If you do not feel comfortable letting him go over to their home, invite them to drop by. But do not deny them access to your child.

Keep in mind that extended-family members often feel awkward talking with you about the divorce and expressing their concern. Give them suggestions on how they can be supportive of your child. For instance, invite them to take your youngster to the park or for a drive. Encourage them to call as often as they would like. Even though you and your ex-spouse are divorced, your child is still a member of both families and should be able to maintain his status within those family units.

Your child may have friends whose parents are divorced, and he may already be talking with them about his experiences. Children from divorced households often compare notes about their experiences and give one another advice, even at this young age. Some communities have formal support groups for children of divorced families, which can make a youngster feel he is not the only one in these circumstances. Although this peer support will not remove the pain that may accompany divorce, it can minimize the shame or embarrassment that youngsters often feel.

Your child's attitude toward you and your spouse may change over time. He might feel a loyalty conflict between the two of you, particularly if you and/or your spouse are trying to pull him to one side of the conflict or the other. Or he might reject the parent he blames for the divorce. In this case, allow your child to have these feelings but still encourage his relationship with that parent. Eventually he will get the message that both of his parents still love him.

Your child may also ask himself: "How can I belong to two people who don't love each other?" Eventually, however, if both parents continue to care for him appropriately, he will recognize that both his mother and father love him.

Although some of your child's emotions—anger, for instance—might be directed at you and your spouse, he may be hesitant to express them. As much as you'd like to know what's going on inside, you may not be able to help ease every hurt. Respect your child and his feelings, and allow him to pick the people (friends, grandparents) he wants to use for support.

MAKING THE DIVORCE
LIVABLE FOR YOUR CHILD

To help your child move through the divorce process as smoothly as possible, keep the following issues in mind:

• Try to make your divorce as amicable as possible. If you and your ex-spouse continue to argue over everything from your divorce settlement to child visitation, this ongoing conflict is going to interfere with the healing process. Both of you should be willing to make some compromises for the sake of your child, and do not overreact to every issue that remains unresolved between the two of you.

Whenever possible, avoid a lengthy legal battle, which can frighten and demoralize your child. Many states require divorcing parents to meet with a mediator before custody suits are heard; try to resolve these matters out of court to save everyone time, money, and aggravation.

Some research suggests that joint custody tends to be a more favorable situation for children than sole custody, but this is true only if both parents can maintain open communication, tolerate their differences, and work cooperatively as a team. Often joint custody arrangements, which force the child to shuttle back and forth and adapt to two households, cause distress and interfere with the child's social life.

• Try your best to understand the feelings of your youngster and your ex-spouse without attempting to change them. Think of your former spouse as a co-parent, and try to maintain a relationship in which you can talk with each other without a lot of discomfort. This may take some time and patience, but eventually you want to be able to work *with* your ex-spouse in raising your child, not to remain adversaries.

Initially, most divorced parents find it easier to discuss parenting issues by phone, since face-to-face contact may raise the emotional climate to uncomfortable levels. But whether you choose to have these conversations by phone or in person, you and your ex-spouse will need to discuss your expectations of each other and establish some ground rules for communicating through the postdivorce period.

At the outset the most important issues to deal with are visitation and access to your child. Make a schedule of when the noncustodial parent will call and visit. At the same time, you and your ex-spouse should set up a regular schedule for speaking by phone about issues pertaining to your youngster; by routinely keeping in touch with each other, the two of you can deal with your child's problems before they become crises.

Of course, these discussions should not only be about problems but should also involve sharing observations about the events in your child's life. As trust builds, you will find it easier to discuss issues related to school, health, morals, religious values, and other important matters. With time you can work out a reasonable co-parenting relationship.

• Respect your child's relationship with her other parent. Allow her to spend time with your ex-spouse, without making her feel guilty because she enjoys doing so. She needs to have a relationship with both her father and her mother. Remember, one of the most important factors in helping children cope successfully is an ongoing relationship with both parents. No matter what you personally may feel about your ex-spouse, unless he or she is abusive to your youngster, it is better for your child to see both parents *regularly* rather than to have only intermittent contact, or none.

If you are the custodial parent, it is your responsibility to persuade the non-custodial parent to maintain this contact with your child. If your ex-spouse breaks off his or her relationship with your youngster, seek professional help yourself to find ways to reach out and include the noncustodial parent in your child's life. Sometimes, former in-laws can help encourage an ex-spouse to take the parenting role more seriously. Court-ordered visits tend to be resented by children and do not promote positive relationships.

• Define clearly for your child any changes in her role in the family. If you are going back into the workplace, for example, you might say, "I need you to be more cooperative with Mommy, and that means helping me a little more. When we get home after I pick you up from day care, I need your help in setting the table for dinner." However, do not make your child feel that he or she has to assume a parenting role—that is, avoid statements like "You are now the man in the family" or "Now I have to depend on you."

Sometimes, you and/or your child can benefit from some emotional first aid during and after the divorce. If you are feeling overwhelmed by the changes in your life, or if your child has long-term difficulties adjusting to the new circumstances, talk to your pediatrician for a referral to a mental-health professional.

During the grieving process every child may have some difficulties—for example, a B student may get C's in her classes for a while. However, if she is cutting school, getting into fights with classmates, and not completing enough work to get even passing grades, then she may need some counseling. Extreme aggression, experimentation with drugs or sex, or signs of depression (irritability, withdrawal, apathy, poor sleep, loss of interest in usual activities) also are signals of a need for help.

The therapist may recommend treating you and your child together on matters that involve both of you. He or she might also suggest that your ex-spouse participate in therapy when problems affecting your youngster are discussed.

The ultimate outcome of divorce for your child depends a lot on how well you can resume a routine life and a normal parenting relationship with your child.

SINGLE-PARENT
FAMILIES

S ingle parenthood can be one of life's biggest challenges.* Seemingly overnight, women and men may find themselves assuming the responsibilities of raising their children on their own.
Although in some ways these new parenting circumstances can be
just as satisfying an experience as sharing parenting with a spouse,
there are problems unique to single parenthood.

More than one fourth of all children in the United States live with
only one parent. Most single-parent situations result from divorce,
but some school-age children have experienced the death of a parent. Others may have been adopted by an unmarried individual.
Children born to a mother who was never married accounted for
36 percent of all children in single-parent families in 1995.

* Because most single-parent households are headed by women, this chapter has been
written primarily from the mother's point of view. However, most of the issues discussed
apply to single fathers as well.

SINGLE PARENTHOOD: SOURCES OF SATISFACTION

Although single parenthood may be a dramatic change from the life you once had or imagined, it can be a workable, rewarding family situation. Particularly when it occurs in the aftermath of a divorce, it may be a more desirable circumstance than the tumultuous marriage that preceded it. Many single parents describe the contentment they feel in having put the tension and dissension of their marriage behind them, and in making a new life for themselves and their children.

Most single mothers work. If they weren't already working before their divorce, most enter the workplace during the postdivorce period. Although looking for work and finding a job to support the family can be stressful, most single mothers report that they enjoy the autonomy associated with bringing home a paycheck. In many cases they also enjoy a strong sense of satisfaction from their jobs.

As children see their mothers succeeding in the workplace, they often develop more respect for them. The children of working mothers also usually have a broadened view of what women can accomplish in life; not surprisingly, then, girls raised in single-parent households tend to see an expanded range of occupational opportunities for themselves later in life.

Although a single mother's work schedule may reduce the amount of time she spends with her children, those hours together tend to become much more precious for everyone. Single parents often develop closer relationships with their children than do parents in more traditional, two-parent families. Other relationships may become more important, too, such as the children's connections with their uncles, aunts, or grandparents.

THE PROBLEMS OF SINGLE PARENTHOOD

These are some of the issues you may experience:

Supporting Your Family

Unless you are receiving alimony and/or child support from an ex-spouse, you are probably the sole source of support for your child. And that can create stress. You and your youngster may be living on less money than when you were married and will need to do some belt-tightening. Some working mothers volunteer to work overtime at their jobs, or take on a second part-time job, in order to make ends meet. Until you find a job that can provide some financial security, economics can be the overriding concern in your life.

This means that your school-age child may see less of you and have less money to buy things he was accustomed to having. That can stress your relationship with him and can add to his resentment of you for getting divorced. Make sure he understands your economic realities and that you need to work more than you would like. Reassure him that even when you are away from him, you think about him. A routine after-school phone call to him from work may ease the distance he feels between you.

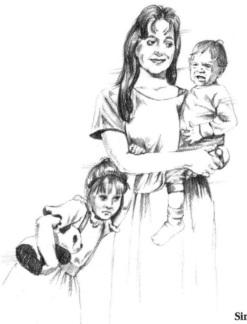

Single parenthood can be one of life's biggest challenges.

Task Overload

A single parent's responsibilities certainly do not stop the moment work ends each day. You may have what seems like a full day's worth of tasks awaiting you at home—from cooking dinner to doing laundry to helping your child with homework. Although these same obligations are faced by working mothers who are married, a single parent has to face these responsibilities alone, without the helping hand of a husband.

For that reason, many single parents feel chronically fatigued. They often feel physically and emotionally exhausted and find themselves yelling more at their children. As their youngsters move through middle childhood and normally become more opinionated and challenging of their parents' points of view, more arguments may develop.

Unless single parents set aside some down time to rest and recuperate, they can experience burnout and depression, feeling hopeless and helpless about trying to transform their lives into something more manageable. Having a little emotional support or help around the house from another adult can go a long way toward helping you to cope.

Reduced Time and Energy for Personal Pursuits

Single parents often feel they have no time for themselves, whether it is to exercise at the gym or to have dinner with friends. Even if they can find time for these individual pursuits, they may be so tired that they have no energy for them. Being deprived of sleep will take a toll on anyone, parent or child. Sometimes the best that you can do for yourself and your child is to get more sleep each night.

For some single parents, during or after the divorce, their lack of energy is dramatic and part of a more serious depression. Persistent sadness, irritability, difficulty sleeping, and weight gain or loss are all signs of depression. A depressed parent has much less to offer a child. If you are depressed, speak to your physician or a mental-health professional.

When Children Become Burdens

Single parents sometimes begin to perceive the responsibilities of child-raising as overwhelming. Even the most routine events in their child's life—carpooling, events at school, or normal oppositional behavior—become burdens for parents struggling to squeeze everything into their day. Single parents experience a great deal of tension and sometimes guilt that comes with not being able to attend to all of their child's needs or to provide all of the opportunities they wish their child to have. At the extreme, these parents feel they can't deal with their children anymore. They may resort to physical punishment and even become abusive if they are pushed too far. Or they may give up altogether and agree too easily to their children's demands. When possible, they may need to turn over more of the child-raising responsibilities to the youngsters' other parent and perhaps get some professional counseling to help cope better.

Childcare

Single parents need to make sure their youngsters are cared for appropriately when they are at work. For middle-years children, many options are available, from commercial childcare centers to after-school programs sponsored by community organizations like YMCAs and Boys and Girls Clubs. Babysitters can also give single parents a break to pursue their own interests for a few hours a week. Sometimes employers or various programs will pay part of the cost of childcare for working parents. (For more information, see Chapter 36, "Babysitters and Other Caretakers.")

Decreased Involvement with the Noncustodial Parent

If you are the primary caretaker of your child, you might find that your ex-spouse has gradually decreased his contact with your youngster. After about the first year following a divorce, many fathers stop seeing their children on a regular basis—and sometimes altogether. That increases the pressure on single mothers and interferes with the child's long-term adjustment to the divorce.

Fathers drop out of parenting for a number of reasons. Since they are no longer in the house, they may feel they have become less important and influential in their children's lives. They may become so dissatisfied with the noncustodial role that, out of frustration or anger, they may decide to give up parenting altogether. In some cases fathers may abandon their fathering responsibilities because they can no longer afford child support. Sometimes they do it in order to avoid paying child support. Or they might have remarried and, in starting a new life, feel they have less time—or no time—to devote to the children of their former marriage. Some fathers feel unwelcome and struggle with how to proceed in developing a separate relationship with their child.

If you are a noncustodial parent, you should remain actively involved in your children's life. In general, youngsters from divorced families who maintain a relationship with both parents tend to be better adjusted than those who have contact with only one parent.

How much time should you spend with your child? As much as possible, given your living arrangements. If you live close to your youngster, maintain regular contact, preferably both during the week and on weekends. It is a good idea to have your child spend at least one night a week at your home in order to give him a sense of his place in your life. This avoids you (the noncustodial parent) developing into a "good time pal" who only visits him to have fun. It also enables him to receive guidance and regular discipline from you.

If you don't live near your child, you need to maintain regular contact via telephone calls, and you should plan visits for extended periods of time (that is, weekends and holidays) so that you both have the chance to stay intimate. Children can accept and adjust to these schedules if they are given appropriate explanations, and if they perceive that they are still important to the non-custodial parent.

Intensified Involvement with the Custodial Parent

Particularly if the noncustodial parent begins playing a smaller role in the child's life, the parent he lives with may develop even stronger ties to the youngster by becoming more emotionally involved and perhaps even overdependent. Sometimes this intensified relationship can be a positive influence upon the child, provided it remains within reasonable bounds and allows the child to pursue friendships and activities outside the home. It can become harmful, however, if the youngster assumes too much of an adult role in the family and therefore gives up his own separate life and privacy for the sake of the parent. This may happen if the single parent asks him to take on more responsibilities around the house or to become the parent's confidant. If parent and child become too closely enmeshed, perhaps because both are lonely in the aftermath of the divorce, their relationship can become so intense that other relationships cannot develop for either of them. At the same time, it may become harder for the parent to maintain authority, even over simple matters like what time the child should go to bed.

While a close relationship with your child is encouraged, avoid the situation in which you are virtually spending all your free time together. Your child is not an adult friend. Both of you need your own friends and outside interests. In some cases, when parent and child have become closely intertwined, jealousy and resentment can surface when one of them develops other relationships—for instance, the daughter who, as an adolescent, finds a boyfriend and leaves her mother home alone on Saturday nights. Such closeness can be confining.

Changes in Children's Behavior

A child's difficult behavior in the aftermath of his parents' separation tends to be temporary and will probably diminish as the crisis of divorce subsides. However, there are a number of troublesome behavioral patterns that, if persistent, are signs of more serious problems. Boys and girls in middle childhood often respond differently in these situations as they adjust to living in a single-parent household. For example, boys may become very aggressive after their father moves out, making it difficult for their mother to assert her authority.

In this situation mothers need to work hard to maintain their authority as soon as this behavior becomes apparent, or matters could get out of control as the child's aggressiveness escalates. At the same time, fathers need to be informed of the child's misbehavior and should support the ex-spouse's position as an authority figure. A phone call or a face-to-face conversation can often be part of this process. Fathers, however, should not be called in to rescue their ex-wives, since this will tend to undermine the mother's authority position and could even cause additional misbehavior by the child as a way of forcing more contact with his father.

Occasionally, boys will develop some of the departed father's behavior and assume a husbandlike relationship with the mother. They may begin to comment on the mother's appearance, try to offer financial advice, become jealous if she starts to date, and otherwise attempt to assume an adult role in the family. Girls, by contrast, tend to become more reserved and withdrawn as their response to the changing family structure. They also sometimes assume a maternal role in relation to their mother and siblings. An eleven- or twelve-year-old girl may actually run the household while her mother is working, which can rob her of her childhood while creating an unhealthy relationship between her and her siblings. If the girl is living with her father, she might also develop some of the departed mother's behavior and function as a "wife" to her father. These are not healthy patterns.

To reduce the stress on an older daughter, involve the grandparents and extended family in helping out; alternatively, when financially feasible, hire a part-time housekeeper to assume some of the household responsibilities. The younger children in the family can also begin taking responsibility for more chores.

WHEN YOU START TO DATE

After the divorce, how soon should you start dating?

Most middle-years children need some time to adjust to their parents' separation before their mother or father begins having new romantic interests. In general, a good guideline is about a six-month wait from the time you separate from your spouse to the time you start to date, although dating will often occur sooner. You should talk with your child about your new adult friends. Allow your youngster to express her feelings and opinions.

Here are some other suggestions to keep in mind:

• **You don't need to introduce your child to all your dates—only to those with whom you are developing a serious relationship.** Although your middle-years youngster may be curious about a man you are going out with, she might form an attachment to him before it is appropriate to do so. She may want you to marry this man immediately in hopes of creating a new, more traditional family unit. Be sure to explain to your child the differences between dating, developing a relationship, becoming engaged, and getting married; she should understand that not all dating and friendships end in marriage.

Also, discuss with your partner the best time for him to meet your youngster. Do not put pressure on your boyfriend to meet your child before she feels ready to do so.

• **Prepare both your boyfriend and your child for their first meeting with each other.** Tell your youngster about this man, and explain why you like him. (Is he smart? Is he fun to be with? Does he have a good job?) Then say something like "I was thinking that you might like to meet John. Would you like him to come over for dinner, or would you like the three of us to go out to dinner together?" Show her that you would like her to participate in arranging this first meeting.

Also, tell your boyfriend about your child. Describe what the youngster likes to do, what sports she enjoys, her hobbies, what she likes in school, and other information you think might help your boyfriend approach her.

• **Don't expect miracles during that first encounter.** There may be some anxiety during the first meeting between your boyfriend and your child. But the goal of that get-together should be only to say hello—not for the two of them necessarily to like each other. Don't rush things. They will need to develop their own relationship over time. Discourage your boyfriend from trying to impress your child, or from attempting to get too close too quickly.

• **Help your child deal with any negative feelings she has.** Sometimes children may see their mother's new love interest as a threat to their fantasy that she and her ex-spouse will someday reunite. When this man becomes a serious enough part of your life that you are introducing him to your child, you also need to deal with any unrealistic ideas your child has ("Daddy and I are divorced, and we really are not going to get back together again").

Your youngster may still prefer her father to your new boyfriend. But with time, she might come to see this new man as a nice fellow with whom she can be friends and have fun. Any jealousy she feels over your dates with another man will probably be resolved after an initial period of adjustment.

Also, let your child's father know that you will be introducing the youngster to your boyfriend. Your child should not feel that this is a secret she has to keep, or that she will have to be the one to disclose this information to your ex-spouse, which she might find painful to do. Children should not be keepers of secrets.

• **Show some discretion about intimate relationships with your boyfriend.** Children learn about the adult world through example—particularly from parents. As you develop a relationship with a boyfriend, keep in mind that your child is learning about intimacy at the same time. Open age-appropriate communication during the development of a sexual relationship with a close friend will allow your child to experience a new level of awareness about grown-up behavior. But direct exposure to frankly sexual conduct is not a good idea.

When school-age children are exposed to these new relationships, they need a clear statement from you about your feelings toward your new friend and your wish to be close to him, and also about the differences between adult relationships and those between children or adolescents. When you have a discussion with your child about a new intimate relationship, encourage her to express her feelings, good and bad, and help her feel comfortable with asking you questions about your new friend and the ways in which you relate.

PARENT-CHILD DISAGREEMENTS

If you and your child are increasingly at odds with each other, creating more stress in the household, you may not have anyone else to turn to for support, now that your ex-spouse is out of the house. If you are beginning to feel overwhelmed by this situation, here is a strategy for regaining control:

Stop arguing. Step back from the problem at hand and try to understand what is really at issue between you and your child. Then, without operating in the heat of the disagreement, try to clarify with your child what is preventing the two of you from getting along with each other.

Perhaps changes in the family circumstances will force both of you to make adjustments. Calmly explain the new situation now that your child's father is no longer living with you. For example: "We cannot afford a housekeeper any longer, so I need your help in keeping your room clean." Or "We just can't afford to send you to soccer camp this summer, but you can get together with your friends at the neighborhood recreation center."

Avoid arguing about situations in which there are no options. Your child may complain that he can't go to the summer camp he would like to, but your budget simply may not make any other choices possible. He needs to understand that everyone in the family has to adapt to the new demands brought on by the one-parent family. Help him take part in the problem-solving; use these trying times as learning experiences.

Parents often become upset with themselves when they are not able to give their children everything they would like, and that sense of failure can cause tension in the household. Single mothers and fathers may need to adjust their expectations about what their child needs in order to be happy, keeping their expectations realistic in order to minimize the amount of stress in their lives.

Children are quite adaptable and will rise to the occasion if you give them the opportunity. The more often you and your child can sit down and talk, the better. Involve him in discussions of what each of you would like to see happen in the future, taking into account your changing circumstances. It is better to *talk regularly*, as well as when issues arise, rather than yell at each other when you reach an impasse.

As one single parent told his child: "When you and I don't agree on something, let's sit down and try to understand what our disagreement is all about. Then let's both try hard to come up with a solution." (For a discussion of family meetings, see page 336.)

GET SOME SUPPORT

It is hard to raise a child on your own. So don't be hesitant to ask for support. Your parents, siblings, and other relatives and friends might be able to care for your child for a few hours a week. So can babysitters. Many parent groups can provide support and information about single parenting, and their meetings are often listed in newspapers or in community and church publications.

In many ways, both you and your child will have to assume new responsibilities and adapt to new schedules. At the same time, do not make too many demands on your youngster, particularly those that may steal part of her childhood from her. Children should have fun, and growing up in a one-parent household does not have to detract from that.

STEPFAMILIES

About 10 percent of children are living in stepfamilies, and the number is growing. Due primarily to the high rate of divorce and remarriage, children often find themselves sharing a household with a new stepparent and his or her children.

Most stepfamilies function quite well. Even so, there are potential problems when two families merge into one.

THE POSITIVE ASPECTS OF STEPPARENTING

After many months or years of single parenthood, mothers and fathers are often relieved to remarry. Most find comfort in the traditional family structure, with two parents under the same roof. In these blended families, mothers and fathers can turn to each other for support and share parenting responsibilities—a welcome relief for some-one who has been handling the parenting chores alone.

Although it takes time and honest effort, stepparents and their stepchildren can develop a genuinely positive regard for one another, and the new family can provide an enriching experience for everyone. Along with a new stepparent may come new stepbrothers and stepsisters, and a new extended family. These relationships require some negotiation, but they broaden each child's experience with people and may introduce him or her to new cultural and ethnic influences. Also, there may be some improvement in the new family's financial situation, as remarriage may make two incomes available to support them.

BECOMING A STEPFAMILY

When you and your new partner are ready for a more committed relationship, discuss these plans with your children to prepare them for the changes that are about to take place. If you are planning to get married, your youngsters will want to be part of any celebration. The wedding ceremony itself is generally a positive experience for children, one in which they should be given a special role. The more that children feel a part of the process of becoming a step-family, the better things will go for all concerned.

Next, a new household will be established, and the blended family will learn to live together. This is a period of establishing who you are, what you are willing to share, and what each individual's role in the new household will be. This process takes some time, conscious effort on the part of all family members, especially the parents, and occasionally some outside help. From the child's perspective, the new stepparent is a "guest in the house." The stepparent needs to develop his relationship with the child gradually and independently from his relationship with the mother.

Once the transition period is over, people settle into routines much as any other family does. Later, there may be changes and transitions that can force adaptations in family life—for example, if the remarried couple has a new baby of their own, or an older child leaves for college.

The success of stepfamilies depends on a number of factors, but especially the quality of the new marriage. If the new spouses begin having difficulties with their own relationship, that will affect nearly every aspect of family life, including how the children fare.

As the children themselves adapt to the new family arrangement, some will do better than others. Sometimes, the fit between stepchild and stepparent is a good one. However, there are many opportunities for problems to arise. Perhaps the child is jealous of the new man in his mother's life. Or he may resent the intrusion of stepsiblings into his home. Sometimes members of the blended family have minimal tolerance for their differences, creating dissatisfaction and tension that can undermine the family's equilibrium.

WHAT YOUR CHILD IS EXPERIENCING

"I'm getting remarried. I think my children are as excited about it as I am."

Maybe so. For a child, remarriage may have many positive aspects, although she may be looking forward to very different things from what her parent is. However, there are also some difficulties that can arise as members of two families begin living under the same roof. Here are some of the most common concerns for school-age youngsters:

Dealing with Loss

As their parents date, develop serious relationships, and eventually decide to remarry, children may be reminded of their original family and of the life they once had with their mother and father. Now, however, with the prospect of this new marriage, they must confront the reality that their parents really are never going to reconcile and that they will never again have their original family back. This can be a source of great sadness.

There are other losses to deal with as well. Children who have built a particularly close relationship with their own mother or father during a period of single parenthood must now learn to share that parent not only with a new spouse but perhaps with stepsiblings whom the youngster barely knows.

As the middle-years child experiences this kind of loss and pain, she may show signs of increased attachment to the parent who is getting married. For instance, she might not want to leave the parent's side in certain social situations; or she might express jealousy when her parent shows attention to the new spouse and his or her children. She might even verbalize some of her hurt and anger ("I don't think he's the right guy for you, Mom").

Some children wonder to themselves: "Where do I belong?" As they see their parent starting a new family, for example, they may feel more like an outsider than part of the new family structure.

With time, however, most children adjust to their new family circumstances. As they get to know their stepparent and stepsiblings better, their level of acceptance will grow too.

Divided Loyalties

Many children feel that if they like and show affection toward their new stepparent, they will be demonstrating disloyalty or a lack of devotion to the natural parent whom this new stepparent, to some extent, is replacing in their home. They may worry that if their mother or father remarries, thus bringing a new father/mother figure into the household, they will lose the love and attention of their other parent.

Your child may still feel awkward for a while, having to get used to two fathers or two mothers. Particularly in the beginning, allow her to view your new spouse in the most comfortable way for her—perhaps as a second father but sometimes just as Mommy's husband. You need to reassure her about these concerns, saying something like "Your stepfather is different from your daddy, and no one will ever replace your own daddy."

Along the way, you can expect your child to make some comparisons between her real parent and stepparent, in both positive and negative ways. She might blurt out statements like "You're not as nice as my daddy." Comparisons are normal during this adjustment period. Eventually, your child will stop making them.

If possible, father and stepfather, or mother and stepmother, should make contact with each other to begin working toward talking comfortably about your youngster. This can begin with a phone call just to say hello and to share observations of the child. Both parties might decide to have lunch or some other informal meeting. Although these two adults may run into each other at special events, such as birthdays and graduations, these occasions may not be opportune times to do much talking.

The more comfortable these two individuals become with each other, the more reassured the youngster will feel that she does not have to choose between the love of her parent and the developing relationship with her stepparent. It will show the child that the adults are pulling together on her behalf, and that they all care and have her interests at heart.

Do not expect your child to solve her loyalty conflicts if you have not resolved your own differences with your ex-spouse. For example, when remarriages occur, the issue of child custody often resurfaces; if a noncustodial father marries a woman with children, he may return to court, requesting that his own youngster now live with him ("I have a wife at home now and I can take care of my child"). In the midst of an ongoing custody battle, the child will find it much harder to deal with her own loyalty conflicts.

Difficulty with New Rules

As children move from a household with a single parent into one that is occupied by a stepparent and perhaps stepsiblings, they will probably be confronted with changes in the way their family operates. Routines will be altered and new chores may be imposed. With more people in the home, privacy issues may become more important. It may be harder for children to carve out a personal space they can call their own.

In a sense, the entire household is in transition, and everyone—including the children—needs to participate in the reorganization and adapt to the way it runs. The majority of family members adapt, but it may take some time.

Unreasonable Expectations

Virtually all couples want their new marriages to be as perfect as possible. Hopefully, having learned from past experiences, they can achieve their expectations. However, within stepfamilies it is unrealistic to hope that the children will immediately respect and love their new stepparents. In the real world, relationships develop more slowly. Children need time to really get to know and feel comfortable with a stepmother or stepfather.

In general, good relationships develop most quickly with younger children. Older youngsters, who are more set in their ways, may rightly feel that their established lifestyles are being disrupted by this new man or woman entering their life.

STEPSIBLINGS

One of the most challenging aspects of a blended family is for the children of each parent to become comfortable living together as brothers and sisters. Children who are brought into the same household with minimal preparation and are expected to function as a congenial, loving family are unlikely to succeed. Storybook relationships may appear to be developing in those first few weeks of getting to know one another, but this is generally only a honeymoon period until the children feel comfortable enough to express their disagreements and conflicts with one another.

As with any siblings, there will probably be some competition between the children in stepfamilies, much of it for their parents' attention. Stepsiblings should not be expected to spend all of their time together, and in fact each child will need some time spent just with his or her own parent.

This is particularly important for the youngster who may live with her

Who Will Handle the Discipline?

All children need discipline. But in stepfamilies, parents often are unsure of who should administer it. Should a stepfather, for example, discipline his wife's children, or should she be the only one to handle it?

Too often, stepfathers attempt to assert authority and directly discipline their stepchildren, rather than letting their wives take the lead with their own youngsters. Particularly in the initial few months, stepparents should play a supportive role in discipline but allow their new spouse to continue being the primary disciplinarian. They should avoid sweeping statements like "From now on, we're going to do things this way!" The new couple should gradually make a transition to shared authority. This transition can be accomplished by a delegation of authority from the biological parent to the stepparent, saying something like "While you're with him, you need to mind what he says—or answer to me."

After years of single parenting, many mothers may welcome having a male authority figure in the house. However, his presence does not relieve her from the responsibility of being the primary caretaker of her own youngsters. If her new husband becomes too assertive in parenting his wife's children, the children may resent him and complain to their mother about their mean stepfather. She may find herself caught in the middle between her husband and her children as conflicts escalate. And if she takes her spouse's side, her youngsters may feel betrayed. It is a position that can and should be avoided.

Also, if the new husband and wife disagree on disciplinary issues, the child may begin undermining and challenging the stepparent's authority, which is not good either for the child or for the marital relationship. When parents disagree this way, they need to negotiate their differences, or problems will escalate.

Over time, stepfathers will develop a closer relationship with the children of their spouses, and they can eventually begin to assert more of their own influence. But at least initially, it is not appropriate for them to become the primary disciplinarian of someone else's children.

mother and whose father remarries. The child may recognize that her dad is now spending less time with her than with the stepchildren who live with him. She may think, "Why do they get to live with Dad and I don't? Does he like them better? I don't get to do as much with my dad anymore because of them."

Children in this situation should have some special time with their fathers on a regular basis. Parents must acknowledge and respect this need, finding afternoons or entire weekends that they can devote solely to their own children, who may live across town or in another part of the state.

Other problems can occur with stepsiblings who live together. Sometimes a child is asked to share a room with a stepbrother or stepsister when, in the past, that same room was hers alone. Or when her stepfather's children come to visit him on the weekend, they may move into her room for a couple of days, sometimes creating anger and jealousy.

Privacy and personal space become important issues in blended families. Whenever possible, children should have their own rooms. Even if they share a room, however, each youngster should have her own toys and other possessions; she should not be forced to turn them all into community property.

In some cases, the remarried couple will have one or more babies of their own, who will become the existing children's half-siblings. While most school-age children generally like having a baby around, they may also complain about the drawbacks. A newborn is often the center of attention of family and friends, and that means a loss of focus on the older children. More important, the older children may feel jealous that their father or mother is starting a new family, and that the baby gets to live with both of her parents, while their own parents are divorced. Even so, most new additions to the family are treated with love by the other children. (See Chapter 35, "Sibling Rivalry.")

With time, stepsiblings tend to become good friends and companions, and their relationships are enriching and rewarding.

SOME ADVICE FOR STEPPARENTS

Stepfathers and stepmothers sometimes feel like throwing their hands up in despair. "I'm really trying to get along with my spouse's children," they may say, "but they just won't accept me."

In most blended families, children challenge their stepparents from time to time. Some youngsters may become openly aggressive; others may keep an emotional distance from their stepmother or stepfather. If this happens in your family, don't take it personally; it is the child's way of testing you and perhaps dealing with his own feelings over having a new adult in his life.

If your stepchild criticizes you, don't overreact; this will become less common as the months pass. In general, the older the child, the more critical and judgmental he is likely to be of you as a stepparent. While letting him express his feelings, you can be comforted by the fact that, if you are fair and making a sincere effort to get along, the negative feelings will eventually be outweighed by more positive ones. It is a sign of progress and a developing relationship that he feels comfortable enough with you to voice his feelings.

To build some bridges, find some interests that you and your stepchildren share, and invite them to join you in these activities. You might hold regular family meetings to pull together on some issues and to iron out differences. (See page 336.) Above all, treat your stepchildren with respect, and you will ultimately win their trust.

Sometimes the difficulty children have within stepfamilies is really a continuation of their anguish over their parents' divorce. Children's responses to the divorce of their parents can take many forms—and those feelings are not easily or quickly resolved. They may linger and then disappear, only to resurface in times of stress, especially the stress present when relationships, like stepfamilies, are formed or broken.

Over the long term, if children are unhappy in stepfamilies, it is frequently because of marital problems between their parent and stepparent. More than one third of children who enter into a stepfamily later experience a breakup of that family. When children sense that their mother or father is unhappy in the new marriage, they are frequently unhappy too.

If you are starting to have difficulties with your spouse, get some counseling to try to smooth out problems before they become serious ones. Also, in most communities, support groups are available to help remarried couples and their children deal with the various issues that can arise in stepfamilies.

45

WHEN YOUR CHILD IS ADOPTED

T oday about 1 percent of the children in the United States are adopted. If you have adopted a child, you are aware of some of the dissimilarities between your family and most others. You certainly prepared for your child in a different way—not with a nine-month pregnancy, but rather by going through the lengthy legal process involved in adoption, usually preceded by years of trying unsuccessfully to become pregnant yourself. Your child has biological relatives outside of your family somewhere in the world. You also have recognized that your youngster is not like you in some ways—that is, her eyes may be a different color, her race may not be the same as yours, and her temperament might be different. She might be outgoing and you might be quiet and reserved; you might be more intellectual, while she might be more athletic and physical. Of course, these latter differences are ones that occur in all families, but they may have special meaning for adoptive parents and their children.

If you did not adopt your child at infancy but rather during the preschool or elementary-school years, her upbringing before you became part of her life could present some problems. Some children may have been denied affection, or even basic nutrition or medical care, in their prior living environment. Others may have been physically abused and thus may have emotional scars from that experience. In some cases a lot of tender loving care is enough to put these children back on track; in other instances children and family members may benefit from some counseling with a mental-health professional. The long-term consequences of these early experiences are often difficult to predict.

No matter what the reasons for and circumstances of the adoption, most of these children are well-adjusted and happy. Nevertheless, adoptive families often feel different and sometimes socially isolated. Indeed, these differences are real, and there are issues unique to the adoptive family that need to be acknowledged and addressed. Like most adoptive families, your own family can learn to deal with them well.

EXPLAINING ADOPTION TO YOUR CHILD

For some parents, telling their child that he is adopted is a formidable, anxiety-provoking task, and thus they put it off or avoid it. However, at some point adopted youngsters need to be told about their origins, ideally even before middle childhood. During their preschool years, children begin asking questions like "Where do babies come from?" That is a good time to begin introducing information about their special backgrounds.

What should you say? Make your explanation simple, direct, and honest. Explain that he was not born to you. Tell him that he was born to other parents who could not take care of him. Then describe why you chose to adopt a child. Talk about how much you and your spouse wanted him, and briefly explain the process you went through to get him.

Allow your child to ask questions. For example, he might want to know "What happened to my first mommy and daddy? Where are they?" You can share a little bit of that information with him, but there is no need to go into too much detail. Your comments should answer his questions in ways appropriate for his maturity level. At the time of the adoption you should have been given some basic information about your child's biological parents—from medical issues (a family history of heart disease, for example) to personal characteristics. (Was the father tall and athletic? Was the mother artistic?) Someday you will want to pass along all of this information to your youngster. One useful way to address all kinds of adoption questions is with a "life-book," a scrapbook of all of the information you have about his past. This can be very helpful to a child with a complicated past of multiple moves. This book can be "read" in more detail to the child as he matures.

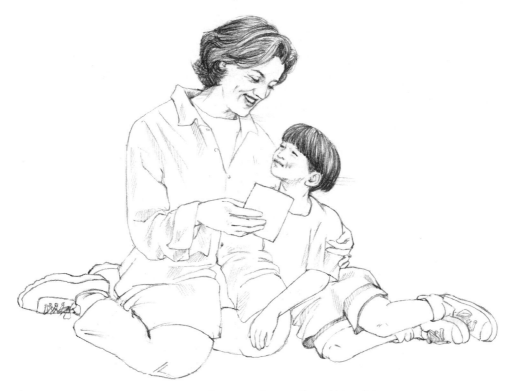

Every adopted child needs to have an honest understanding of his origin.

If your child is already of school age and has not been told that he is adopted, you need to talk with him about it, as early during this time of life as possible. Adoption should not be a secret. Every youngster needs to have an honest understanding of his origin. Adopted children who have not been told seem to sense that somehow they are different; this nagging intuition can influence their self-image. The longer you wait, the harder it will be to discuss it with your child. Also, he is liable to find out from someone else—perhaps by overhearing the conversations of relatives, or from teasing by neighborhood children who have learned from their own parents that he is adopted.

If you have waited until the middle years of childhood to tell your youngster that he is adopted, he may be upset, but that is a natural reaction. Allow him to express his feelings. Talk about why he is sad or angry, and let him know that you acknowledge and understand those feelings. Remind him that you and your spouse love him, that this is his family and always will be.

Often parents who are reluctant to tell their youngster about the adoption may have difficulties of their own in accepting that their son or daughter is not their biological child. Sometimes they might feel ashamed or inadequate because they could not have children of their own, and they avoid explaining the adoption to their youngster so that they will not have to revisit that issue.

Sometimes parents are hesitant to talk about the adoption because they are trying to be protective of their child's feelings, sensing that he might be hurt at finding out he was adopted. They might also be afraid of being rejected by their adopted youngster. They might think, "What if my son says, 'I don't want to live with you anymore; I want to go live with my real mommy'?" That, however, is an uncommon reaction, and not one that children are really serious about pursuing.

Keep in mind that it is important for the child to know about his adoption by the time he enters school. Your honest communication about this important issue early on can strengthen the relationship you have with him, building a strong bond of trust. So if you have any apprehensions about telling your child, try getting beyond them.

After you've told your child, he will have more questions about it in the days, weeks, and years ahead. His questions are normal and do not reflect a lack of affection toward you. The more your child talks about it with you, the more comfortable he will feel with the idea, and the stronger his relationship will become with you.

Your answers to these questions should be direct but still sensitive to the emotional maturity level of your youngster, and what he has already learned and understands about the adoption. Do not dismiss these questions and concerns, but do not overreact to them either. Acknowledge the fact that his family situation is different from that of many or most of his friends. At the same time, do not magnify the significance of his special circumstances, nor dwell upon them. Your child's basic needs are the same, regardless of whether he is living with biological or adoptive parents, and most aspects of his life will be the same as those of his peers.

If your child becomes quiet about the adoption after you have talked about it, give him some time alone with his thoughts. Then, if he hasn't raised the issue again within a few weeks, you might say something like "Since we talked about the adoption, you haven't said anything more about it. You must have some feelings about it. Do you ever think about your other mommy and daddy? Do you have any other questions you want to ask me?" Make sure he feels as comfortable as possible with the way he became part of your family.

You should not leave it to your child to continue the conversation. Raise issues naturally and gently. For example, at his birthday you might say, "I wonder if your birth mom is thinking about you today? She would be proud if she knew you." Another time you might comment on a physical characteristic, as in, "I bet those broad shoulders came from your birth dad. I remember when I met him. . . ."

There are some normal stages through which your adopted child is likely to pass. During the ages of five to seven years, for example, he may understand that he has "two mothers" and "two fathers," but the social customs and the full meaning of adoption are probably still a bit unclear. He is likely to ask questions about why his birth mother did not keep him. And he may have anxiety-generating thoughts like "Since my first mother left me, maybe my second one might too."

When your adopted child is a little older—between the ages of seven to nine years old—he will develop a better understanding of being adopted. You can expect to be asked specific questions about his biological parents. In a sense, he will be trying to construct a more accurate "memory" of his original family, which of course is really just a fantasy about his first mother and father and how he came to be adopted.

Later in the middle years—during ages nine through twelve—all children, including those who are adopted, become increasingly concerned with their appearance and fitting in. Your adopted youngster may become more curious about and sensitive to differences in his own hair color or eye color if it differs from your own. He will also become even more interested in his biological parents, and what his original cultural origins may have been. Expect many more questions about both his biological and adoptive relatives, and his family tree.

"SHARING" YOUR CHILD

As you raise your adopted child, she is yours in every sense of the word. At the same time, however, there is an aspect to her life—the fact that she has biological parents elsewhere—that may make it necessary for you to "share" her at some point with her past.

The majority of adoptions of older children and many infant adoptions are "open," and the adoptive parents have met or even know the birth parents, who may live nearby. Sometimes birth relatives have continuing contact with the children.

During middle childhood your youngster will probably have questions, fantasies, and feelings about her biological parents. Most adoptive families can deal with these matters well. Children at this time tend to feel more psychological and emotional conflict about being adopted. At various times they may test and challenge their adoptive parents with statements like "My real parents wouldn't . . ." But adoptive parents often become anxious if their child says this. During the school-age years, children sometimes say such things in the heat of an argument, to manipulate their mother and father and to try to get their way. Don't panic over these kinds of challenges; they are a normal part of your child adapting to and accepting her unique family circumstances. Nonadopted children test their parents with similar kinds of statements too.

In adolescence and young adulthood, your child may become interested in learning more about her biological mother and father and even may consider searching for them. This may be a function of curiosity, or she may want to get

> ## *Discipline and Your Adopted Child*
>
> Some parents are hesitant to discipline the child they have adopted. They may set fewer limits than they would for a birth child. They might react less strongly to misbehavior.
>
> What are the reasons for these patterns of parental inaction? Some adoptive parents are afraid their youngster might stop loving them if they disciplined her. Or they may doubt their own right or ability to parent this child fully.
>
> If that is your attitude, you are not fulfilling some of your parenting responsibilities. One of your tasks is to help your child grow and mature by disciplining her and helping her adjust to the limits you set. You need to look at the obstacles that may be preventing you from assuming this parental role, such as being fearful of losing her affection to a birth parent who is in close proximity.
>
> Keep in mind that even though you did not give birth to this boy or girl, he or she is your child. That means you have the right and the obligation to say, "It's time to go to bed now," or "No, you can't have your brother's toy right now." Your child's well-being depends on your willingness and ability to function as a full parent.
>
> If your child ever says to you, "I don't have to mind you; you're not my real parents," respond with a statement like "We *are* your real parents. We just aren't your biological parents." A parent is someone who parents and who loves his or her child, and that is what you have been doing for years.

a sense of completion about her own identity. There are avenues available for pursuing this search, usually through support groups, state-mandated confidential intermediaries, or the adoption agency or lawyer. Although you might feel threatened by her desire to learn more about her birth parents or even to meet them, remember that her interest is normal and appropriate for her developmental stage. We all want to know where we came from, and what our roots are. Most adopted children and young adults understand that they do not really belong with their biological parents.

Children from Other Countries

A significant number of families adopt children from other countries. If you have made this conscious decision to become a multi-racial or multicultural family, there are things you can do to assist your adopted child's adaptation and development. You have the responsibility as a parent to instill in your child pride and knowledge about his ethnic origins. This will also help give him tools to combat discrimination and stereotyping.

Here are ways you can incorporate his heritage and customs into the family:

- Have multiethnic toys, clothes, objects, artwork, food, and music in your home as a part of daily life.

- Follow news and events and celebrities from his country of origin.

- Visit ethnic restaurants, stores, cultural programs, and exhibits as an ongoing part of family life—not as special events.

- Make adult friends in the ethnic community as an example of how you value your child's origins.

- Select nonadoption, multicultural books to read to your child or to give to him or to the school library.

HOW HAVE YOUR RELATIVES REACTED?

When you adopt a child, it is important for your relatives to accept him as a part of the family. Most do, but unfortunately there are exceptions to the rule.

For a child to feel loved and welcomed, he needs to be treated like a full member of the family. If your parent, brother, sister, or other relative has difficulty relating to your child as part of the family, you need to talk with this relative about it. Explain how important it is for your child to feel accepted. Do not settle for anything less.

SIBLING RIVALRY

Some families are composed of both adoptive and biological children. And that can sometimes create conflict, anger, and hurt feelings. Remember, all children will find reasons to argue.

Each child in your family should understand her own origins, and those of her brothers and sisters. But no matter what her background, every youngster should be treated the same by you, your spouse, and the other siblings.

Sometimes academic or athletic differences between your children can seem exaggerated because of their different origins. For instance, if your adoptive child does not do as well in school as your biological child, their differing backgrounds can heighten any tensions that might emerge because of their respective school performances. Having a chronically ill or physically impaired child in the home will add to the usual stress within families. Sometimes the adoptive child may feel "different" to begin with, and if her sibling excels in areas where she doesn't, she could feel that she is less than a full member of the family.

With all of your children—whether they are adopted or biological—look for their strengths, and focus on those as much as possible. As one mother told her child: "Yes, you are having a hard time with math right now. But I know you will be able to learn it. And there are many other things you can do that make you very special."

As you raise your adopted youngster, keep in mind that adopted children are, first and foremost, children. In the same way, adoptive parents are parents. There is a lot of joy and satisfaction in raising children, and your relationship with your adoptive child can be as deep, loving, and long-lasting as any parent-child relationship.

A DEATH IN
THE FAMILY

By school age, children understand that death is an irreversible event. Yet even though youngsters recognize that death is something more than going to sleep for a long time, they still may have many unanswered questions that they may not verbalize: Where did grandmother go when she died? What is she feeling? Is she in pain? Why did she die? Can we ever see her again? Are you going to die too? Who will take care of me if you die?

Offer opportunities for your child to ask these questions. The more clearly and honestly you answer them, the better he will fare through the grieving process.

The reactions of children to death are highly personal. One child might quietly and sadly express his grief. Another might become rambunctious and oppositional. Still another might become extremely anxious. Youngsters often take their cues from watching the reactions of other family members, particularly their parents. In some families, death is a taboo subject, and children sense that they

A Child's Reaction to Death

What can you expect your child's response to be to the death of someone in her life?

Death of a Pet. If a child is attached to her pet, she may find its death quite difficult. Even so, this event will prepare her for later encounters with death by giving her some understanding of the experience.

Death of a Grandparent. When a grandparent dies, children may not find it as devastating as the loss of a parent or a sibling. To them, their grandparent is an older person, and when people get old, they often die. However, if the grandparent has provided day-to-day companionship for the child, perhaps even living with the family or residing nearby, the death will be much harder.

Also, with the passing away of a grandparent, children often think, "Now that my daddy's daddy is dead, does that mean that my daddy is going to die next?" If you sense this kind of reaction, reassure your child that you and your spouse are healthy and will probably live for a long time.

Death of a Parent. Whenever a child loses a parent, the event is traumatic and alters the course of her development. You cannot protect the child from what has happened, but you can help her face the reality of it.

If you are a surviving parent, in addition to dealing with your own feelings of loss, you need to help your child through this experience. Expect reactions ranging from regression and anxiety to anger and depression.

should not talk about it; in others, death is discussed openly, and children feel comfortable expressing their sadness.

Some adults believe that children should be shielded from death. They keep children away from funerals. They try not to cry in front of their youngsters. They may make up stories in an attempt to protect children from pain ("Grandma had to go away for a long time; we won't see her for a while"). They may avoid all discussions of the deceased.

Despite the good intentions of these actions, they don't work and are counterproductive. As with most topics, communicating with children about death

Be honest and open about what has taken place. Provide your child with a lot of comforting, both verbal and nonverbal. Reassure her that you are not going to leave her, too, and that life will get back into a routine as soon as possible.

If the primary caretaker (usually the mother) has died, and the father must return to work, he should find someone to assume a caretaking, nurturing role for a while—perhaps a relative or a nanny. Even so, while these substitutes can assist with day-to-day functions, the surviving parent will still need to spend more time with and give more attention to his child to help her adjust to their new life.

Death of a Sibling. When a brother or a sister dies, children can find it just as difficult as losing a parent, sometimes even more so. In some ways a sibling is the person to whom a child is closest. They have been constant companions, sharing many life experiences. Perhaps they even shared a bedroom.

When a sibling dies, children may feel guilty, particularly since at some point nearly every youngster wishes that her sibling were dead. Or they may have survival guilt ("Why did he die and I didn't?"). They may even feel guilty because of the jealousy they experienced if their sibling was ill and got extra parental attention.

If one of your children dies, do not ignore the others during the grieving process. Even though you may be overwhelmed with your own sadness, your other children need a lot of attention, comforting, and understanding. Mobilize other extended-family members and friends to help give your children support. Try to avoid putting the deceased child on a pedestal, or your other children may feel they can never be as perfect or as good in your eyes.

should be honest and direct. Children need to grieve as much as adults do. They need to be able to share their feelings and talk about how they are going to miss the person who has died. By school age they have already been exposed to death, even if only indirectly, by watching television or hearing about it from friends. Death should not be covered up and hidden.

To help your child, you need to feel comfortable with your own grief reaction over the death of a loved one. It is appropriate for your child to see you cry when you feel sad; he will take comfort knowing that you are expressing your feelings so openly. This will make it easier for him to do the same.

How Is Your Child Reacting?

Unlike adults, children usually learn about the death of a loved one from others. They probably were not at the hospital when the deceased died, and they must rely on adults to tell them what happened.

Give your child prompt and accurate information, and answer her questions in language she can understand. If possible, as in the case of a terminal illness of someone she loves, give her a chance to prepare for the death in advance. You might say something like "Grandma is very, very sick and may not get better; the doctors think she might die soon." By contrast, if the death is sudden and violent—for example, in an automobile accident—your child's grieving process will be more difficult.

Children grieve in a manner similar to adults. They may experience a variety of feelings—sadness, anxiety, anger, guilt, shock, and helplessness. They may be confused and disbelieving. They may be restless and have trouble sleeping. They might cry, lose their appetite, and withdraw from friends. Especially during the first months of acute grieving, many children are fearful and anxious both about their own safety and that of their surviving family members.

Some younger school-age children may view death as something reversible or temporary. They might even deny that the person has died at all. In their play and fantasy they may continue to speak about the deceased individual as though he or she were still alive.

In the later years of middle childhood, however, as youngsters are better able to understand the death and what caused it, they will be able to deal with it more directly. They may express their feelings about the death openly (through crying, for example), or in their play or daydreams. At times, their reactions may be quite severe.

The intensity of your child's grieving also will depend on her relationship with the individual who has died. If the deceased is an aunt or uncle whom the youngster was not particularly close to, your child may not have much of a reaction. However, if she has lost someone whom she was dependent upon—for example, a parent or, in some cases, a grandparent who frequently cared for her—she will be more devastated by the death, and it will take her longer to get over the passing away of this person. Children who lose a parent or a sibling often end up dealing with that death for the rest of their lives.

Once a death occurs, accept your child's response, whatever it is. If she is upset, be respectful of that reaction. If she is quiet, that should be respected as well. These individual responses will reflect the child's own development and maturity, the circumstances of the death, and her own personality.

Some factors seem to make it more difficult for the child to cope with the death of a parent. The death of the primary caretaker (usually the mother) is harder on children. When the surviving parent's functioning becomes chronically impaired, children lose a critical source of support. Unanticipated deaths are more difficult to cope with than when the family has time to plan and the child can say goodbye.

Grieving is a process. It takes time. Don't expect it to come all at once and be over with quickly. However, since grieving is a healthy process, you can help it along by talking to your child about what she is feeling, answering her questions, and not hiding your own grief in order to protect her from pain.

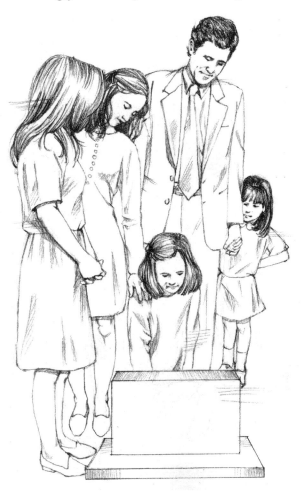

WHAT ABOUT THE FUNERAL?

Many parents are hesitant to take their children to funerals. However, by the time a child reaches school age, he should be given a choice as to whether he wants to attend the funeral. Explain to him what a funeral is—that it is the time when the person who has died will be buried, and when those who knew her get together to remember her. Step by step, describe what will happen, from the time you arrive and greet people in the chapel, to the burial at the gravesite. Tell him that people will be sad and crying.

If the child decides to go, an adult should stay with him during the entire funeral. If he becomes too upset to remain (especially a younger school-age child), the adult accompanying him should go with him out of the ceremony. At the funeral he will see other people grieving, which will make it easier for him to express his own feelings. And despite parental fears, he won't be traumatized by attending the funeral.

GETTING BACK TO NORMAL

After the death of someone close, like a parent or a sibling, your middle-years child may want to stay home from school for a few days. She may need to be close to you and other people who can provide her with comfort and support.

Before long, however, you need to get the family back into a routine. While allowing the grieving process to continue, also try to redirect your child's attention to the normal life events that can give her a sense of continuity. Returning to school can make her feel that her life is getting back to routine. Some children, in fact, work extra hard at school as a way of dealing with their grief.

Make sure you sit down with your child each day to talk about what she is feeling. Some symptoms related to the loss can continue or resurface after many weeks and even months. Perhaps holidays or the anniversary of the death will remind children of their loss. Youngsters are sometimes afraid to go to sleep. They may have fears of separation from their surviving parent. They might refuse to go to school, or become chronically depressed.

When these conditions linger, you may need to get your child some professional counseling to put the healing process back on track. Family therapy may be useful if family members feel so overwhelmed by grief that they cannot get their lives into a regular routine. Also, ask your doctor for a referral to a support group for children whose siblings have died.

PART VII

CHILDREN IN SCHOOL

MAKING SCHOOL CHOICES

For most parents, seeing that their child has a good education is one of their highest priorities. They recognize that education is not only an important part of growing up but is also a crucial factor in their child's future. In our society a good education is often equated with success in life.

Your child may have already attended preschool for one or more years. There he socialized with other children and perhaps got a start on learning the alphabet and other fundamental skills. Even so, as you contemplate signing up your child for kindergarten, you may have questions about his readiness for what lies ahead. Is he mature enough to begin school? Does he have the knowledge and skills he needs? Or would he benefit from another year of preschool instead?

EVALUATING YOUR
CHILD'S READINESS

By law, children must be enrolled in school or an approved alternative program by a particular age. In most parts of the country, these age requirements are five years old for kindergarten and six years old for first grade. Even then, cutoff dates, after which children must wait until the next school year to enter class, vary greatly.

The idea that because of their birth date some children are "ready for school" and others are not has become controversial. Just as children begin to work or talk at different ages, they also develop the psychological and social aptitudes necessary for school at varying ages. In addition, many parents and educators feel that schools need to be ready for children. This newer approach emphasizes how school programs can be designed so that all children of the chronological age to enter school can benefit from the program. Of course, the reality is that a match between your child's development and the school's resources and adaptibility may not exist.

When you're deciding when your child should start school, consider your child's unique abilities and local circumstances. Gather accurate information about your child's development, especially communication skills, including language development and the ability to listen; social skills and the ability to get along with other children and adults; and physical skills from running and playing to using a crayon or pencil. Talking with your child's pediatrician, preschool teacher, and/or childcare provider can provide some useful, objective observations and information.

Some schools may conduct their own tests to evaluate your youngster's abilities. So-called readiness tests tend to concentrate on academic skills, but most usually evaluate other aspects of development. These tests are far from infallible; some children who do poorly on them still fare well in school. Even so, you can use them as one of the yardsticks in determining how your child's development has progressed relative to other children of the same age. Often, your own parental intuition about your child's capabilities is an accurate measure of how well she is prepared to enter school, particularly if you have an older child with whom you have had experience.

When you or the school identify some areas of your child's development that seem to lag behind, use this information to help you and the school plan for the special attention that your child may need. By sharing information with your child's teacher and other school staff, you can help the school be ready for your child. At the same time, you are establishing a partnership for your child's education that can and should continue throughout her childhood.

Parents can encourage their children's cognitive, physical, and emotional development before they enter school. Kindergarten teachers appreciate having children who are enthusiastic and curious in approaching new activities, can follow directions, are sensitive to other children's feelings, and can take turns and share. Some specific skills that will make your child's first year at school go smoothly include her ability to:

- Play well with other children with minimal fighting or crying.

- Remain attentive and quiet when being read a story.

- Use the toilet on her own.

- Successfully use zippers and buttons.

- Say her name, address, and telephone number.

There are great benefits to reading to your child beginning in infancy. Help your child acquire some basic skills, like recognizing and remembering letters, numbers, and colors. Expose her to enriching and learning experiences like trips to the museum, or enroll her in community art or science programs. To promote social-skills development, encourage her to play with other children of both sexes in the neighborhood and to participate in organized community-sponsored activities.

Some parents consider purposefully delaying their child's entrance into kindergarten. They believe that their child may gain some advantage and be more likely to succeed in academics, athletics, or social settings if she is older than average for her grade. Delaying school entry in order to obtain some advantage is not necessarily a winning strategy. Although there is some evidence that being among the youngest in a class may cause some academic problems, most of these seem to disappear by the third or fourth grade. On the other hand, there is evidence that children who are old for their grade are at significantly greater risk of behavior problems when they reach adolescence.

REGISTERING YOUR CHILD FOR SCHOOL

To enroll your child in school, you will need to demonstrate that he meets the school district's age requirements for kindergarten. Some schools require that a child be five by September of his entry year. Others use different cutoff dates. If proof of age is requested, bring a birth certificate, religious (baptismal) certificate, or a physician's record. If you feel convinced that your child is ready for kindergarten and you want him to attend, but he has not reached the designated chronological age, find out the exemption process that may be offered in your school district.

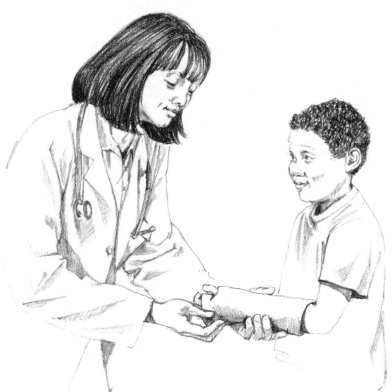

Before your child begins school each fall, check with his pediatrician for recommendations on sports participation and other school issues.

Visiting the Doctor

Before your child enters school, make an appointment for your youngster with your pediatrician. The doctor will make certain your child is properly immunized and can discuss with you the various issues related to this important transition.

Since many schools register new kindergarten students in the spring, schedule this doctor's visit for late winter or early spring so the important readiness issues discussed earlier can be addressed well in advance, and so that you avoid the late-summer logjam in the physician's office. Ask for a copy of your youngster's immunizations to bring with you to school during registration.

Immunizations

When you register your youngster, you will be asked for his immunization record. Specifically, the school staff will want to see either a copy of the record from your child's pediatrician or the clinic where the immunizations were given, including the doctor's signature, or a summary copy from the physician's office.

If you do not have a record but are sure your child has had all the necessary shots, the school will usually give you some time to obtain the records. In many places they will not be able simply to take your word for it; the immunization requirement is a state law, and the state dictates which types of records are acceptable.

A fully immunized child who has had a four- or five-year-old checkup will have had one or two MMR (measles, mumps, rubella), five DTP, DTaP, or DT (diphtheria, pertussis, tetanus), four polio vaccines, and three to four *Haemophilus influenzae B* conjugate vaccines. He may have also been immunized against hepatitis B and chicken pox. All these immunizations are not necessarily required for school entry, so check with your school to find out which ones are needed. (See page 25 for immunization information.)

If your child does not have the immunizations required by your particular school district, your pediatrician will likely recognize this and can address the problem during the prekindergarten appointment you have made. The needed immunizations can often be given at that visit. Even if additional immunizations are needed, your child will probably be admitted to school with a note from your pediatrician that the immunizations are "in progress." School personnel are aware that time intervals (such as six weeks) are often needed between some of these immunizations, but may allow only that amount of time, so be prompt.

If your child has not been immunized because you have moral or religious objections to immunizations, ask the school staff about the exemption process. Some parents who have not had their children previously immunized decide to have immunizations done when their children start school because their youngsters will now be exposed to large numbers of children and diseases. Talk it over with your pediatrician if you have questions or concerns.

CHOOSING A SCHOOL

In your school district you may have a choice of which school your child will attend. In addition to public schools, there may also be private or parochial schools to which you might decide to send your youngster at extra expense. It is important for you to familiarize yourself with the schools from which you are choosing. Once you understand the differences among the schools, you will be better able to make an informed decision. No school is a perfect fit for each child. Knowledge about your child's school is important both to prepare her for the year ahead and to equip you to work with the school as an advocate for your child to assure that she receives the best education possible.

Elementary schools have traditionally included kindergarten through the sixth grade (K–6) or kindergarten through the eighth grade (K–8). In recent years, children have been grouped in different ways to accommodate their developmental needs, as well as to make better use of the school district's resources. In some districts students may be attending schools with structures such as K–2, K–4, K–5, or a 3–4–5 combination.

Educators are also becoming increasingly aware that pre- and early adolescents (ages ten to thirteen) have particular educational needs. These youngsters can benefit from more autonomy and an increased ability to experiment than is available in most elementary schools, yet they need a safer, more structured, and more overtly supportive environment than that of the usual high school. Educational programs for these children, called middle school, are becoming a specialty of their own, with students grouped in grades 5–6–7–8, 6–7–8, 7–8, or 7–8–9 combinations.

What to Look For

When selecting your child's school, here are some questions to ask and some information to obtain.

Expectations. What are the school's academic, athletic, and social expectations for students in the grade your child is entering?

Individuality. Is learning individualized? That is, are each child's individual skills and needs considered by the teachers, or is the entire class taught the same material at the same pace at the same time? Some children simply do not fare well in a high-pressure, highly organized atmosphere, while others thrive in it. You need to assess what environment is best for your child. Keep her out of classroom situations that may lead to frustration, poor performance, and a dislike of school and learning.

Disabilities and Special Needs. Is the school able to meet the special needs of your child and in compliance with the federal statutes protecting individuals with disabilities? Are special education services available? Most important, do you feel your school is welcoming of those with different physical, educational, and emotional needs?

"Grouping." Are children grouped by ability, or do all classes have children at different levels?

"Climate." What is the climate at the school? If you visit the school during the academic year, you will learn a lot. Do students and teachers treat one another with respect? Do teachers communicate a love for and an excitement about teaching and learning? Is the school an orderly, but not repressive, environ-

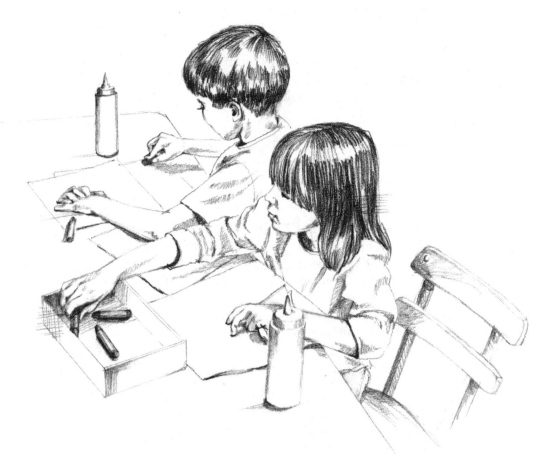

ment? Are the children well behaved but still allowed to be playful individuals? Is the work of students displayed on the classroom walls and bulletin boards, showing that their efforts are valued? Is praise from teachers commonplace? Do you sense a positive relationship between the school and the surrounding community?

Cultural Variety. What is the school's racial, ethnic, and socioeconomic composition? There are many lessons that a child can learn from developing friendships with youngsters of different backgrounds and cultures. Does the school consider differences in race, religion, and culture to be assets of which everyone is proud? Does the school handle holidays with religious significance sensitively?

Do programs exist for meaningful study of different cultures (curriculum units, appropriate educational trips)? Are students provided with opportunities to interact with students from different backgrounds, through visits, school-to-school pen pals, and the like? Are parents from the school interested in working together to provide their children with these experiences?

Are children treated equally regardless of their family's income? For example, do all children go on field trips regardless of their ability to pay? Are children who receive free or reduced-cost lunch made to stand in separate lines?

The Principal. Is the principal a visible presence at the school? Do you see him or her welcoming children in the morning, visiting classrooms, or walking through the halls? The principal's leadership is one of the most important factors in contributing to a school's effectiveness and sets the tone and standards for the school.

Student-Teacher Ratio. What is the student-teacher ratio? Most educators believe that, from kindergarten through the fifth grade, a ratio of twenty-five-to-one or less is adequate. When the ratio exceeds thirty-to-one, the ability to teach can be seriously impaired. Even so, there is more to the story than these numbers: In a classroom with many children who need a significant amount of individualized attention to help them control their behavior, a ratio as low as fifteen-to-one may still be too high and might be improved by, for example, the presence of a teacher's aide. Conversely, if the majority of children are capable of independent work, then a higher ratio might be acceptable.

Teachers. How do teachers and children interact? Do teachers spend most of the classroom time lecturing? Or does the teacher coach the students' learning, and does the school day consist of a mixture of talking to and with the students, and include lots of student input? Are small-group activities encouraged, with or without direct teacher participation? Students can learn a great deal by helping one another within a structured setting.

Resources. In addition to academics, what is the quality of other aspects of the school, such as the library or resource center, art and music classes, guidance counseling, and physical education programs? Is there access to computers and the Internet? Physical education classes should be more than a time to blow off steam. There should be a balance between fitness activities and skill development. In some schools, classroom teachers are responsible for PE classes, while in others, where formal PE instruction is provided, classroom teachers may supplement it with coordinated activities that have been designed by the PE teacher.

In its athletic activities does the school emphasize cooperation, or is the atmosphere competitive? Is winning emphasized over participating? If competition is too intense, it can result in injuries or emotional stress.

With reductions in school budgets, physical education programs are often one of the first areas to be cut back or even eliminated. In schools where this

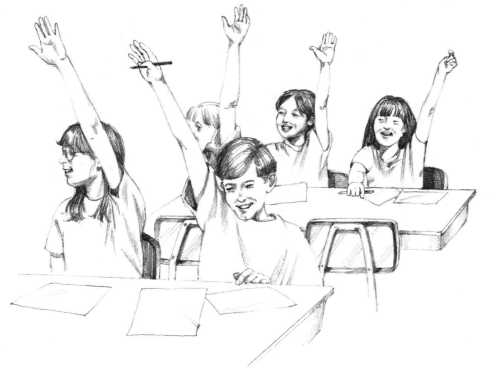

is occurring, classroom teachers frequently have taken on more responsibility for these programs, particularly those teachers who have some training in this area. Also, parents have come together in groups after school to organize physical activities.

Nutrition. How seriously does the school take good nutrition? Is the food served in the cafeteria consistent with the principles of good eating that are taught in the classroom? Unfortunately, this may be difficult to accomplish. The surplus food made available to schools at a discount is often high in fat and salt content; by contrast, fresh vegetables for salad bars tend to be more expensive, harder to keep, and more time-consuming to prepare.

With parent and community support, however, many schools have implemented innovative, cost-effective programs to decrease fat and salt content in cafeteria meals. For example, schools have reduced the number of times they serve fried foods each week. They have made low-fat milk available to students. Multiple school districts have joined together to purchase fresh fruit and vegetables in bulk at lower prices. Schools have also encouraged students to bring healthier snacks to school for birthdays and other classroom celebrations.

Some schools have initiated a government-funded breakfast program in order to help low-income families supplement the nutrition of their children. The presence of this kind of program can indicate the school's commitment to students' nutritional needs.

Year-Round Schools

As a way to increase achievement, some school districts are experimenting with an increase from the usual 180 days to 220 days of school a year. These districts are trying to avoid the loss of students' skills and learning momentum that occurs during the ten-week summer vacation. This experiment is different from that of schools that are rearranging their schedules to stay open all year to relieve overcrowding, with each student still attending only 180 days a year.

The main drawback to the 220-day, year-round program is financial. Teachers have to be paid more for their increased workload. In a time when many school districts are already financially strained, these additional costs may be prohibitive.

Whatever happens to this movement, parents should give some thought to helping their own children maintain skills over the summer, especially children having difficulty in school. Although there may be formal programs in which you can enroll your child, most youngsters will also be helped with a regular reading time and by playing numbers games with their parents. (For example, how much will this vacation cost? How many miles will we cover on this trip, there and back? What percentage of the trip will we take today? What is the total amount of money we are spending shopping today?)

Safety. Are the children physically safe at school? Safety should be a paramount concern in the classrooms, the playgrounds, the kitchens, and parking lots. Many schools keep a daily log of injuries and accidents on playground equipment and elsewhere on the school grounds and review these records to try to implement programs for greater safety.

Inquire about other safety and environmental issues. Is there a nonsmoking policy in the school buildings? Are arts and crafts materials safe for children? Is ventilation adequate, and are room temperatures kept at moderate levels? If appropriate, have radon levels in the school buildings been evaluated, and has the water been tested for lead? Has asbestos still present in the ceilings or walls of classrooms been appropriately dealt with?

How are health services delivered in the school? Who provides emergency first aid? How do children or parents gain access to the nurse or health aide? (See "Dealing with Health Problems at School," page 534.) Does the school have a clinic? A dental screening program?

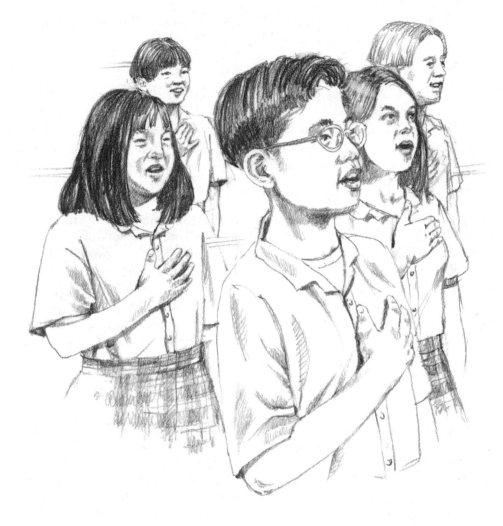

What is the school's policy in creating a healthy environment? Is it striving to become a model as a health-promoting institution?

Before- and After-School Programs. Are early morning activities or an after-school program available at the school? If not, are there any school-based resources to help parents find this needed childcare? If programs are scarce in your community, consider joining with other parents and approaching YMCAs or other agencies to encourage them to start an after-school program.

If your efforts to find out more about a school—public or private—are not met with open arms or do not answer most of your questions, do not allow yourself to be put off or intimidated. If you show some flexibility, such as making an appointment for a day that is less busy than others, the school staff should be willing to accommodate your visit. Most principals, in fact, will be proud to show you their school, and will welcome your interest and involvement in your child's education.

NEW LEARNING STRUCTURES

Maintain an open mind about learning situations with which you might not be familiar. For example, some schools have an open structure, in which classes are all under one roof without walls between them. Teachers might have their own distinctive style of teaching. While some prefer having their students in assigned seats, others work best with an approach that seems less structured, with students free to roam through the room during particular assignments. Some teachers utilize learning centers for independent learning or solitary study. To some degree, your child's success will hinge on the match between his need for structure and choice, and the teacher's own approach to teaching. Even if your child is growing up in a fairly structured home setting, you might be surprised to find that he does quite well in a relatively unstructured classroom environment. In any event, a high-quality teacher will adapt his or her own teaching style so that students are more likely to learn.

In addition to teaching style, evaluate how well your child's teacher communicates and resolves conflicts in the class. Also, what are the teacher's areas of special skill or interest?

If magnet schools are available in your community, consider them as another option. As their name implies, these schools attract students from surrounding areas. They tend to emphasize a particular area of the curriculum—for instance, science, the arts, foreign languages—and students may choose them because of a special interest or talent. In some school districts students are assigned to these magnet schools. Free transportation may be provided.

DOES A PRIVATE OR RELIGIOUS SCHOOL MAKE SENSE?

Private and religious schools come in different sizes, philosophies, and affiliations. Parents consider a private or religious school for their child for many reasons: a particular educational philosophy and method of teaching; a reputation for high student achievement and academic success; a religious affiliation and an education with a religious orientation; a military orientation; or a family tradition.

If you are deciding whether this type of school is right for your child, there are other issues to consider besides the factors mentioned above. For instance:

- What are the expectations of the school's staff and students?

- What are the educational styles and characteristics of the principal and teachers?

- What is the student-teacher ratio?

- What additional educational and student service resources—such as special education, nursing, physical and speech therapy, and audiology—are provided?

- What safety and nutritional services are available?

- Is financial assistance available to help meet tuition fees?

While comparing private/religious and public schools, other criteria may help you make your decision. Ask about licensing requirements for teachers, administrators, and health-care personnel, since they are sometimes less stringent in private and religious schools. Check to see whether the private or religious school has fewer resources and teachers trained specifically in art, music, physical education, guidance counseling, and special education. Determine whether high tuition costs keep the private or religious school from attracting a mix of students from different backgrounds. Finally, find out if parents are required to make a substantial time commitment to volunteer at and fund-raise for the school.

PREPARING FOR A
NEW SCHOOL YEAR

T he start of each school year can be a particularly exciting—
and anxious—time during middle childhood. While youngsters
may look forward to seeing their old friends again, they might
be apprehensive about a new teacher and, in some cases, a new
school.

In the days and weeks immediately preceding the first day of
school, make an effort to find out some basic information about
what awaits your child. For instance:

- What will her daily schedule be like? What time does school begin and when does it end each day?

- Should your child bring a bag lunch and a snack to school, or
  are meals provided, or does she have the option to purchase
  them? If lunch is scheduled relatively late, your child may want
  a larger morning snack.

- Are certain clothes required for physical education classes and recesses? Some parents forget that children go outdoors for recess, and in the winter that may mean hats, gloves, boots, and maybe snow pants, even if the children do not need to wear them in the car or on the bus. Inquire as to whether your child should bring shoes to change into.

If it is possible in your school district, visit the school with your child to see her new classroom and meet her new teacher before school officially starts.

SAFETY

If your child will be walking to school, walk the route with him to assess its safety. Find out about traffic patterns and crossing guards. Instruct your child to stay on sidewalks and main roads rather than cutting through alleys and wooded areas that may be somewhat deserted.

Although safety rules will probably be discussed in class, do not wait for that instruction: Make your own rules specific to your child's situation. In a low-key but firm manner, tell your youngster: "These rules are one way we take care of ourselves." Reassure him that he can keep himself safe. Review these safety issues several times during the year.

If an older sibling goes to the same school, have the children walk together. Otherwise, you might find a responsible older child from your neighborhood who would be pleased to be invited to walk your youngster to school. As your children grow older, remember to look around your neighborhood for young children to help in this way.

What is the school's policy regarding checking on students who are absent? Particularly if the school encourages it, call early in the morning whenever your child is absent. This will provide an additional measure of safety for your child, since if he does not show up for school, the school secretary will be more likely to check with you.

Does the school have rules regarding bikes and/or skateboards? Some schools require helmets and locks for cyclists. Before the first day of school, review the basic safety rules with your youngster. By insisting your child wear a helmet and abide by all bicycle safety guidelines, for example, you will be encouraging a behavior that is potentially lifesaving and can become a lifetime habit. Ask the school staff if your community has a program offering low-cost or even free helmets for children; if there is no such program in your area, talk with other parents about starting one to increase the number of children wearing helmets and thus make it more socially acceptable for your own youngster to wear one. Wear your own helmet whenever you bike or skateboard to model appropriate safety behavior.

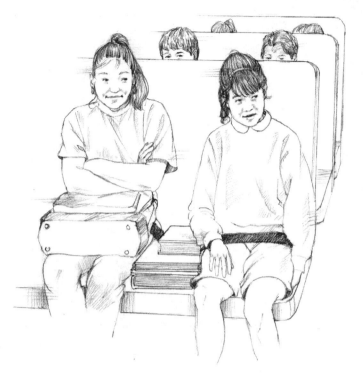

THE SCHOOL BUS

Is bus transportation available for your child? Many parents have particular concerns about bus rides on the first day of school, and also when older youngsters riding the bus start to cause trouble. Also, what happens if a child misses the afternoon bus or is detained after school?

On your child's first day of elementary school, you might be tempted to drive her to school, particularly if she seems apprehensive about the bus ride or about starting school in general. However, except under unusual circumstances, strongly encourage your child to ride the bus that first day. Your youngster should be there if seats on the bus are assigned, and the driver needs to get used to the stop where your child will be picked up. You can take your child to the bus stop and meet her there when she returns. If your work schedule doesn't allow you to be there, arrange for another adult or an older sibling to take on this responsibility.

Review the basic bus safety rules with your youngster: Wait for the bus to stop before approaching it from the curb. Do not move around on the bus; this will help avoid injuries if the driver needs to stop quickly. When disembarking, cross at least ten feet in front of the bus and only when it is fully stopped, the red lights are flashing, and the driver has signaled that it is safe. Of course, the child should also check to make sure that no other traffic is coming.

WHERE WE STAND

Recent surveys show that 22 million students ride school buses to and from school each day. Seat belts, however, are not mandatory for larger school buses.

Thousands of students are injured, and dozens of others are killed every year riding these buses. The American Academy of Pediatrics would like to see changes in present laws to reduce the number and seriousness of these injuries. We believe that seat belts should be required on all newly manufactured school buses, regardless of their size and the number of students they transport. We also urge that seat backs be elevated to 28 inches—four inches above the federally mandated height—so as to support and cushion a child's head and neck. In addition, padding designed to adequately absorb impacts during crashes or fast stops should completely cover the rears of seats and the top rails.

In most cases, you won't be allowed to ride on the bus with your child, even on the first day of school. Although some parents feel better following the bus to school in their car and making sure their child finds her classroom, the school staff is usually prepared to help youngsters navigate through the school grounds on opening day.

If your child complains about trouble occurring on the bus, caused by older and/or rowdy youngsters, find out what the particular problem is and take appropriate action. If your child is being teased or harassed, encourage her to suggest some potential solutions in hopes that she can resolve the difficulty herself. If she is being hurt or is afraid for her safety, call the principal for some assistance. To minimize problems, discourage your child from bringing expensive or popular toys to play with on the bus, since they can easily become damaged when other children want to try them. Bear in mind that drivers need to concentrate on driving the bus; they have neither the time nor the training to serve as disciplinarians.

EXPECTATIONS

As you help your child get ready for the new school year, look back on your own school days at your youngster's grade level. If you had some negative experiences, make certain you do not project them onto your own child. For example, the mother of a third-grader reflected upon her own year in the third grade and recalled having problems with reading that her teacher confused with "laziness" and "motivation problems." The mother realized that because of her own experience, she had been passing negative expectations on to her child. When she recognized the message she was conveying, she made an extra effort to put her old feelings aside and approach her youngster's situation afresh and optimistically.

Expectations can be a powerful influence on the kind of school experience your child has. Even when they are communicated in casual conversations, they can have a significant effect on your child's outlook. Past experiences can also influence a child's outlook and expectations. While he may have had some problems in the previous year, you and he should try to approach the new school year with a clean slate and a positive attitude.

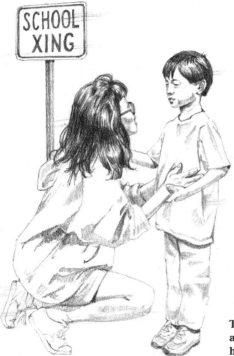

Talk with your child about his feelings about his first day of school.

MAKING THE FIRST DAY EASIER

Most children are anxious and excited on the first day of school each year. You can help make the day easier for your youngster by keeping the following guidelines in mind:

- Point out the positive aspects of starting school: It will be fun. She will see old friends. She will meet new friends. Refresh her memory about previ-

A Checklist for the First Day of School

As you and your child prepare for the first day of the new school year, use this checklist to help make sure you have taken care of the necessary tasks and learned the information you need.

- Is your child registered? (If he attended the same school the previous school year, he is already registered.)

- When is the first day of school?

- What time does school start?

- How is your child going to get to school? If your child is biking, does he know the school rules for bicycles? If he is walking for the first time, with whom will he walk? Have you reviewed safety precautions with him, regarding traffic and strangers?

- Does your child know his teacher's name?

- What will his daily schedule be like?

- Will he need to bring a snack? What kinds of snacks are allowed and encouraged? Does he need to bring something to drink, or can he buy something? Will water be available?

- What time is lunch? Can your child buy it at school, and how much will it cost?

ous years, when she may have returned home after the first day with high spirits because she had a good time.

- Remind your child that she is not the only student who is a bit uneasy about the first day of school. Teachers know that students are anxious and will be making an extra effort to make sure everyone feels as comfortable as possible.

- Review all your child's accomplishments from last year, and talk about the kinds of interesting things she will learn in the months ahead.

- Buy her something (perhaps a pen or pencil) that will remind her you are thinking of her while she is at school, or put a note in her lunchbox.

- What clothes will your child need to wear? Are there any restrictions on what can be worn? Will he need a different set of clothes for physical education or art classes?

- Does your child need to bring pencils, paper, notebooks, and other supplies? (Often, the teacher will announce these requirements on the first day.) Does your child have something in which to carry his books and supplies back and forth to school? Will he have a place (besides his desk) to keep his things at school?

- Have you filled out all health forms or emergency contact forms that have been sent home?

- Have any new health problems developed in your child over the summer that will affect his school day? Does the school nurse know about this condition, or is an appointment set up to discuss it?

- If your child will need to take medication at school on the first day, have arrangements been made for this?

- Does your youngster know where he is going after school (e.g., home, babysitter)? Does he know how he will get there? If you will not be there when he arrives, does he know who will be responsible for him, what the rules are, and how to get help in an emergency?

- Does your child have your work telephone numbers in his backpack?

- Reassure your child that if any problems arise at school, you will help resolve them. (If problems do occur, get involved as soon as possible.)

- Find another child in the neighborhood with whom your youngster can walk to school or ride with on the bus. If your child is older, have her offer to walk to school or wait at the bus stop with a new or younger child.

- If your child is not going to ride a school bus and you feel it is appropriate, drive your child (or walk with her) to school and pick her up the first day.

- Encourage her to look for new students in her classroom or in the playground, invite them to join the group for a game, and ask them about their interests.

- After school, show your child some special attention and affection. Give her a hug and ask what happened at school. Did she have fun? Did she make any new friends? Does she need any additional school supplies (notebooks, rulers, erasers) that you can shop for together?

In addition to the suggestions listed above, your child may need some extra support if she is starting a new school. Here are some suggestions to make the transition easier.

- Talk with your child about her feelings, both her excitement and her concerns, about the new school.

- Visit the school with your child in advance of the first day. Teachers and staff are usually at school a few days before the children start. Peek into your child's classroom, and if possible, meet the teacher and principal. You might be able to address some of your child's concerns at that time. She may have no questions until she actually sees the building and can visualize what it will be like. (When you formally register your child in the new school, bring her immunization record and birth certificate; usually school records can be sent directly from school to school once you sign a "release of information" form.)

- Try to have your child meet a classmate *before* the first day so they can get acquainted and play together, and so your child will have a friendly face to look for when school begins.

- Do not build up unrealistic expectations about how wonderful the new school will be, but convey a general sense of optimism about how things will go for your child at the new school. Remind her that teachers and other students will be making an extra effort to make her feel welcome.

- If your child sees another student or a group engaged in an activity she is interested in, encourage her to ask if she can participate.

- As soon as you can, find out what activities are available for your child in addition to those that occur during school itself. Is there a back-to-school picnic or party planned? Can she join a soccer team? (For community sports programs, sign-ups often begin weeks or even months before the start of the season.)

During the first few weeks at a new school, your child's teacher will probably conduct some informal assessments. You should be able to get some idea of how your child's academic and social adjustments are going at that time.

(See also "Family Moves," page 343, and Chapter 47, "Making School Choices.")

GETTING INVOLVED IN YOUR CHILD'S SCHOOLING

One of a child's greatest assets is parents who are involved in his education and his school. When parents care and become active participants and partners in the educational process, their own child—and all other children at the school—benefit enormously.

COMMUNICATING EFFECTIVELY WITH SCHOOL PERSONNEL

Parents should be knowledgeable about the educational program their child is receiving and should be actively involved with the school. The first step toward productive involvement is to know the members of the school staff. After all, these are the people with whom your child spends a large percentage of her life and on whom you and she depend for her getting a good education. Many parents meet their child's teacher, principal, and the school secretary during an open house at school or at the first parent-teacher conference. However, you might find it helpful to meet these individuals earlier in the school year. Demonstrate your interest and involvement early.

Nevertheless, keep in mind that the first few days and weeks of the school year are quite busy. So if you need more than just five minutes to introduce yourself and exchange brief greetings, respect the demands on the teacher's time by calling and setting up an appointment beforehand. Teachers cannot stop their classroom activities when a parent arrives.

During the first week of school many teachers explain their expectations for the child's work and classroom behavior, as well as the consequences of not complying with these rules. If you make sure your child understands the guidelines early, you can help her get off to a good start in the class. If she does not know what the teacher's expectations are after a week or two, contact the teacher. (Some teachers have the class participate in setting expectations for classroom behavior and consequences, so there may be a natural delay.)

Teachers vary in the way they communicate their plans for the year to parents. Some will send out a memo in the first two weeks. Others do not present that information until parents' night. Ask when you will be receiving information about the curriculum and plans for homework and various projects. If you feel you need the information sooner, set up a meeting or perhaps a phone call for a quick overview.

While most schools will encourage you to stay in touch with your child's teacher, be aware of some of the difficulties involved in doing so. There are effective ways to deal with these problems. Sending a note to the teacher is an excellent way to establish contact about many issues. Let the teacher know specifically what you need. (This is preferable to "Please give me a call.") Teachers may have limited access to telephones. They must remain with their students most of the day, and many schools have only one phone in the office. Many times, teachers can send home a note with the information you want. If you would like to be called instead, let the teacher know your phone number and convenient times to reach you. During your first contact, ask how the teacher would prefer to be reached in the future.

BECOMING AN INVOLVED PARENT

Fortunately, the relationship between parents and the school staff is usually quite good. In most instances teachers and principals welcome your input and your hands-on involvement in the school. Active involvement in the parent-teacher association (PTA) or parent-teacher organization (PTO) is an excellent way to provide the school with your help and input in an organized way. In these days of budgetary restraints and two-career families, a parent who is able to volunteer even an hour or two a week is much appreciated.

Some parents enjoy volunteering in the classroom, working with students at a regular time each week, perhaps helping a small group with reading, arts and crafts, or computers. If you can volunteer in your child's classroom on a weekly basis, let the teacher know early in the year, and work out a convenient time for both of you—a time when the children you will be working with are readily available and will not be out of class for a special education program or band practice.

Schools often need help preparing and serving meals or refreshments for special events. Make sure your volunteer efforts coincide with the curriculum or the philosophy of the school or the teacher. If you have agreed to bring refreshments for a class party, the teacher might want them to be healthy snacks to reinforce the nutrition education going on at school. Rather than cupcakes, the teacher might prefer a fruit platter.

Field trips and educational trips have become important means of giving children diverse experiences in the community which they can then use as springboards for writing and discussions. However, without parent chaperons, these excursions may not be possible. If you are able to volunteer, you will probably be responsible for a particular group of children. If you need lead time to plan your participation in these trips, ask the teacher for as much notice as possible.

Even if you cannot help out at your child's school very often, try to do so at least once in a while. Even participating in one activity a year—accompanying a class on a field trip or helping out backstage on the day of a talent show—can mean a lot to your youngster. It will make him feel that his activities at school matter to you.

Many parents try to attend school events of which their children are a part. However, if there is an important event in your child's school life that you simply cannot attend because of work or other commitments, try to have someone else there—a grandparent, an uncle, or a friend—who can give your youngster moral support and maybe even take pictures for you to look at later.

Some parents are getting involved in the schools in another way—namely, on the policy-making level. Many schools have "site councils," "parent advisory councils," or "Healthy School Teams," which help determine the direction of each school. Also, school boards need candidates for their seats, as well as volunteers to serve on special committees that evaluate everything from curriculum to school safety.

Occasionally, the relationship among teachers, administrators, and enthusiastic mothers or fathers becomes strained and frustrating for all parties. Whether parents are lobbying for a new program for their child's school or are trying to serve as an advocate for their own child, who might be having difficulty with a particular subject area or teacher, their input can sometimes be perceived as more disruptive than helpful, no matter how well-intentioned it may be.

To make your relationship with the school productive, show the staff respect, listen to their point of view, exhibit some flexibility, and find compromises whenever possible. Both you and the school have the same goal in mind—to educate your child—so try to work *with* the teacher and staff rather than assuming an adversarial stance.

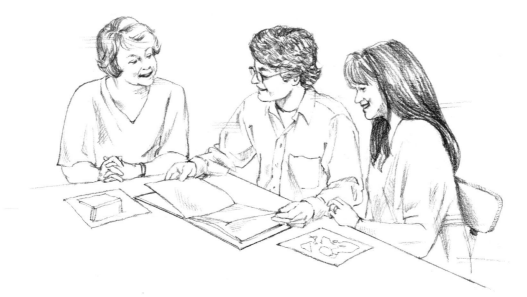

THE PARENT-TEACHER CONFERENCE

You may remember that when you were a child, your parents were called to school when you had misbehaved or had serious academic problems. But there are other reasons for parents to come to school. Once or twice a year you will have a routine scheduled conference with your child's teacher—an opportunity to discuss your youngster's capabilities and progress, and your mutual goals for her for the school year. Together, you and the teacher can develop plans to make the school experience as positive as possible.

Before these conferences, parents sometimes worry that they themselves are being evaluated and judged as parents, or that they might ask a silly ques-

Does Your Business Support the Schools?

Parents are finding ways to participate actively in their child's education through more than just volunteerism. A growing number of businesses are affiliating themselves with local schools, giving time, money, and professional expertise to improve the educational system.

What is the reason for this trend? Business leaders are recognizing that the schools alone cannot solve the complex problems that affect today's children and families. They also are increasingly concerned about the quality of the workforce of the future. As a way to improve their own employee pool down the road, businesses are actively helping out in the following ways.

- Adopt-a-school plans provide a variety of resources to a specific school in the business's own community.

- Financial and other incentives are given to children for staying in school.

- Investments have been made in teacher-training programs.

- Employees are given time away from work to attend parent-teacher conferences.

- Students are being invited to spend a day at a business in the community to see how it operates.

- During lunch hours, businesses offer parenting and health-related classes to their workers.

- Businesses that hire students as part-time after-school employees are taking greater responsibility for the possible negative effect this work may be having on the students' performance at school.

tion or embarrass themselves in some other way. They may even experience the same type of general anxiety that they feel when visiting the doctor's office, anticipating that something is wrong.

If those feelings sound familiar, remind yourself of the positive nature and intent of these conferences. You are in a partnership with the teacher and other school personnel. You are an expert on your child and family, and certainly have information to share with the teacher that can be helpful in enhancing your youngster's classroom experience. At the same time, the teacher can tell you what is going on in the classroom, as well as suggest appropriate plans and goals for the remaining school year and possibly for the next year.

Before each conference think about the questions you have and the issues you want to raise. For instance:

- Are there areas in which my child is not working up to her capabilities?

- What can I do at home to help her improve in the subjects in which she is weak?

- Does my child get along well with her classmates? Does she tend to be overly shy or overly aggressive?

- Have you noticed any learning problems or behavioral difficulties?

- Is there a need to formally assess my child's capabilities or further explore the course of her difficulties?

- Has my child had any unexplained absences or tardiness?

- Are her homework assignments being turned in, and are they well done? Am I supposed to help my child do homework or correct it?

- What are my child's strengths and interests, and are they being nurtured?

Since the time allotted for the conference may be short, you may want to make a list of your questions in their order of importance. If both parents cannot attend, talk about the conference with the other parent in advance, and go over the issues he or she thinks should be raised.

Ask your child, too, if there is anything she would like you to discuss. Are there particular reasons she is continuing to have difficulty with math, for example, or science? Is she having any problems with classmates? Reassure your child that the conference is designed to help her do better at school, and for you to better understand her school experience, not to find things about her to criticize. In some schools the students attend all of these parent-teacher conferences; find out your school's philosophy about this in advance, and if you would like a conference without your child, it can usually be arranged.

Arrive on time for the conference. Meetings with parents usually are scheduled at precise intervals. If you feel you need more time with the teacher, request the last conference of the day, or ask for a special time of sufficient length so all of your questions can be discussed. Also, if your time is up and you still feel there is more to discuss, schedule a second meeting or a phone call to continue the dialogue. Between meetings, if there is a problem with your child that you are trying to resolve, collect as much information as possible and come to the next meeting with some ideas and solutions in mind.

After the conference, discuss it with your child. Tell her what you learned and what you and the teacher decided about future plans and strategies.

Consider sending the teacher a note of thanks, particularly if the conference proved helpful or you sensed a special thoughtfulness or commitment to your child's educational progress and well-being.

QUESTIONS COMMONLY ASKED BY PARENTS

"My child is having continued difficulty with his schoolwork. We've tried things the teacher has suggested. Should I consider having him tested for special-education services?"

Schedule another meeting with the teacher with this specific question in mind. Review with the teacher any extra help your child is now receiving and other strategies that have been tried. Talk about the problems that still exist and what other approaches might be considered. If the conference does not produce any significant new directions to pursue, be prepared to request that your child receive further evaluation including consultation with the special-education teacher, the school nurse, a guidance counselor, and your child's pediatrician. You might also request that the principal and/or special-education teacher join you at this meeting to answer your questions and provide input.

At the end of the conference, make sure that a plan has been established and that you are clear about the next step. If testing or other evaluation or consultation meetings have been scheduled, tell your child about it and why it is being done. He should understand that the testing is designed to determine additional approaches to help make learning and schoolwork easier for him.

"Why does my child's school give standardized tests?"

In many school districts, children routinely undergo a battery of standardized tests, designed by university, state, or private educational services and scored by computer. They are intended to provide a measure of a child's achievement or skill level in certain subjects. In other districts the results may be used to place children in particular classes or programs, and to measure their need for extra services. Some schools report that the collective test scores are used only to examine the school's overall direction and needs and to evaluate teacher performance.

Opponents of these tests argue that they measure only certain components of a child's achievement and intelligence and neglect other important ingredients of success, such as creativity, motivation, and a practical approach to life.

You need to know what your child's scores are and how they are being used in his school. If he does not do well on these types of tests, and your school makes extensive use of their results, you should consider several options. If your child learns well, despite his test scores, you might have him tutored in taking tests. Also, ask that appropriate information be added to your child's file about his strengths and successes.

"Should my child be allowed to use a calculator?"

All children need to be able to perform the mechanics of math without a calculator. Once they have mastered these skills and can set up problems, then the use of a calculator may be appropriate—but only if the teacher approves. Talk with the teacher about it, and ask the reasons for his or her decision.

Bear in mind that whether or not children use calculators for school and homework, they need to learn how to use one. Also, it is always appropriate to play number games with the calculator. For example, you can compute a problem in your head while your child checks your answer on the calculator; switch roles for the next problem.

"Should I buy my child a computer?"

It is important that your child learn basic keyboard and computer skills. Many schools are training elementary-school students in computer skills, and have found that the youngsters have an aptitude for developing these skills. There are many computerized learning programs that students use at school to practice and review math and language art skills.

Even if having a home computer is an option for your family, there is no consensus among educators that it is essential. Here are some factors to consider:

- Does your child have a special learning problem that could be helped by working with a computer? For example, does he have a muscle or neurological problem that makes it difficult for him to write with a pencil and paper, and thus could a computer make it easier for him to do his homework and term papers?

- Do you have the time and money to find, buy, and teach your child educational programs?

- Will the computer be used almost exclusively for video games?

- Will it interfere with family time?

Parental time and interest, and not the availability of a computer, are the critical ingredients for learning at home. If you do have a computer in your home, you need to carefully monitor its use—supervision is a must. First, computers can absorb too much of your child's time, consuming time otherwise available for homework, play, and physical activity. Second, the Internet's chat rooms can be easily accessed by children, and some have violent or sexual content that is entirely inappropriate for school-age children.

PROBLEMS AT SCHOOL

Sometimes your child's teacher will ask you to come to school to discuss a specific concern about your child. When that happens, schedule the meeting as soon as possible, since most problems are best dealt with early.

During this parent-teacher meeting, some parents feel they are on the defensive and are unsure of just how to react. Here are some guidelines to bear in mind:

- Do not feel threatened. The development of most children is uneven, and thus there is often one area of a child's performance that could use improvement. Withhold judgment and listen carefully to what the teacher has to say.

- Ask for specifics. For instance: "Could you give me an example of what is taking place? How often is this happening? How do the teacher and the other students respond to this particular behavior? Is this an isolated episode or a pattern of behavior?"

- Be open to the idea that situations within your family might be contributing to your child's difficulties, and share them as you deem appropriate.

- As you discuss the problem and possible solutions, try to approach the situation as a partnership, and look for ways to work together for improvement.

- If the problem is relatively uncomplicated, you and the teacher may decide during your conversation what action needs to be taken.

- Before the meeting ends, determine how and when you will follow up with one another to evaluate the success of the interventions and the progress of your child. What are the things you will be looking for to judge her progress (for instance, misbehaving less in class)? And how will this progress be communicated to you?

- If you feel that the opinion of another professional would be helpful in evaluating the problem or suggesting possible solutions, speak with the principal or another member of the support staff (counselor, nurse, psychologist), either with or without the teacher present. You also might decide to seek out an independent opinion from someone outside the school system. Ask your pediatrician for his or her opinion or for a referral.

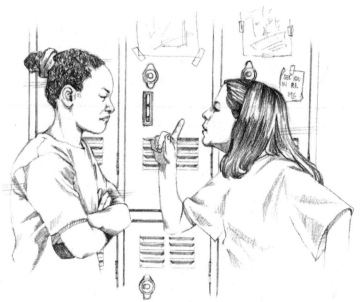

Problems with peers can make school difficult for some children.

SPECIAL CONCERNS ABOUT PEERS

Many difficulties can arise at school that will require your intervention. One of the most common is when a child feels rejected by classmates.

If your youngster comes home upset and crying that "everyone is being mean to me at recess and in the cafeteria," keep in mind that at some time most children have conflicts with their friends and end up feeling pushed away. Parental reassurance can comfort these youngsters until things return to normal at school.

However, if a pattern of rejection exists, let your child know that you are sensitive to how difficult this situation is for him, and that you are going to help him figure out ways to make things better. Give him a clear message that you are on his side and are going to help.

Rejection by a child's peers may be a group reaction to someone they see as different. It may also result from inappropriate behavior on the part of both parties and need to be modified.

Ask your child for more facts about the situation. Schedule an appointment with his teacher. Consider requesting that the principal or guidance counselor attend the meeting. Have them obtain information from the recess and lunch aides about what is happening.

Follow the steps described in "The Parent-Teacher Conference," page 486. After this initial meeting, or whenever you feel you have enough information, you may want to consult with your pediatrician, who is familiar with your child's developmental pattern. (See also "Friends," page 152, and "Children Without Friends," page 157.)

ACADEMIC/TEACHER PROBLEMS

At one time or another, nearly every child does poorly on a particular test or has difficulty with a subject or two in school. These situations can often be dealt with successfully by working one-on-one with your child, or through a three-way interaction involving you, your child, and her teacher.

On occasion, a concern persists despite your best efforts to resolve it. Perhaps you are unhappy with certain aspects of the learning environment in your child's classroom. Maybe you feel she is not receiving the proper help with a particular subject. Or perhaps your child has complained that the teacher has humiliated her in front of her classmates.

In situations like these, approach the teacher first with your concern. Explain the problem without being accusatory or insulting. (Avoid statements like "You're not doing your job!" or "I cannot believe you said that to my child!") Give the teacher a chance to explain what is taking place, to share another perspective, and to suggest a solution. If you are dissatisfied with that encounter, or if you feel that sufficient progress is not being made after trying the teacher's plan, then bring your problem to the attention of the principal. The principal may suggest a meeting with you and the teacher. In many instances the difficulty can be resolved with input from the principal.

The principal can become your ally in other situations too. Approach him or her for problems unrelated to the classroom—for example, difficulties with a bus driver or a playground aide. At times, other school personnel—such as guidance counselors or psychologists—may be helpful.

If the principal and teacher, or others, have initiated a specific plan to improve the situation, give things a reasonable chance to improve. (It will not change in a couple of days.) However, if the problem still remains unresolved, then continue up the educational hierarchy, which may lead you to the superintendent's office. For an issue involving school district policy, the superintendent and his or her associates will be the decision makers. If you still remain dissatisfied, approach the school board members. They may be able to get action on your problem, or put you in touch with the person who can.

As you move up the administrative ladder, gather, organize, and stay focused on the facts; save your emotional reactions for someone else who can acknowledge them. Be persistent and remain as pleasant and objective as possible. You will not make progress by losing your temper and by alienating the people who might help solve the difficulty.

At some point along this path of seeking help, consult your child's pediatrician for advice or for a referral to another professional outside the school system.

REPEATING A GRADE: DOES IT HELP?

Teachers and parents are sometimes faced with the question of whether to have a child repeat a grade because he seems unprepared to learn the material in the next grade. When making this decision, keep in mind that research shows that low-achieving students tend to progress at the same rate, whether they are retained or promoted. Retained students do not necessarily score better on achievement tests at the end of the repeated grade, compared with similar students who are promoted. Even if retained students improve on standardized test scores, their overall learning does not appear to increase.

You must also consider the negative effects of grade retention on social and emotional development. Quite often these students have fewer friends and a poorer self-concept. If a child already has emotional or social difficulties and has an academic deficit only in a particular area, he might benefit more from special services rather than retention.

Usually teachers will mention a child's immaturity when they recommend retention. Ask for specific examples of this problem. Is it in the physical, emotional, or social realm? Ask if retention is the only or the best solution. If your child's schoolwork is on track, but he has difficulty controlling his impulsive behavior with his friends on the playground, then a consistent home-school approach to helping him change his behavior may be appropriate.

Other issues also must be considered. Rigid, test-based policies regarding promotion and retention often do not take into account issues beyond the student's control, such as the poor quality of teaching, poor teaching environments, learning disabilities, emotional problems, or family difficulties that may cause students to miss school.

In general, then, retention does not help children learn and, in fact, may contribute to a poor self-concept, diminished self-esteem, and emotional or social difficulties.

Other practical solutions may be alternatives when retention is being considered for your child, whatever the reason.

- Some schools have instituted a policy that prevents students from entering the first grade before they are ready to read and write. By creating a "readiness first grade" for six-year-olds who are not quite ready for the usual first grade, they have eliminated the need for students to repeat the same first-grade curriculum. For example, the content of the reading materials varies between the readiness class and the regular class, so students do not repeat the same work. Teachers report fewer behavior problems in the more positive learning environment of this approach.

- Multi-age grouping, or mixing children from two or more grade levels in the same classroom, can be beneficial. In this way, a child stays in the same classroom with his friends—continuing to develop socially and emotionally—but receives the appropriate academic work that he needs. It also allows the youngster to do grade-appropriate work in those areas in which he is capable.

- Some schools make adjustments during the school year itself, moving the child to a different class or involving a tutor if it is obvious he will need extra help.

- Sometimes children are permitted to repeat a failed semester instead of a full year, which requires the teacher and student to be flexible.

School staffs tend to be very knowledgeable and experienced in decisions about retention, and do not lightly make the recommendation to hold a student back. Some students do benefit from retention, particularly those who already have strong self-esteem and are emotionally healthy but are still having difficulty keeping up academically with their classmates. Some educators argue that if a student is continually moved ahead without acquiring the basic academic skills he needs, he will not develop the literacy or problem-solving abilities required in today's job market. This can be counterproductive to your child's education. If you suspect that this process is occurring, schedule a meeting with the teacher.

However, when retention is recommended and you are not comfortable with it, seek an additional opinion. Talk it over with your child's pediatrician, another teacher, or a psychologist. Consider whether an outside evaluation would be helpful.

If you and the teacher ultimately decide that it is necessary to retain your child, ask for the teacher's suggestions on the best way to explain it to your youngster. Also, inquire about the program that will be in place next year to address your youngster's problems. In preparation for the next school year, help your child figure out positive ways to discuss his grade retention. Role-play how he can answer the inevitable questions from his friends and classmates.

For the middle-years child, the optimal times to retain him are at the end of kindergarten or first grade, or upon moving to a new school or a new city.

SCHOOL DISCIPLINE

Many classes have a student who constantly talks out of turn, or chews gum in class when it is clearly prohibited, or gets into fights with classmates, or peeks at another student's paper during a spelling test. All of these situations warrant some disciplinary action. Most schools have a policy about discipline, and in many cases it is available in writing, often published in the school handbook. Although both students and parents tend to think of discipline as a form of punishment, it actually means to teach in a correct way and has a highly desirable purpose: providing an orderly, safe environment to promote learning.

Disciplinary efforts work best when clear explanations are given to both children and parents about:

- the behavior that is expected

- the behavior that is unacceptable

- the consequences of unacceptable behavior

The American Academy of Pediatrics feels strongly that while departures from expected behavior should be dealt with appropriately and firmly, teachers and school staff should also take into account each child's individual temperament, attention span, and cognitive abilities. For example, a youngster with an attention deficit hyperactivity disorder (ADHD) may have more difficulty sitting still in class than most of the other children. This disorder should be kept in mind when discipline is being considered.

In all cases disciplinary actions should show respect for the youngster and take into account the student's capabilities, effort, and ability to improve and respond positively. While discipline may include an extra homework assignment or a loss of privileges, physical punishment should *never* be used, nor should a child ever be humiliated in front of others.

If your own youngster has disciplinary problems at school, you need to take a more active role in determining the reasons and ensuring that she behaves appropriately. Make certain she understands the type of behavior you and the school expect from her in the classroom and on the playground.

On occasion you might be unhappy with the school's approach to discipline. In that event, address your concerns directly to the teacher, principal, or other school personnel. Do not make derogatory comments about the school to your child. Your own attitudes and behavior are a powerful role model for your youngster, and if you do not appear to have much respect for the school, your child will not either.

For example, if your youngster is being kept inside at recess as a form of punishment, and you feel she really needs to get outside and burn off some excess energy, be careful how you express your dissatisfaction to your child. Do not say something like "That is really a stupid form of punishment, isn't it?" Instead, talk to the teacher and suggest another form of punishment that might be more appropriate. You and the teacher should try to find a common ground so your child receives a consistent set of expectations and positive reinforcement both at home and at school.

In general, a child should not be kept from play at recess to complete classroom assignments at her desk. She will dislike her work even more if she misses out on outdoor activities that she enjoys. And since her attention will probably be on the playground, she may not learn much from what she is doing. It is very important for children to be outside playing with others at times during the day.

In all cases ask the teacher and/or principal to keep you apprised of disciplinary problems with your youngster. Some principals call home immediately upon the child's first visit to their office; others believe that by the upper grades of elementary school, the youngster should take more responsibility for her own behavior, and thus these principals may try to help the child work out the problem without parental intervention.

If there is a serious problem, you probably will be notified at once; but for more routine behavioral difficulties, you cannot necessarily count on being called. If your child tells you she has been to the principal's office and you want to know exactly what happened, feel free to call the principal. On the other hand, many issues can be resolved effectively without your involvement and without your also punishing your child at home for something that she is already being disciplined for at school.

Finally, keep in mind that behavior problems are often a signal of stress or a call for help or attention. Consider the causes of the behavior difficulties as well as the problems themselves.

Does Your Child's School Practice Corporal Punishment?

When you were a child, did your school principal sometimes paddle students who misbehaved? Or were youngsters slapped with an open hand or struck with a strap or ruler at school?

Physical punishment remains a part of the disciplinary policy of many schools, sanctioned by laws in twenty-three states. At least 470,000 students were subjected to corporal punishment during the 1993–94 school year, according to the most recent statistics available.

Nevertheless, studies consistently show that physical punishment of school-age children is not effective. The American Academy of Pediatrics believes that corporal punishment can actually have a negative influence upon a child's self-image and thus interfere with his academic achievement. Punishment does not teach more appropriate behavior or self-discipline and may even cause a youngster to behave more aggressively and violently. Antisocial behavior is lowest among children who have never been spanked.

In a very limited number of circumstances a principal or other school official may need to physically restrain a student to protect that child or other students from physical injury or to prevent property damage. The Academy is working to encourage school boards and legislatures to ban corporal punishment in the schools of all states and to adopt alternative approaches for managing student behavior.

51

HOMEWORK

During the elementary-school years, virtually all children begin to have homework. Precisely when it starts will depend on the school and the teacher, although in general it will begin between second and fourth grades. When homework is assigned, it will average about fifteen to twenty minutes per night in the early elementary-school years, but depending on your child's capabilities, he may need more or less time to complete it, sometimes up to about an hour.

As a general guideline, some educators believe that the number of minutes a child should spend on homework is equivalent to his grade level times ten. Thus, a third-grader should complete his nightly homework assignments in about thirty minutes; a fifth-grader in about fifty minutes. Find out early in the school year about the teacher's philosophy regarding homework, and plan accordingly. Ask the teacher questions about how much homework is assigned, how often, and how involved the teacher prefers parents to be.

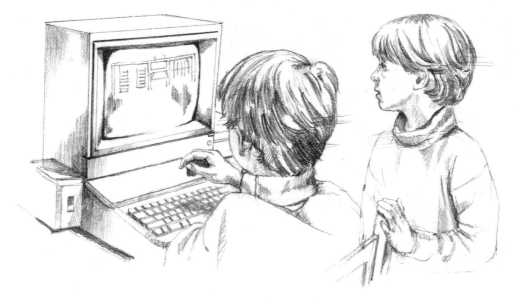

DEVELOPING GOOD HOMEWORK HABITS

Help your child develop good homework habits. That means designating a regular location and time to work on daily assignments. She does not necessarily need a desk in her room; the kitchen table can work just as well. No matter what place you choose, it needs to be well lit and quiet, without the distractions of the television set, other children playing, or people talking on the telephone. Keep your child's materials (paper, pencil, dictionary) nearby so she can get started quickly and on her own each afternoon or evening.

Some children get right down to work without much encouragement. Others need help making the transition from playing to a homework frame of mind. Sometimes providing a ten-minute warning is all it takes to help a child get ready mentally as well as to move to the place she intends to work.

There is no universally right time to do homework. In some families, children do best if they tackle their homework shortly after returning home from school in the midafternoon; other youngsters may do best if they devote the after-school hours to unwinding and playing, leaving their homework until the evening, when they may feel a renewed sense of vigor. Let your child have some say in the decision making. Homework can often become a source of conflict between parent and child—"Johnny, why can't you just do your homework without arguing about it?"—but if you agree on a regular time and place, you can eliminate two of the most frequent causes of homework-related dissension.

Some parents have found that their children respond poorly to a dictated study time (such as four o'clock every afternoon). Instead, youngsters are given guidelines ("No video games until your homework is done"). Find out what works best for both your child and the family as a whole. Once this is determined, stick with it.

Some youngsters prefer that a parent sit with them as they do their homework. You may find this an acceptable request, particularly if you have your own reading or paperwork to complete. However, do *not* actually do the homework for your child. She may need some assistance getting focused and started and organizing her approach to the assignment. Occasionally, you may need to explain a math problem; in those cases, let your child try a couple of problems first before offering to help. But if she *routinely* requires your active participation to get her everyday homework done, then talk to her teacher. Your child may need stronger direction in the classroom so that she is able to complete the assignments on her own or with less parental involvement. One area where children may need parental help is in organizing how much work will have to be done daily to finish a long assignment, such as a term paper or a science project.

If your child or her teacher asks you to review her homework, you may want to look it over before she takes it to school the next morning. Usually it is best if homework remains the exclusive domain of the child and the teacher. However, your input may vary depending on the teacher's philosophy and the purpose of homework. If the teacher is using homework to check your child's understanding of the material—thus giving the teacher an idea of what needs to be emphasized in subsequent classroom teaching sessions—your suggestions for changes and improvements on your child's paper could prove misleading. On the other hand, if the teacher assigns homework to give your child practice in a particular subject area and to reinforce what has already been taught in class, then your participation can be valuable. Some teachers use homework to help children develop self-discipline and organizational and study skills. Be sure to praise your youngster for her efforts and success in doing her homework well.

In general, support your child in her homework, but do not act as a taskmaster. Provide her with a quiet place, supplies, encouragement, and occasional help—but it is her job to do the work. Homework is your youngster's responsibility, not yours.

As the weeks pass, keep in touch with your child's teacher regarding homework assignments. If your youngster is having ongoing problems—difficulty understanding what the assignments are and how to complete them—or if she breezes through them as though they were no challenge at all, let the teacher know. The teacher may adjust the assignments so they are more in sync with your youngster's capabilities.

Talking About Your Child's School Day

"What did you do in school today?"

"Nothing."

This is a familiar exchange between parent and child. And it can be a frustrating one for an interested parent who genuinely wants to keep abreast of a child's activities at school and yet not appear nosy. (This issue of intrusiveness becomes more of a problem with the ten- to twelve-year-old child and certainly with adolescents.)

Youngsters will usually be more responsive about their day at school if they are asked fairly direct questions at a time that is appropriate. For instance, when a child first arrives home from school, he might be tired and want a snack, or want to relax or play with a friend rather than rehash the day. It might be better to talk with him about school later in the day or evening. Or begin the conversation with a statement like "You look pretty hungry. Let's have a snack and then you can tell me about your day."

Make your questions as focused and nonjudgmental as possible. For instance:

- "What new thing did you learn in school today?"

Whether or not your child has homework on a particular night, consider reading aloud with her after school or at night. This type of shared experience can help interest your child in reading, as well as give you some personal time with her. Also, on days when your child does not have any assigned homework, this shared reading time will reinforce the habit of a work time each evening.

To further nurture your child's love of reading, set a good example by spending time reading on your own, and by taking your youngster to the library and/or bookstore to select books she would like to read. Some families turn off the TV each night for at least thirty minutes, and everyone spends the time reading. As children get older, one to two hours may be a more desirable length of time each day to set aside for reading and other constructive activities.

As important as it is for your child to develop good study habits, play is also important for healthy social, emotional, and physical growth and development. While encouraging your child to complete her assignments or do some additional reading, keep in mind that she has already had a lengthy and per-

- "What questions did you ask in class?"

- "How is that book you've been reading in class? What's happening in the story?"

- "Do you have any papers or artwork in your backpack that we could look over?"

- "Is learning long division getting a little easier?"

- "Tell me about the spelling test. Was there a word or two you had trouble with?"

Knowing that their students may have trouble remembering everything that happened in school, teachers often communicate about class and school issues through written notes. Ask your child each night if he has any notes for you.

At times your child might want to talk about school when you're right in the middle of something else. As much as possible, try to be responsive, perhaps saying something like "I want to hear about school, but right now I'm very busy fixing dinner. Let me get this casserole in the oven, and then we can sit down and really talk." Or "Why don't you hop on this stool and help me make this salad while we talk."

haps tiring day of learning at school and needs some free time. Help her find the play activities that best fit her temperament and personality—whether it is organized school sports or music lessons, free-play situations (riding her bike, playing with friends), or a combination of these.

HOMEWORK FOR CHILDREN AGES TEN TO TWELVE: DEVELOPING RESPONSIBILITY

As children enter the fourth grade, the purpose of homework changes to some extent. In grades one to three, students are learning to read; thereafter, they are reading to learn. In fourth grade both schoolwork and homework become more challenging. Learning tasks require more organization and more sustained attention and effort. Because of this change, homework becomes a more integral part of children's learning and is reflected more in their academic record. This shift comes at a good time, since at about the fourth grade, children are ready for and want more autonomy and responsibility and less parental hovering and interference.

Homework for older children has a number of purposes. It provides an opportunity for review and reinforcement of skills that have been mastered and encourages practicing skills that are not. Homework also is an opportunity for children to learn self-discipline and organizational skills and to take responsibility for their own learning.

Many of the same suggestions for approaching homework that were recommended for younger children apply to older children as well. Homework is best done when the child has had a chance to unwind from school or after-school activities, is rested, and is not hungry. You and your child should agree upon a regular schedule for when homework will be done, and the length of time that should be devoted to it. This schedule should provide predictability and structure but should be sufficiently flexible to respond to special situations. Some children do best if their homework time is divided into several short sessions instead of a single long one.

Usually parents can be helpful by assisting their child in getting settled and started. You can look together at each day's homework assignment and decide what parts might require help from you, a sibling, or a classmate. The most difficult parts should be done first. Reviewing for tests and rote memorization tasks also should be done early and then repeated at the end of the homework session or first thing the next morning. As is the case for younger children, homework should be done in a location with few distractions (no television, radio, telephone, video games, comics, toys, or conversation), and where all the necessary supplies and reference materials are available.

Here are some specific suggestions on how to approach homework of different types:

Reading Assignments

1. Divide chapters into small units or use the author's headings as a guide.

2. Find the topic sentence or the main idea for each paragraph and underline it or write it down.

3. Write a section-by-section outline of the reading assignment, copying or paraphrasing the main points; leave some room to write in notes from class discussions.

Writing (Composition)

1. Begin by recognizing that the first draft will not be the last, and that rewriting will produce better work.

2. Make a list of as many ideas as possible without worrying about whether they are good or correct.

3. Organize these "brainstorm" ideas into clusters that seem reasonable, and then arrange the clusters into a logical sequence.

4. Write down thoughts as to why these clusters were made and why the order makes sense.

5. Use this work as an outline and write a first draft; at this stage, do not worry about spelling or punctuation.

6. Revise the first draft, paying attention to detail.
   Check the

Meaning: Does it make sense and meet the purpose of the assignment?

Paragraph formation: Does each paragraph have a topic sentence and are the other sentences logically related?

Sentence formation: Does each sentence express a complete thought? Are capitalization and punctuation correct?

Word: Was the best word chosen? Is it spelled correctly?

Neatness: Is the paper easy to read? Does it follow the format and style the teacher expects?

Math

1. Work toward mastering the basic facts and operations (addition, subtraction, multiplication, and division) until they become automatic. Do this work in small doses, and limit the number of facts to three to five each session. Use writing, flash cards, and oral quizzes.

2. Be sure the basic concepts of computation are well understood. Do computation homework slowly and check the results, since if the facts are understood, most errors come from being careless.

3. Use money examples when learning decimals.

4. For fractions, use visual or concrete aids rather than oral explanations.

Studying for Tests

1. Gather together homework assignments, class notes, outlines, quizzes, and handouts, and arrange them chronologically (by date).

2. Four days before the test, read the information through in a general way.

3. Three days before the test, look at major titles of sections in notes and books.

4. Two days before the test, review the titles of sections and read the information and organize it into related clusters.

5. The night before the test, repeat the process of the night before and recite as much as you can from memory.

OTHER WAYS TO REINFORCE LEARNING

In addition to doing homework, your child should spend time reading not only with you, but on his own as well. If a child finds pleasure in reading, it will become a lifelong habit. His teacher or school librarian can help you and your youngster select some books for leisure reading. Make sure he has a card at the public library as well. Also, if he would like and if you can afford it, join a children's book club or subscribe to a magazine for children in the appropriate age group (such as *Boys' Life, Highlights for Children, National Geographic World, 3-2-1 Contact, Stone Soup*). If your youngster sees you reading regularly, there is a good chance that he will follow your lead and sit down with a book himself. Set aside some time to talk with him about what each of you is reading. If you have been regularly reading aloud to your youngster, by school age he'll probably want to read aloud to you, too, perhaps alternating chapters in a book you both enjoy.

Also, find time to converse with your child about your respective days, including what he did at school. Even on a night when you are particularly busy, you should still be able to find a time and place to talk. (See Chapter 13, "Communicating with Your Child.")

You should also encourage your child to write and/or draw without any educational purpose in mind other than to express himself. Perhaps he can compose original stories, or write cards, letters, and invitations to friends and relatives. Keep paper, pencils, crayons, markers, and tape in a convenient location so he can sit down and use them without advance planning. Many researchers believe that writing improves a child's reading skills, and vice versa.

Plan some activities—an art project, for example—that you can do with your child. Keep phone call interruptions to a minimum during this period;

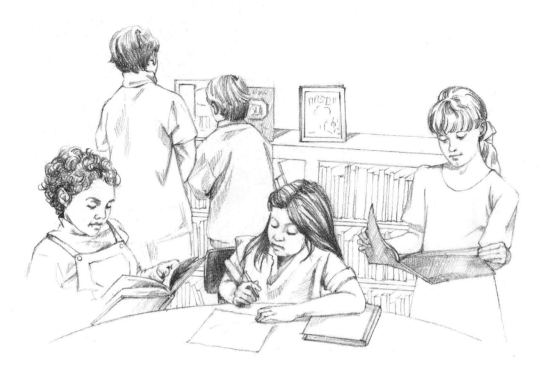

make it a time you are spending with each other. (Some children say they wish they could call their parents on the phone, because a phone call always gets first priority.)

Put a map on the wall in your child's bedroom and refer to it frequently. You might ask, "Where does Aunt Linda live? . . . Can you find the city where the President lives?" You can also use the map to talk about history, especially around a historical holiday.

Many children enjoy going to the library too. Because they use the school library frequently, children almost instinctively feel at home when they go to the community library. (In schools, libraries are now often called *learning centers,* because they have video and audio materials as well.)

Also, find some community activities that are pure fun. Despite their recreational nature, they can still be viewed as providing support for what is being taught in school, since they will broaden your child's base of experience and give him something new to write about.

Try reinforcing your child's health education at school in a number of ways—for instance, by making healthful food choices when you shop. No matter what is taught in the classroom and served in the school cafeteria, these influences are much less likely to have an impact upon your youngster if you do not follow the same health-promoting guidelines in your own food selections. Actively involving your child in the process by having him read recipes and measure ingredients can reinforce nutrition education. (See Chapter 5, "Nutritional Needs.")

Capitalize on your child's physical education program at school, too, by scheduling some weekend or after-school activities that are appropriate for the entire family. Swimming, tennis, bicycle riding, and skiing are some of the sports that children can participate in for their entire lives and that can keep your child fit long after he has left school. Do not overlook walking, either, as a perfect way for the family to enjoy physical activity together. (See Chapter 7, "Physical Fitness and Sports," for a thorough discussion of fitness and exercise.)

LEARNING DISABILITIES

I n the middle years of childhood, youngsters leave the protective confines of the family and enter the world of school and peers. As that happens, they need to "make it" in the outside world in many ways, an important one of which is being successful in the classroom.

Unfortunately, early school experiences are not always positive. When children learn slowly—or if they need to work too hard to learn—both children and parents can feel disappointed, frustrated, sad, and confused.

If your child experiences school failure or appears to be under-achieving, you need to consider the possibility that she has a learning disability (also called learning disorder, learning difference, or learning difficulty). This developmental disorder is quite common, affecting 20 percent or more of children. When it is present, it can cause emotional, social, behavioral, or family problems, especially if the disability is not diagnosed or is misdiagnosed, or if the interventions or treatments used are not appropriate or do not achieve results.

The earlier you become aware of a possible problem, and the sooner your child is evaluated and helped, the better the chances for a positive outcome.

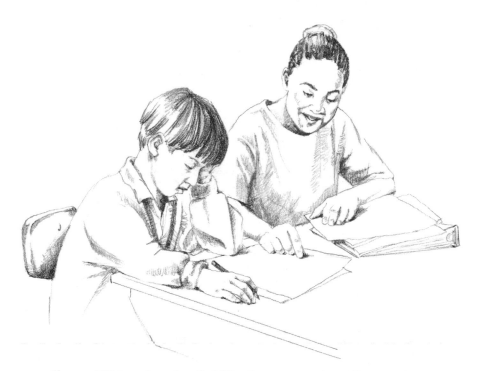

If your child has a learning disability, there are a variety of interventions or supportive services available to assist him.

WHAT ARE LEARNING DISABILITIES?

Learning disabilities result from a variation in your child's central nervous system functioning. This does not mean that your youngster has "brain damage" or is mentally retarded, although in some cases, a previous head injury or brain infection might cause learning difficulties. In most instances, children are born with the tendency for learning problems; the cause is "invisible" and hard to pin down, and the affected children look and act like other children and are in other ways no different from them.

Learning disabilities tend to run in families. About 50 percent of these children have a parent, sibling, or extended family member with a similar difficulty, although in the past it was much more frequently misdiagnosed or mislabeled.

The Impact of Common Learning Disabilities

When learning disabilities occur, they generally affect three general skill areas:

- academic skills, such as reading, writing, spelling, and arithmetic

- language and speech skills, encompassing areas such as listening, talking, and understanding

- so-called motor-sensory integration skills, such as coordination, balance, and writing

When problems exist in any of these areas, there is a breakdown in one or more stages of learning. For instance, the child may have difficulty taking in information through hearing or sight. Or he could have problems remembering the information he has heard or read. Finally, he may be unable to utilize this knowledge in a productive way.

Learning disabilities can vary in severity, from mild to severe. They may affect a single learning task like spelling, or they can influence many of them, like reading, writing, and listening comprehension. In some children, their presence may be very obvious even before school age; in others, they may become apparent later and then only in subtle ways. Parents may not even be aware that their child has a learning disability until his learning capabilities are challenged and he is unable to keep up with classroom demands and expectations.

Learning disabilities can last a lifetime, becoming more or less obvious depending on the academic and other learning demands that the youngster faces. With help, however, they often do improve.

When a child does poorly in school or seems to lose his motivation to learn, he might be responding to other problems in his life. He might be experiencing problems with peers, or there may be family problems that he finds distracting. As with learning disabilities themselves, social and emotional problems that mimic learning disabilities require immediate and appropriate help.

Does Your Child Have Attention or Learning Problems?

Attention deficit hyperactivity disorder (ADHD) is a problem closely associated with learning disabilities. About 25 percent or more of youngsters with learning disabilities also have attention difficulties, which can affect their academic, language, speech, and writing skills, as well as all other areas of learning.

If your own child has been diagnosed with a learning disability, you need to consider whether attention problems are present as well. If he has been diagnosed as having ADHD, he might also have a learning disorder.

For more information on attention problems, see Chapter 22, "Attention Deficit Hyperactivity Disorder."

DIAGNOSING A LEARNING DISABILITY

Learning disabilities are traditionally diagnosed by conducting two tests and noticing a significant discrepancy between their scores. These tests are an intelligence (or IQ) test and a standardized achievement (reading, writing, arithmetic) test. Most children found to have a learning disability have normal or above-normal intelligence but do not fully demonstrate that potential on achievement tests. For example, a youngster might score 112 on the full-scale IQ test, but her math score might be 90; this discrepancy of 22 points between her potential ability (IQ) and actual achievement (in math) might qualify her for special services at her school. Some states, for example, define a learning disability as a difference of 15 points, but the criteria for services vary from one part of the country to another. As a result, state-mandated definitions sometimes exclude a range of learning difficulties that do not produce wide discrepancies.

When a learning disability is not detected early, diagnosed correctly, and treated effectively, it can cause a number of other problems. These additional difficulties may be emotional, and a child can show signs of sadness, frustration, or disappointment. Behavior problems like acting out might occur. Or the learning problems may show up within the family, causing, for example, misunderstandings, increased stress, or blaming others. Studies show that among children whose families seek professional help for emotional or behavioral problems, 30 to 50 percent of them have learning disabilities.

COMMON LEARNING DISABILITIES

Language and Speech Disabilities

These are among the most common learning problems and can be quite significant, because most learning is dependent on language. If your child has such a disability, it can affect his reading, spelling, writing, speech, and ability to understand what he hears or reads. It may also affect his memory or comprehension—that is, the ability to recall or understand information previously heard or read. Your child may have difficulty following instructions, understanding explanations, or expressing himself. These problems can not only affect his learning but also may impede his social interactions, which require good listening and speaking skills. As a result he may become embarrassed, confused, or quiet and withdrawn. He might even resort to acting out his feelings, thoughts, or frustrations with inappropriate behavior.

Writing Difficulties

Like children with other types of learning disabilities, children with writing problems may be bright and creative but may have difficulty expressing themselves on paper in a coherent manner. This may cause frustration or even a writing phobia. Since any written document is a semipublic, permanent display of one's work, these children sometimes feel extremely embarrassed or self-conscious and often try to avoid writing assignments or don't make much of an effort when doing them. Writing is a complex task that requires the simultaneous use of many skills, including letter formation, grammar, vocabulary, spelling, the mechanics of writing (punctuation, capitalization), and organizing ideas into sentences and paragraphs. While some children may master each of these skills separately, carrying all of them out at the same time may prove difficult. Writing problems are complex and may have several causes, including visual, fine motor, language, and/or memory difficulties.

Visual Learning Difficulties

When youngsters have a weakness or disability in understanding visually presented information, it may affect their ability to read, spell, interpret, or remember the printed word, graphs, tables, illustrations, and maps. These are learning problems; the children's vision is normal and unrelated to the specific problem.

Sometimes visual learning difficulties occur along with another weakness—for example, in conjunction with fine motor difficulties—which can affect handwriting. When that happens, the child's writing may be illegible. He may have difficulty forming letters or numbers, or keeping numbers properly aligned in columns. He may write letters or numbers backward. This can affect not only his writing ability (including legibility and speed) but also his proficiency in mathematics, causing him to make miscalculations.

Memory and Other Thinking Difficulties

As children move through elementary school, they are increasingly asked to remember, retrieve, and use more and more information rapidly. They need to recall specific information in a very detailed manner, as well as to recall and assemble information in a creative and open-ended way. The first, more specific memory (called convergent) is useful in short answers or multiple-choice tests and in analytical, fact-oriented reasoning. The second, more general memory (divergent) is useful in essay writing, retelling a story, interpreting a poem, or describing a character in one's own way.

Memory involves taking in information, classifying it, associating it with previously learned information, and consolidating it. Many children understand what they read or are taught but can't remember it later on, perhaps for a test, or they can't recall it in a different context. While a memory problem can be subtle and difficult to assess, you should suspect this type of difficulty if your child is underachieving.

Some youngsters have particular trouble remembering several pieces of sequential information, such as multiple instructions or a series of words or numbers (like a telephone number). As a result, a school-age child may have difficulty doing a three-step math problem, organizing events, learning the alphabet, remembering multiplication tables, or recounting a story in the proper sequence. Even learning the days of the week, months of the year, and class schedules can be hard.

A number of factors can make memory problems even worse. These include too much or too complex information being presented at one time, or an excessively rapid rate of incoming information. Attention problems, emotional disorders (depression, anxiety), boredom, loss of motivation, and fatigue (poor nutrition, inadequate sleep, mental exertion) can also contribute to memory difficulties.

Difficulties can occur with other higher-level thinking as well. Some children have problems with a skill called abstract reasoning, meaning that they are unable to determine the general meaning of a particular word or symbol—perhaps the symbol for an unknown quantity in a math problem. They also cannot make inferences by going from a specific, concrete fact to a more general type of thinking.

Youngsters may also have difficulty with organization and thus be unable to assemble information into a usable form. Good organizational skills can also help children associate newly learned information with their existing knowledge, making it fit in with something familiar so it can be more easily retrieved and utilized.

Summarizing skills are another possible problem area. Children may have trouble taking a large amount of information and condensing it to a more manageable size so it is easier to remember and use. Youngsters with this skill are able to separate major facts and concepts from lesser ones, ascertaining which ones are most worthwhile.

Inadequate Social Skills

These often occur in conjunction with learning disabilities and usually result in difficulties interacting with other children or adults. Children with this problem may have trouble interpreting the messages or intentions of others and responding appropriately to others, even to parents and teachers who are trying to be helpful. Recognizing and alleviating these difficulties are critical, because peer acceptance and a successful social life are extremely important to the youngster in middle childhood and greatly affect his self-image and self-esteem. (See Chapter 9, "Developing Social Skills.")

WHAT PARENTS CAN DO

If your child is performing below grade level, is failing or struggling to maintain barely passing grades, or is not achieving to the degree to which you think she is capable, here are some suggestions for beginning to get her the help she needs:

- Trust your instincts. You know your child best, and if you suspect something is wrong, it should be investigated. Don't assume that learning disorders don't matter or that your child will "grow out of it." Early recognition and treatment are important.

- Ask the teacher for his or her opinion about the possibility of learning disabilities in your child. Listen to any concerns the teacher may have. Rely on his or her experience and training.

- If your youngster appears frustrated, unmotivated, or bored, or is acting up in school, these could be signs of a learning problem that needs diagnosis and treatment. Also, if your child is failing, underachieving, or working extremely hard just to keep up, this could also be a symptom of a learning difficulty.

- Ask your child questions relevant to her situation. Here are some suggestions of areas to pursue, often with the help of the teacher's input:

    Reading: "How well do you read? Do you like to read? Do you understand or remember what you read?"

    Writing: "How is your handwriting? Is it difficult copying from the chalkboard or a book? How is your spelling? Grammar? Punctuation? Do you finish tasks and written assignments after everyone else?"

    Arithmetic: "Are you having any problems with adding? Subtracting? Multiplying? Dividing? Can you perform these tasks with double digits? Do you understand why you carry and borrow? Do you sometimes forget the rules of math, or get partway through a problem and then forget what you were trying to do? Can you perform word problems?"

    Language: "When the teacher is speaking, do you have difficulty listening, understanding, remembering, or keeping up? Do you have trouble organizing your thoughts before you speak? Are you sometimes unable to find the word you want to use? Do difficulties like these arise in class? With friends? With other adults?"

- Although the answers to these questions may indicate that a learning disability is present, also consider whether other issues may be contributing to the problem. Is your youngster devoting adequate time and energy to her schoolwork? Is she interested and involved in the learning process? Could your family's everyday functioning and expectations be affecting her adversely? Is she preoccupied with peer relationships or with problems at home? Are academic and emotional stresses causing frustration and a loss of confidence and motivation, almost to the point of helplessness ("No matter how hard I try, I still can't learn")?

- Think back to your own childhood. Many parents experienced similar learning difficulties when they were youngsters, and these problems tend to occur in families. Your own empathy, understanding, and acceptance will influence the course of your child's learning problem, as will your attitude toward schools and learning.

- Speak with other adults and professionals. Seek out information and guidance from your child's principal, guidance counselor, school psychologist, coach, or the parents of her friends.

- Your pediatrician's advice will also be helpful, because he or she understands child development, knows your child, and has experience in these common childhood problems. He or she may also be able to send questions to school to try to clarify an apparent problem with learning.

Your pediatrician can also determine whether any physical problems (including a vision or hearing deficiency) could be playing a role in your child's learning difficulties. He or she can refer you and your child to the appropriate professionals, perhaps suggesting that your youngster have a formal learning-disability evaluation, either by the school or by private psychologists and educators not affiliated with the school system. In most states, if a child is failing or otherwise performing below grade level, the public schools are obligated to conduct such evaluations and may be required to provide special services (for children with ADHD, see Chapter 22, "Attention Deficit Hyperactivity Disorder").

Your pediatrician can also serve as an advocate within the school system, ensuring that your child gets the appropriate services to which she is entitled.

YOUR RIGHT TO SPECIAL SERVICES

Once a learning problem is suspected, ask your child's school staff about the free, special educational services (evaluation and, if appropriate, treatment) mentioned earlier. Sometimes teachers or principals are reluctant to request a consultation or make a referral. If you feel strongly that your child's needs are not being met, persevere. Public school systems must make special services available under the Individuals with Disabilities Education Act, a federal statute enacted in 1975. In order to receive federal funds, every state and school district must have a procedure for identifying, assessing, and planning an educational program for these youngsters, from age three to twenty-two. This law covers not only children with learning disabilities, but also those with perceptual problems (hearing or visual impairments), cerebral palsy or other brain injuries, mental retardation, orthopedic problems affecting mobility, and serious behavioral and emotional difficulties that can interfere with the process of education.

This law provides five basic rights: the right to

1. a free, appropriate public education

2. an individual educational plan (IEP) based on a complete developmental assessment and approved by parents

3. access to records or the right of parents to review the child's educational records

4. due process, or giving parents the right to participate in the evaluation and decision-making process

5. the least restrictive educational environment (placing the child in a learning situation that is as normal and convenient as conditions allow)

THE EVALUATION

A minimal evaluation includes a psychological assessment of cognitive function (an IQ test) and an educational assessment of academic achievement (a standardized test). Other testing might evaluate so-called neurodevelopmental functions (such as language, memory, attention, and motor skills), the emotional status of your child, and a social assessment (family and environment).

This evaluation process can be complicated, time-consuming, and difficult for parents and child to understand. Sometimes it is quite expensive if you obtain the evaluations outside the school system. In most cases, you should start with the full evaluation provided by your child's school. If it cannot be done within a reasonable time or if specialized testing is needed, request payment from the school system before you get a private evaluation. However, regardless of where they are done, these evaluations can be both informative and productive.

Because the entire evaluation process may be complex and involve many people, a case manager or services coordinator (like a pediatrician, psychologist, or learning-disability educator) may be helpful. The coordinator can also assist you in planning appropriate interventions or treatments, making referrals, monitoring the effect of treatment upon your child, and arranging for follow-up evaluations. Frequently this takes a team effort.

Once an evaluation is completed, schools usually arrange a meeting to fully discuss the findings and your child's educational plan. This meeting might be attended by your youngster's teacher(s), guidance counselor, the special-education teacher, the principal, the school psychologist, and nurse. Sometimes children attend the meeting. Occasionally you may want to ask your pediatrician to attend to provide support for you and your perspective. If you wish, bring someone with you who might serve as the child's advocate and who is familiar with these evaluations and meetings and understands the implications of the findings and interventions. Make sure the results are explained to you in terms you can understand.

In explaining the learning problem to your child, avoid simplistic, negative labels such as *learning disabled, handicapped,* and *hyperactive;* instead, help him look at himself in a comprehensive and positive manner that acknowledges weaknesses but also emphasizes strengths and special attributes.

Children with learning disabilities generally respond well to a sensitive and appropriate evaluation and treatment plan. This is particularly true if this plan is supportive, removes blame from both child and parent, focuses on the present problems, attends to other associated concerns, allows the youngster to achieve at a higher level than before, and results in his feeling more confident, self-reliant, and motivated. It can be helpful to point out successful adults who also have learning disabilities.

WHAT INTERVENTIONS ARE AVAILABLE?

After you and your child understand the results of the evaluation, ask the school for a description of the various interventions or supportive services it can offer. This will begin to provide you with a clear, comprehensive view of what may lie ahead for your child.

Your decision about interventions will depend on the evaluation results and the school district's resources, including the specific resources of your youngster's school.

Resource Room. Your child may qualify for part-time or full-time special services in a resource room for certain specific academic subjects, while being "mainstreamed" for other subjects and activities. Make sure goals and expectations are set appropriately, with a timetable for achieving them. If needed, your child may also receive help for language problems (speech or language therapy) or motor problems (physical or occupational therapy).

Inclusion Mainstreaming or Full/Partial. This is a system in which a handicapped youngster is educated alongside her nonhandicapped peers to the greatest extent possible. For students who do not meet the discrepancy criteria for special services under federal law but still need some help, their regular classroom teachers should make changes in the classroom to meet the child's needs, such as modifications in the youngster's curriculum, the manner in which subjects are taught, homework assignments, and overall expectations. Throughout this process it is essential that the child's strengths, including extracurricular activities, are nurtured and maintained.

"Bypass" Interventions. Besides direct intervention, "bypass" strategies also are quite effective for some children. This is a method in which weaknesses are circumvented or bypassed. For instance, a child with writing problems might use a word processor to write reports. If she has good oral expressive skills, she could be allowed to give oral reports rather than written ones, and take tests orally.

Home-Based Support. At home you can modify the environment or the emotional climate, keep expectations realistic, and generally be supportive of your child. Develop homework routines, be available for help, maintain quiet in the house during homework hours, and if necessary, reduce your child's commitment to extracurricular activities to allow more time and energy for studies. Again, nurture and maintain other avenues of success and gratification.

Hiring a tutor may be very helpful and often can reduce or eliminate homework-related tensions between parent and child. However, be realistic and do not overload a youngster's capacity to perform, or deprive her of time to pursue interests and activities unrelated to school.

Children and Learning Disabilities

Here are some points to keep in mind about learning disabilities.

- Children with learning disabilities are a very heterogeneous group. Their disabilities vary in degree, nature, and complexity.

- Learning disabilities may affect more than just learning. Some of these children also have poor social and athletic skills. Behavior problems, emotional difficulties, low self-esteem, and family stresses can also occur.

- Learning disabilities change with time. They may diminish or resolve themselves with intervention and maturation; they may appear when certain demands are placed upon the child in a vulnerable area; or they may last a lifetime.

- Children with learning disabilities are often misunderstood. They are sometimes accused of being lazy, retarded, or not trying. They may be subjected to humiliation and inadequate teaching methods. They, their parents, and their teachers frequently do not really understand their learning problems, and thus these difficulties need to be clarified and explained by a professional in a nonjudgmental manner. Emphasize that these problems are not the fault of the child, parent, or teacher.

Other Interventions. If your youngster is feeling depressed, anxious, or discouraged, psychological counseling may be appropriate. Sometimes family counseling is very helpful so family members can better understand each other's feelings and needs, reassign roles and responsibilities, and diminish intense sibling rivalry.

If your youngster has serious attention problems, or hyperactive-impulsive tendencies, she might be helped by medication that reduces distractibility and increases attention span. This medication should be part of a therapeutic package that might include educational and behavioral intervention and psychotherapy. (See Chapter 16, "Seeking Professional Help.") Also, any medical conditions that may be contributing to the learning difficulties or that cause school absenteeism need to be treated. These might include central nervous system illnesses or injuries (such as seizure disorders) or a hearing or vision impairment.

Controversial Treatments. There are many unproven treatments for learning problems, including megavitamins, patterning exercises, eye exercises,

- Learning disabilities affect families, and families affect learning disabilities. Children who are failing or struggling too hard feel confusion, disappointment, anger, anguish, and guilt, as do their parents. Parental attitudes and parenting style affect the children and their attitude toward learning.

- Determine whether emotional, social, or family problems are causing or contributing to your child's academic problems, or conversely, if his academic and learning problems are really the root cause. Professional help for family or emotional difficulties needs to be sought, but it should not divert attention away from the learning disability.

- Children with learning disabilities are entitled to the full support of the school system and require a good advocate and long-term follow-up.

- Be sure your child has other activities and interests that serve as avenues for success and gratification.

- To ensure the best results for your child, recognize learning disabilities early, arrange for the appropriate intervention, and make sure that he is followed over the long term. Also, instill a sense of optimism and hope in your child that together you will work toward a solution to these difficulties.

special glasses, and diets that eliminate certain types of foods or additives. The American Academy of Pediatrics does not recognize any of these treatments as being effective and therefore does not recommend them. Seek the advice of your pediatrician and other professionals about any treatment you are considering.

MONITORING YOUR CHILD'S PROGRESS

Your child's status should be reevaluated periodically, since development is an ongoing process, changing over time and in the face of new demands. In some cases a learning disability may be obvious only in specific situations when the child is called upon to perform a particular function. Also, as some children mature, they outgrow or learn to compensate for their difficulties. These youngsters may develop excellent coping skills and develop an unusual degree of insight about themselves. On the other hand, some learning disabilities may become more significant and disabling as the child matures or faces greater challenges. Once identified as having learning disabilities, children are entitled to a reevaluation every few years (this varies by state) to determine their current situation and need for services.

Regular meetings with teachers are an effective way to monitor your child's status and discuss his progress. It also is a way to let the school and the teacher know that you remain an advocate for your child and that you appreciate what the school is doing. Furthermore, your involvement sends a strong message to your youngster that you are willing to stand up for him and seek appropriate services and support. In some cases change and improvement may not fully raise your child's abilities to age- or grade-appropriate levels, even though the situation may improve. Many children eventually experience success once they complete high school, because they can then select the higher education, vocational training, or job that best suits them and provides them with gratification.

A number of educational and parent associations can provide you with information (reading material and conferences on learning disabilities), as well as moral support and advice. School personnel and other professionals can provide you with a list of these organizations. One such group with state and local chapters is Learning Disabilities Association, 4156 Library Road, Pittsburgh, Pennsylvania 15234.

OTHER EDUCATIONAL HANDICAPS

MENTAL RETARDATION

About 2 percent to 3 percent of children are considered mentally retarded. Their general intelligence is significantly below average, and they have difficulty adapting to their environment.

As measured by standardized tests, the average IQ (intelligence quotient) is 100; normal ranges from 90 to 110. The degree of mental retardation depends upon how far below this normal range a child's IQ falls. Experts use these lower IQ scores to label a child as mildly, moderately, severely, or profoundly retarded. The majority of children with below-average IQ scores are not considered to be mentally retarded, but below average, with test scores between 70 and 89.

The diagnosis of mental retardation can be made only by a certified psychologist capable of administering, scoring, and interpreting a standardized intelligence or cognitive test. The psychologist must also be able to observe and assess adaptive behavior.

Adaptive behavior enables children to interact with, adjust to, and meet the demands of other people and day-to-day living. Specific adaptive behavior includes a child's motor skills, communication abilities, self-help and independent living skills (eating, dressing, toileting), and other everyday skills (using public transportation, maintaining an appropriate job, taking care of a house).

Mental retardation can have a variety of causes, including hereditary disorders such as phenylketonuria (PKU), early alterations in the embryo's development (Down's syndrome), and exposure to toxic substances (alcohol) or infections while the child is in the mother's uterus. Problems in labor and birth that put stress on the baby, or problems after birth like injuries to the brain, can result in retardation and/or loss of specific functions, such as memory or language abilities. In most cases the cause of retardation is not known, having no specific identifiable source.

By middle childhood most youngsters with mental retardation have already been assessed and provided with an appropriate school setting. If you have a mentally retarded child, she is entitled to an education just as any other youngster is. Federal law mandates evaluations to identify children with suspected handicaps and to provide appropriate services for them.

Although screening for developmental delays and retardation is a central part of pediatric care from birth onward, some children with mild retardation and developmental disabilities are not identified until the early school years. Early identification is critical to a better outcome, because a child's developmental handicaps are not necessarily fixed or set, and in fact they are often responsive to appropriate treatment.

As mentally retarded children progress through the school system and through their own developmental stages, they require an evolving training and/or educational program that is appropriate for their abilities and responsive to their needs and the needs of their families. Initially, these children may need help in acquiring the basic developmental skills (fine and gross motor skills, speech, and language skills) that are within their capabilities. As children acquire competence in these areas, they are better able to learn academic and other school-related skills.

Even so, these children still require a special educational setting with more individual attention and support. This is especially true of youngsters who also have behavior problems. However, some of these children can engage in nonacademic activities, such as sports, physical education, art, and singing, with their nonretarded peers. Increasingly, children with mild cognitive impairments (i.e., mild mental retardation) are being mainstreamed into inclusion classrooms.

Preparing retarded children for both lifelong vocational pursuits and as much independence as possible is the major goal of their education. Even in the elementary-school years, a child with a particular interest or talent might benefit from special training in or exposure to relevant vocations. Specialized vocational training is a major goal in the high school years.

Children with severe and profound degrees of retardation constitute a small percentage of mentally retarded children. These youngsters lack self-care skills. They communicate poorly and often have behavioral problems including repetitive or self-stimulating behavior. Home care is frequently difficult or impossible for parents, and these children are often placed in residential settings and receive special education. Nevertheless, with new trends and philosophies, many experts feel that these children, especially as teenagers or adults, are best served in smaller, more normal environments such as group homes within the community.

Parents can obtain information, support, and services through medical centers, community schools, respite care programs, family support networks, and their pediatricians.

AUTISM

Autism is a relatively rare, lifelong developmental disability that is quite variable in its severity and associated problems. It is approximately four times more common in boys than in girls, and usually appears in the first three years of life, occurring in about 10 to 20 of every 10,000 births. It is considered to be one of several pervasive developmental disorders, as is a similar condition known as Asperger's Syndrome.

Autism is characterized by a variety of unusual behaviors, including communication deficits and difficulty interacting with others. It is usually, though not always, accompanied by mental retardation. Children with autism have great variability in their developmental skills. Often motor skills are relatively normal, but language, social, and self-help abilities are usually impaired. Sometimes these children do not acquire speech; other times their language may be significantly delayed or unusual. If they are able to talk, they may use words without attaching the usual meanings to them or may merely echo what they have heard. They often are not able to understand other people's speech, facial expressions, or perspective.

Children with autism often interact with other children and adults in unconventional ways, and they may not use toys and other objects as intended. Their play tends to be rote and repetitive; pretend and imaginative play is very limited. Some children are subject to self-injurious, repetitive, self-stimulating, and occasionally aggressive behavior. They may engage in various forms of oppositional behavior such as tantrums. Other children may be socially withdrawn or even unaware of their surroundings. They may appear not to hear well, but hearing tests are usually normal.

There is no single cause of autism, but genetics play an important role. Children with autism are at increased risk for epileptic seizures and for attention deficits.

The diagnosis of autism should be made by a multidisciplinary team that has experience with autistic children. These specialists are usually found at major medical centers, but community subspecialists, in collaboration with educators and other professionals, can also provide this service.

Children with autism require specialized services within the community and within the school system. Contrary to previous beliefs, early and ongoing intervention can significantly improve the functioning of many children with autism. Their families need and should seek out information and support. These services can be obtained from medical centers, community agencies, advocacy groups, family support networks, Internet sites, and the family's pediatrician.

Keep in mind that all children have essential needs, regardless of their levels of intelligence and knowledge. Children with mental retardation or autism may not always be able to demonstrate or communicate their love or their need for love and affection, but they need as much love as any other child.

IF YOUR CHILD
IS GIFTED

Gifted and talented children have outstanding abilities and are potentially capable of high performance. Their giftedness can occur in a variety of areas, including general intellectual aptitude, specific academic capability and achievement, creativity (such as in art, music, or the performing arts), leadership, and athletics. Gifted children deserve special educational programs and services beyond those normally provided by the regular school curriculum in order for them to realize their potential talents and to help make their greatest contributions to society.

In middle childhood, gifted children are often noted to have superior abilities in reading, language, math reasoning, science, literature, and the arts. They often have a variety of interests and tend to read more, read more difficult books, and be involved with collections, activities, and hobbies; they tend to have more knowledge of a variety of games. These traits tend to be of long standing and may become more apparent with age.

IDENTIFYING A GIFTED CHILD

Parents are usually aware that their gifted child has unique abilities or talents. Occasionally, however, teachers are the first to point out that a youngster is exceptional in some way. Unique aptitudes may not be apparent until the child is in a setting that shows them off. Then they can be documented through intelligence and achievement testing by qualified professionals, as well as by high levels of proficiency and achievement. A child who is gifted in a non-academic domain (such as music) often requires the support and advocacy of the teacher. Parental support is critical for a gifted child to receive appropriate services and opportunities.

PROVIDING SERVICES FOR THE ACADEMICALLY GIFTED CHILD

To meet the needs of gifted and/or highly intelligent students, schools should include programs to help them master the important concepts and various content fields; develop skills and strategies that allow them to become more independent, creative, and self-sufficient learners; and develop a joy and enthusiasm for learning. Some may also benefit from being with similarly talented peers so they have a social group with which they are comfortable.

Specifically, programs and classes for gifted children should provide them with stimulation and challenge in their areas of strength and should encourage more creativity and originality.

Of course, these are the very same things that should be provided to all children. What distinguishes educational programs for gifted children is their accelerated pace of learning and the increased breadth and depth of topics covered.

However, both schools and parents often find it a challenge to provide the appropriate services and stimulation for gifted children. Teachers are faced with a diverse group of students and must meet the needs of all of them; thus, teachers may not have enough time to devote special efforts to the gifted students in their classes. Also, teachers may not be trained to stimulate the higher thinking and productivity levels of gifted children. Some teachers find the superb critical thinking and analytical skills of many gifted children to be an annoyance and a challenge they prefer not to face. The youngsters' verbal skills, large vocabulary, and ability and eagerness to question traditional facts and conclusions may be perceived as irritating and dominating by some teachers and fellow students. This can lead to social problems that require developing better social skills.

If possible, schools should hire teachers who are trained to work with gifted students in a variety of fields. Often, gifted students are brought together for several hours a day to allow them to work with other gifted students and with a mentor. Independent study, advanced special classes, and taking advantage of resources outside the school (such as college courses) are other possibilities. Some gifted students prefer to go to schools that specialize in the field in which they excel, such as a performing arts school, a math and science school, or a school that emphasizes sports.

If your school does not offer specific services for gifted children other than advanced courses, you may need to seek out extracurricular activities and situations for your gifted child.

THE GIFTED UNDERACHIEVER

Despite their high intelligence and talents, some gifted children do not live up to their potential in the classroom. These are the gifted children who also have a learning disability. More boys than girls fall into this category. Approximately 10 percent of gifted children are delayed in reading by two or more grade levels, and approximately 30 percent of gifted children have a significant discrepancy between their potential, as measured by intelligence tests, and their achievement.

When an educational specialist diagnoses a gap or underachievement, he or she will look for signs like a significant discrepancy between the verbal and nonverbal portions of an IQ test, or between scores on an IQ test and a standardized achievement test. The assessment may also include aptitude testing, as well as emotional, behavioral, and family evaluations.

In some cases parents may hold especially high or unrealistic expectations of a gifted child. These parents may have difficulty understanding why a child of superior intelligence or talent is underachieving. They may blame the school for not providing adequate stimulation and challenge through its curriculum and teaching. They may criticize the school for emphasizing conformity rather than originality and creativity.

Gifted underachievers are especially prone to developing a poor self-concept. They may grow increasingly negative about themselves and feel increasingly incompetent, unaccepted, and isolated. Their expectations of themselves tend to decline as they meet with continued frustration and a long-term lack of success.

Talk with your school principal, a learning specialist, or a professional who works with gifted children to help an underachieving gifted child get back on track. Perhaps your child would be better off in a regular classroom receiving some special attention than in a special class for gifted children. Do not ignore the problem and merely hope that it resolves itself. Again, early recognition of the situation and appropriate intervention makes for the best outcome.

SCHOOL AND YOUR CHILD'S HEALTH

THE SCHOOL AS A HEALTH EDUCATOR

Many parents are keenly interested in the basic academic education of their youngsters—reading, writing, and arithmetic—but are not nearly as conscientious in finding out about the other learning that goes on in the classroom. A comprehensive health education program is an important part of the curriculum in most school districts. Starting in kindergarten and continuing through high school, it provides an introduction to the human body and to factors that prevent illness and promote or damage health.

The middle years of childhood are extremely sensitive times for a number of health issues, especially when it comes to adopting health behavior that can have lifelong consequences. Your youngster might be exposed to a variety of health themes in school: nutrition, disease prevention, physical growth and development, reproduction, mental

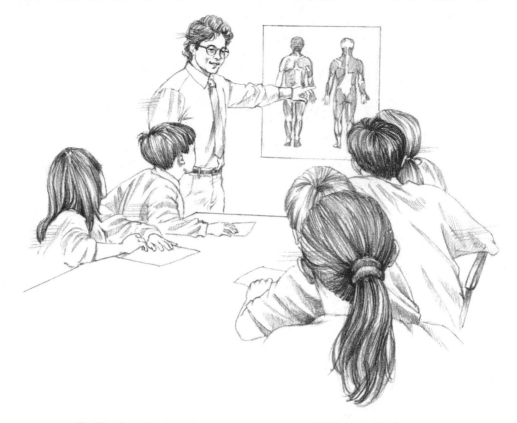

Health education is an important part of your child's overall education.

health, drug and alcohol abuse prevention, consumer health, and safety (crossing streets, riding bikes, first aid, the Heimlich maneuver). The goal of this education is not only to increase your child's health knowledge and to create positive attitudes toward his own well-being but also to promote healthy behavior. By going beyond simply increasing knowledge, schools are asking for more involvement on the part of students than in many other subject areas. Children are being taught life skills, not merely academic skills.

It is easy to underestimate the importance of this health education for your child. Before long he will be approaching puberty and adolescence and facing many choices about his behavior that, if he chooses inappropriately, could impair his health and even lead to his death. These choices revolve around alcohol, tobacco, and other drug use; sexual behavior (abstinence, prevention of pregnancy and sexually transmitted diseases); driving; risk-taking behavior; and stress management. Most experts concur that education about issues like alcohol abuse is most effective if it begins at least two years before the behavior is likely to start. This means that children seven and eight years old are not too young to learn about the dangers of tobacco, alcohol, and other drugs, and that sexuality education also needs to be part of the experience of elementary-school-age children. At the same time, *positive* health behavior can also be learned during the middle years of childhood. Your child's well-being as an adult can be influenced by the lifelong exercise and nutrition habits that he adopts now.

Health education programs are most effective if parents are involved. Parents can complement and reinforce what children are learning in school during conversations and activities at home. The schools can provide basic information about implementing healthy decisions—for instance, how and why to say no to alcohol use. But you should be a co-educator, particularly in those areas where family values are especially important—for example, sexuality, AIDS prevention, and tobacco, alcohol, and other drug use.

Many parents feel ill-equipped to talk to their child about puberty, reproduction, sex, and sexually transmitted diseases. But you need to recognize just how important your role is. With sexual topics—as well as with many other areas of health—you can build on the general information taught at school and, in a dialogue with your youngster, put it into a moral context. Remember, you are the expert on your child, your family, and your family's values.

Education seminars and education support groups for parents on issues of health and parenting may be part of the health promotion program at your school. If they are not offered, you should encourage their development. Many parents find it valuable to discuss mutual problems and share solutions with other parents. Although some parents have difficulty attending evening meetings, school districts are finding other ways to reach out to parents—for instance, through educational TV broadcasts with call-in capacities, Saturday morning breakfast meetings, and activities for parents and children together, organized to promote good health (a walk/run, a dance, a heart-healthy luncheon).

In addition to providing education at home on health matters, become an advocate in your school district for appropriate classroom education about puberty, reproduction, AIDS, alcohol and other substance abuse, and other relevant issues. The content of health education programs is often decided at the community level, so make your voice heard.

As important as the content of a health curriculum may be, other factors are powerful in shaping your child's attitudes toward his well-being. Examine whether other aspects of the school day reinforce what your youngster is being taught in the classroom. For example, is the school cafeteria serving low-fat meals that support the good nutritional decisions encouraged by you and the teachers? Is there a strong physical education program that emphasizes the value of fitness and offers each child thirty minutes of vigorous activity at least three times a week? Does the school district support staff-wellness programs so that teachers can be actively involved in maintaining their own health and thus be more excited about conveying health information to their students?

In addition to school and home, your pediatrician is another health educator for you and your child. Since your child's doctor knows your family, he or she can provide clear, personalized health information and advice. For instance, the pediatrician can talk with your child about the child's personal growth patterns during puberty, relate them to the size and shape of other family members, and answer questions specific to your youngster's own developmental sequence and rate.

For most school-related health concerns, your pediatrician can provide you with specific advice and tailored guidance. You and your pediatrician may also consult with the school staff on how to deal most effectively with schooltime management of your child's health problem.

WHERE WE STAND

The American Academy of Pediatrics supports sexuality education in the schools, with content that is developmentally appropriate for particular age groups and that focuses on responsible sexual behavior and decision-making. Polls consistently show that parents approve of sexuality education in the schools, and the AAP believes that parents should participate in the development and the evaluation of this curriculum. Qualified teachers should be assigned to teach these programs, and the curriculum should be revised and updated at regular intervals.

DEALING WITH HEALTH PROBLEMS AT SCHOOL

There is wide variation in the health services offered by schools. For instance:

- In some schools there is a full-time certified school nurse who spends most of his or her day attending to the acute and chronic health needs of students. He or she handles acute health problems, administers medications, and performs health assessments and screenings as well as special procedures ordered by a child's personal doctor; he or she also refers children to their physician for physical exams, diagnosis, and treatment. School nurses can also play a central role in promoting a healthy and safe school environment.

- In some communities, a full-time school nurse is responsible for several schools and thus spends only a limited time in each school. He or she is responsible for training other staff members (teachers, administrators, secretaries, health aides) to handle acute health situations when the nurse is not on site.

- A full- or part-time nurse practitioner is available in some schools, working with consulting physicians, school nurses, social workers, or health educators in a school-based health center where routine medical care is delivered in the school. This has been an important and successful way to provide care to students in areas where care has been limited because of a lack of health-care providers, an absence of insurance, or transportation problems. The American Academy of Pediatrics believes that all children deserve a "medical home" and supports the implementation of school-based clinics, especially in areas where children do not have access to health care.

Acute Health Problems

Most illnesses and injuries that arise during school are minor (bumps, scrapes, headaches) and can be cared for by the school nurse. In many instances the child can return to class. When the problem is more serious, a parent will be called to come and take the child home. If the situation is extremely serious or life-threatening, the child will be transported by ambulance to the hospital emergency room or nearest physician. In many but not all schools, one or more staff members have been trained in CPR (cardiopulmonary resuscitation) and first aid. Parents should know how these situations are handled at their child's school.

Seeing the Nurse

Most students can go to the school's health office and speak with the nurse whenever they need to during the day, usually just by asking their teacher. If you would like your child to consult with the nurse, send a note to school with your youngster, or call the school early in the day. Let your child know the reason for the visit so that she will not be confused or surprised when she is called to the office.

Short-Term Health Problems

Sometimes your child may have a health condition that does not last long but still interferes with her functioning at school. This kind of problem should be brought to the attention of the school nurse, the teacher, or the principal. For instance:

- Hearing loss related to an ear infection could require a temporary change of seats to the front of the classroom.

- Some infections—especially an ear infection, strep throat, bronchitis, and sinusitis—may necessitate the administration of medication for a week after your child is well enough to return to school. Ask your pediatrician if a medication can be prescribed that can be given before and after school and then at bedtime, thus not requiring it to be taken at school. Ask about your school's policy about medication before your child's first illness. Your school may require a written order from the doctor before it will administer the medication, plus require that the medication be in its original, labeled container. It will be easier to take care of this during the visit to the doctor's office.

- If your child has a readily visible problem—like a rash, conjunctivitis (pinkeye), or unusual bruises—that has already been evaluated by your pediatrician, let the school staff know about the doctor's diagnosis and treatment. Thus, school personnel will not have to pursue further evaluation of your youngster, which may disrupt her classroom work and unnecessarily concern her.

- If your child has an injury or illness that requires immobilization or limitations on physical activity, ask the school about alternative activities available during physical education classes and recess. When the child is unable to participate in PE for months or even years, a formal adaptive PE program—one that is appropriate and safe—needs to be designed for her. Discuss this with the school principal.

CHRONIC ILLNESSES

If your child has a chronic illness, you need to ensure that he receives proper medical care and supervision at school and also participates fully in the educational program. Make certain the school nurse and your child's teacher have enough information to understand how his health problem affects your youngster and how it may influence his school performance.

Talk with school personnel about what steps they should take if your child develops symptoms at school. These guidelines should be written in the form of an individual health plan that the school should follow, based on directions from you and your pediatrician. When the school staff is familiar with this plan and the health problem, they will be better able to make sure your child's ac-

When to Keep Your Child Home from School

If your child is not feeling well, your physician is the best person to consult about whether she can go to school. Common sense, concern for your child's well-being, and the possibility of infecting classmates should all contribute to the decision about whether your child should stay home.

As general guidelines, keep her home if:

1. she has a fever

2. she is not well enough to participate in class

3. you think she may be contagious to other children

If your child has been ill but is feeling better, yet has still awakened with a minor problem, such as a runny nose or slight headache, you can send her to school if none of the three circumstances listed above is present. Even so, make sure the school and your child have a phone number where you can be reached during the day if more serious symptoms develop and she needs to return home.

tivities are not restricted unnecessarily. If your child does experience difficulty, the school staff will be able to provide immediate and appropriate attention. Be certain they have emergency numbers to reach both you and your child's doctor during the day.

When your youngster needs to take medication at school, it should be kept in a locked cabinet. In some schools, inhalers for older children with asthma may be carried and self-administered under well-defined guidelines. Medication should be administered in a private place to avoid any embarrassment your youngster may feel. If this is not happening—for instance, if your child is required to take his medication in a busy school office and feels uncomfortable doing so—you or your child should consult with the school nurse or principal to identify an alternative.

If major changes occur in the status of your child's condition, including modification of his medication schedule, let the school know, particularly if it is relevant to his school functioning and routines. During this time of change, since your child spends so many hours a day at school, the teacher and/or

Health Screenings in School

In most schools, children in the middle years are routinely screened for a number of common physical conditions. Hearing and vision tests are two of the most frequent evaluations, important because difficulties with these senses are often subtle, and neither parents, teachers, nor children may even recognize that a problem exists. While most difficulties with hearing or vision should have been identified prior to entering school, some may have been missed and others develop later. A child who has difficulty reading the blackboard may not know that she is seeing differently from anyone else. Nevertheless, even mild deficiencies of sight can significantly affect a child's ability to learn.

In some states these screening tests are mandated by law and may also include dental checks, scoliosis evaluations, blood pressure readings, and height and weight measurements. In school districts in which nurses are available for more thorough assessments, testing for tuberculosis and even physical exams may be conducted.

If the school notifies you that these screenings have turned up a potential problem in your child, have her checked by your pediatrician. In the meantime the school nurse should be able to tell you what the school's findings may mean, and whether there is any urgency in obtaining an evaluation by your doctor. In some cases you may be able to wait until your youngster's next well-child visit for a repeat screening or a more comprehensive evaluation.

Sometimes your youngster's pediatrician will find that the suspected abnormality is not serious after all. Even so, this does not mean that the screening was inaccurate. Screening tests are designed to identify children who *may* have a problem, but a more thorough examination by a doctor is always necessary to determine the extent and severity of the condition.

school nurse can often provide you with helpful feedback on how your child seems to be doing.

When you switch schools or if a new illness develops, the nurse may find it helpful to talk directly to your child's doctor. For this conversation to occur, you may have to sign a "release of information" form, which the school nurse will send to the doctor prior to their discussion of your child.

Sometimes, with both the child's and parent's permission, a disease like diabetes can be explained to the youngster's class so that his classmates will become more knowledgeable and supportive of their fellow student in an open and comfortable way. A similar kind of class education about seizure disorders can make the situation less embarrassing for a student with frequent seizures and minimize the disruption if he should have a seizure in class. Elementary-school children are frequently quite accepting and supportive in these circumstances.

Even though your child has a chronic illness, he should still participate in all educational trips and other activities. If special arrangements need to be made to accommodate your child (such as special food, transportation of essential medical equipment, bee-sting kits), you might want to offer to help organize these things for the first trip of every year to ease the transition for the new teacher.

At each parent-teacher conference, make sure that your youngster's educational program is not being adversely affected by his condition.

(For further information, see Part VIII, "Chronic Health Problems," as well as the comments on specific diseases that may require special considerations at school.)

OTHER HEALTH PROBLEMS AT SCHOOL

When potentially contagious health problems appear at school, the health of your child must be considered along with the health of other children and school staff. Some health disorders are of particular concern in schools. Problems like head lice can spread from one child to another rather easily and thus can become mini-epidemics in classrooms. Other conditions, like AIDS, are much more serious, but concerns about the transmission of the AIDS virus in school have created more anxiety than is warranted. Some childhood disorders (including colds, sore throats, chicken pox, and impetigo) are dealt with in more detail elsewhere in this book.

Head Lice

Head lice are crawling insects, only about one-sixteenth of an inch long, that live and multiply in human hair. Lice are not a major health problem, since they do not transmit diseases or cause permanent problems. Nonetheless, the reaction of parents, and sometimes of school staff, has made them a significant health issue.

Lice make their home in human hair, nourishing themselves with blood from the scalp. They can cause reddened, rashlike areas. The average number of lice on an infected child's head is about ten. Their eggs (called nits) stubbornly attach to the hair shafts—most often in the back of the head or near the ears—and cannot be shaken or brushed off.

When should you suspect lice? Your child may complain of a very itchy scalp, although lice may be present for weeks or months without causing an itch. If you look carefully at her head, you should be able to see the eggs, although some parents may confuse them with dandruff. (Dandruff, however, tends to be loose flakes of skin, while nits firmly attach themselves to the hair.)

Lice are quite contagious and can be spread quickly by close contact with a friend or classmate, almost always by head-to-head contact. Routine head inspections by school personnel usually miss all but the worst cases.

Lice can be difficult to treat. Your doctor may prescribe a treatment or recommend a nonprescription anti-lice shampoo or rinse containing a substance called pyrethrins. Follow the instructions carefully. Your child will probably need to vigorously scrub in the shampoo, working up a good lather, and then rinse thoroughly. This treatment can often take care of both the lice and their eggs, although a second application may be required several days later. Do not treat longer than the manufacturer or your physician recommends. Unfortunately, many lice have developed resistance to most pesticide medication in common use.

Although lice move quickly away from any disturbance in dry hair, thoroughly wetted, their mobility is much reduced. Fine-tooth combing after ordinary shampooing is a simple way to lift out lice. Repeating this process every three to four days for two weeks is usually effective in ridding a child of head lice. Combing your child's hair with a fine-tooth comb can also remove some nits, as can pulling them off with your fingernails. Be sure to wash the comb thoroughly or soak it in anti-lice shampoo before anyone else uses it.

The presence of lice does not mean that your child has poor hygiene habits. Anyone can get lice, even if she bathes or shampoos every day. As a preventive measure, discourage your child from sharing combs, brushes, towels, or hats with friends.

Many schools have policies about children with lice. In most of these schools, students with live lice are sent home when the lice are discovered; those students who have only nits and no live lice are usually sent home at the end of the day with a note, although it is likely that if nits are present in a child who has not received treatment, live lice are also there. Students can be readmitted to school once they have been treated. Some schools have "no-nit" policies, stating that students who still have nits in their hair cannot return to school; however, since many anti-lice shampoos effectively kill the nits, many schools do not feel this extra restriction is needed.

Cooperate with the elementary or middle school by notifying the staff if your child has become infected. Although school personnel and parents used to overreact to the presence of head lice in the classroom, this type of response is hopefully a thing of the past. Most people now recognize that lice can happen to anyone and do not pose an emergency situation.

Fifth Disease

Fifth disease (Parvovirus B19) is a viral disease that causes a lacy-appearing rash on the arms and creates a "slapped cheeks" look on the face. Since children rarely feel sick with this disease and are contagious only before they develop the rash, there is no reason to exclude them from school unless they feel too ill to attend class. This disease can be dangerous for a developing fetus, so whenever a case is detected, all female school employees should be notified. It can also be more serious for people with some hereditary disorders, such as sickle-cell disease, that affect red blood cells.

AIDS/HIV Infection

AIDS/HIV infection is an increasingly common, life-threatening infection that affects children as well as adults. Unfortunately, there is widespread but unwarranted anxiety among parents whose children attend school with a youngster with AIDS, fearing that their own child may contract the disease. The AIDS virus (human immunodeficiency virus, or HIV) is transmitted only through blood, blood products, and sexual contact. Casual physical contact—including touching or holding hands with someone with AIDS, or sharing a drinking glass—will *not* transfer the AIDS virus.

Your child will *not* be in danger if she attends school with someone with AIDS, even if she plays with the same toys or is exposed to coughing or sneezing. There is not a single documented case of the transmission of AIDS from child to child, or teacher to child, in the school setting. To allay parental concerns and to significantly lower the risks, schools have implemented procedures for dealing with the blood and other bodily fluids of all staff and students. Children with AIDS whose pediatricians have approved their attendance pose no danger to their peers and should attend school.

Hepatitis

Hepatitis is an infection of the liver, spread by a virus. Its symptoms include jaundice (yellowish discoloration of the skin), loss of appetite, nausea, weakness, and abdominal pain. There are several major types of hepatitis—types A, B, and C—and while all are cause for concern, hepatitis A tends to occur most often among children. These viruses are present in the blood and in bowel movements; thus, children should wash their hands after every bowel movement and before eating. As with AIDS, precautions should also be taken around the blood of infected individuals.

Children infected with acute hepatitis A should remain at home until one week after the onset of their illness and until jaundice (yellow skin color) has disappeared. Youngsters who are hepatitis B or C carriers but are symptom-free can attend school.

Chicken Pox

Chicken pox is a common viral disease among children. Although youngsters are contagious before they break out with skin lesions, they should not return to school until the sixth day after the rash has appeared, or sooner if all the lesions have dried and crusted. Vaccines to prevent chicken pox are available and safe. All school-age children who have not had chicken pox should be immunized. Widespread use of this vaccine will make chicken pox much less common in school-aged children.

PART VIII

CHRONIC HEALTH PROBLEMS

IF YOUR CHILD HAS A CHRONIC ILLNESS

As a child matures, parents often need to modify their hopes and expectations in light of their youngster's developing skills, interests, and values, which are not always the same as their own. Mothers and fathers often worry also about their child's well-being and happiness and puzzle over what their role should be in helping the youngster achieve his full potential. Certainly parents should become their child's most devoted advocate and conscientious guide through life, helping him overcome the array of obstacles that each child must face.

In terms of their physical well-being, most children are healthy. Their illnesses, while frequent, are minor and short-lived. Parents need to obtain appropriate medical care for them, help them develop health-promoting habits, and comfort them through their episodes of illness.

For some children, however, illnesses or health impairments are not self-limited but may continue indefinitely. These youngsters

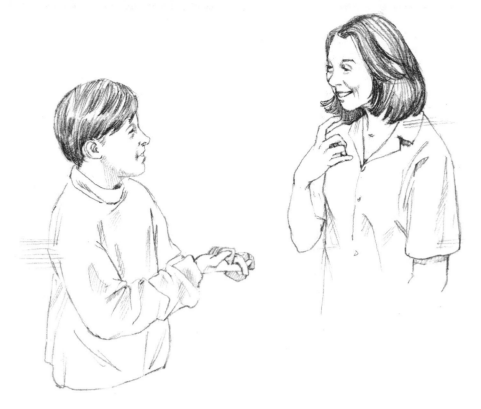

may have a serious physical disability, such as spina bifida or an injury-related disability; a sensory deficit such as blindness or deafness; or a chronic condition like asthma, epilepsy, diabetes, or literally hundreds of other chronic diseases of childhood. The parents of these children have a much more difficult task.

Studies show that between 10 percent and 20 percent of children have some type of long-term illness, disability, or other type of health impairment. Most of these conditions are neither life-threatening nor severely limiting in terms of activity. However, about 2 percent of children have chronic illnesses that do seriously impair their ability to accomplish the usual activities of youngsters their age, or that increase the number of days they miss from school or spend in the hospital.

Most children with chronic illnesses do well in school, develop appropriately, and achieve their goals in much the same way that other children do. Most are healthy children who happen to have a chronic illness. While their illness may create certain difficulties, with the support of their parents most lead effective and exciting lives and grow up to become productive adults.

If you are the parent of a chronically ill child, the following chapters are designed to help you and your youngster cope with the difficulties you may be facing and reassure you about what may be normal and expected behavior and responses. Equipped with information and guidance, you can minimize the obstacles facing your child, yourself, and your family.

PARENTS' INITIAL REACTIONS

When you first learn that your child has a disability or a chronic disease, the news is often unexpected and can seem devastating. Many families experience a sense of powerlessness at the prospect of dealing with an unexpected illness and facing a future filled with unknowns.

As a first step to coping with your child's special needs, find out as much as you can about her condition and its care. The more information parents and children have, the less frightening the present and future will seem. Knowledge is empowering. It can help both you and your youngster feel more in control of, and less a hostage to, the condition you both must face. Information will also help you guide your child—and serve as her advocate—through the potentially complicated medical-care system.

The type of information you convey to your child should be appropriate for your child's age. You can gauge this best by listening to her questions. Studies show, for instance, that kindergarten-age children typically view illness as quite magical: One child, when asked "How do you get better from an asthma attack?" simply responded, "Don't wheeze."

Young children who have diabetes may sometimes attribute their illness to eating too much candy. Some youngsters believe they have become ill and been hospitalized as punishment for disobeying their mother or father.

Beginning at about ages ten to twelve, children begin to grasp the complex mechanisms that can contribute to disease. By the fourth grade, children tend to believe that germs cause all illness. These older children may be capable of understanding more straightforward information about their disorder.

Remember that as children grow up, their ability to understand information and assume responsibility for their own care increases. Every year or so, someone should check out what they understand about their illness, fill in the gaps, and correct misperceptions. All too often, the explanations stop at the time of diagnosis.

FINDING A DOCTOR

Of course, your youngster will need to be under a doctor's care. Choose a physician who is accessible, whom you trust, who you believe is knowledgeable, to whom you can relate easily, and who can coordinate your child's treat-

What Do You Need to Know?

When your child is diagnosed with a chronic condition, you will want to inform yourself thoroughly about it. Here are some questions to pursue through reading and talking with your child's pediatrician and other health-care providers.

- Is this going to be a lifelong illness, or may your child outgrow it?

- What is the expected course of the illness, and what is the usual regimen of medication and diet required?

- How can you explain the condition to your child appropriately?

- Will the illness require expensive treatment, frequent disruptions of school or vacations, and restrictions of activities?

- In what ways is the illness likely to alter your family's daily routines?

- Who and where are the specialists in your geographic region who treat this condition?

- What are the currently accepted ways of caring for this illness?

- Are there any controversies in the area?

- Which of the costs associated with this condition are covered by your health insurance?

- What additional funding is available for children with this condition?

- What books and other literature should you read? What are good books for your child to read?

- Are there local or national parent groups or advocacy groups?

- Are there local groups of children with this or related conditions? Are there groups of siblings of children with chronic conditions?

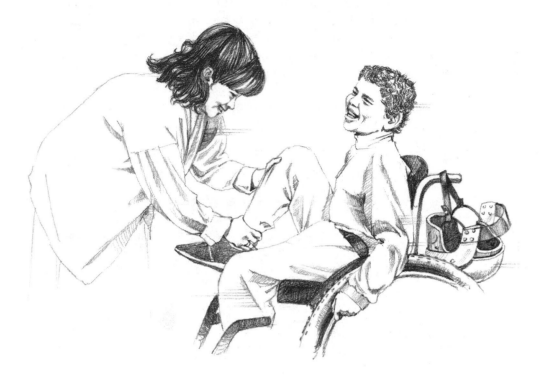

ment with other health-care providers. You are choosing a professional partner for a relationship that may last many years.

The pediatrician who has already been caring for your child is the first choice to consider. Stay with a physician who is not only well-informed about your youngster and his condition but knows something about your other children and the family. Also, look to him or her for guidance when selecting other health-care professionals and specialists who will work with you and your child. If you feel you would like a different primary-care provider, ask for a recommendation. (See Chapter 2, "Keeping Your Child Healthy," or Chapter 16, "Seeking Professional Help.") Alternative sources of care (such as emergency rooms) are not satisfactory substitutes for comprehensive care.

Many children with chronic health conditions have special health-care needs and require care from multiple physicians such as allergists, neurologists, rheumatologists, hematologists, endocrinologists, or surgical subspecialists. Whenever possible, a child with special health-care needs should receive specialty care or consultation from a pediatric subspecialist rather than an adult medicine specialist. Many will also benefit from services provided by occupational therapists, physical therapists, speech and language therapists, or mental-health professionals. Sometimes the various health professionals involved with your child's care will offer conflicting advice, leaving you uncertain which professional's advice to follow. Parents are also often uncertain about which health professional to turn to with a specific concern or question.

You should have one professional you can call upon to coordinate your child's care and to help make sense of any conflicting advice. If you are com-

Questions to Ask Your Managed-Care Organization

If you have joined a managed-care organization (MCO) for your child's health care, here are some questions to consider:

- Does your child's physician belong to the MCO's provider network?

- Can families choose their primary and specialty providers?

- Does your child's physician have any financial incentives to limit your access to care?

- Are pediatric subspecialists available through the MCO?

- Do benefits include enabling services: transportation, care coordination, home care, unusual or experimental medications or treatments?

- How is health care paid for while traveling out of town?

- Is a specialty hospital part of the managed-care network?

- Who actually makes health-care decisions: families, physicians, gatekeepers?

- If you disagree with a benefit decision, what resource do you have to resolve your grievance?

- Are there limitations on the amount of services a child can use in a year? In a lifetime?

- What will you pay for each visit and prescription?

- Does the managed-care plan provide family-centered care?

fortable with your child's pediatrician in this role, then explore how to establish open communication and collaboration with this physician most effectively. In some instances it may make sense to have a medical subspecialist play this role. Parents should seek assistance from professionals who are knowledgeable about their child's illness, are aware of common side effects and consequences of treatment, and know about the natural course of the illness and about long-term effects of medical interventions. Such a person can anticipate or at least identify common problems at an early stage.

A clear understanding of how best to reach this individual (for instance, the best times to call with nonemergency concerns, how to set up conferences or extended appointments for extensive discussions, how to reach him or her for emergencies, whom to turn to when he or she is unavailable) will greatly improve your child's care.

Consider yourself, your child, and to some extent the rest of the family as partners with the physician or physicians, sharing the responsibility for your child's well-being. Even when you feel your youngster is under the best of care, do not be afraid to ask questions or challenge recommendations. You and your child should participate in making plans and decisions as much as possible.

Parents and professionals sometimes get so wrapped up in a child's chronic health problem that they forget his other health-care needs. Remember that routine health issues such as immunizations, dental care, injury prevention, good nutrition, and regular exercise are as important for your child as they are for children without a chronic condition.

HELPING YOUR CHILD COPE

The Stress of Illness

Stress is part of life. It motivates us to succeed, but it can also interfere with life's joys and accomplishments. Children with chronic illnesses often deal with more stress than other youngsters. For example, they may have to cope with an imperfect body, frequent hospitalizations, painful injections, surgery, or even premature death.

A child with kidney disease who requires dialysis three times a week faces predictable and repeated periods of stress. A youngster with cancer, who must undergo repeated chemotherapy, copes with the fears and anxieties of each approaching treatment. A child with epilepsy may feel apprehensive about the possibility of having another seizure.

Unfortunately, there are no simple ways to help your child avoid these stresses. Here are some suggestions that may make the situation a little easier.

- Listen to your child. Whether she is feeling sadness, frustration, or rage, it is helpful for her to express her emotions. She should feel that she can share her thoughts and fears without your overreacting or becoming upset. Ask how she is feeling. Be available and supportive. Listen not only to what your child says, but also try to hear what is left unspoken.

- Inform your child about what lies ahead. Anxiety is often based on the unknown or on inaccurate presumptions about the future. Find out what your child does and does not know. Explain exactly what will happen during an upcoming doctor's appointment or hospital visit; if you are unable to answer all your child's questions, both of you should talk to the doctor. Do not expose a child to a frightening procedure unless she has been informed of it beforehand. Conversations with other children who have gone through the same experiences can be invaluable.

- "Rehearsal" can help children cope with frightening situations. Many hospitals can now arrange for youngsters to spend time in the children's ward *before* they undergo surgery or other procedures. These visits can familiarize children with the hospital setting and what to expect.

- Encourage your youngster to spend time with other children with a chronic illness.

- Frequently talk about the illness or condition so that your child feels comfortable being open about it.

- Emphasize your child's strengths—the things she can do well despite the condition.

- Help your youngster feel that she can be in control of some aspects of her situation. Try to find choices that can be given to her, such as which arm to have blood drawn from, when a procedure will occur, or what reward she will get for cooperating.

Maintaining and Building Self-Esteem

Children with different types of special health-care needs share many of the same life experiences and problems, irrespective of their particular illness. For example, they often are anxious about medical treatments and hospitalizations. They may be absent from school more frequently and, as a result, suffer academically. Their illness may keep them from participating in some school and social activities, either because of physical disabilities or from a simple lack of energy. In turn, their self-esteem and self-confidence may suffer.

Especially when there are visible signs of their disorder—such as the loss of hair from chemotherapy, obesity due to medications (such as cortico-

Common Problems Faced by Children with Chronic Illnesses

- Accepting limitations caused by the health condition
- Anger
- Anxiety
- Embarrassment
- Fear
- Feelings of inadequacy
- Frustration
- Guilt
- Inappropriate reactions or expectations of family members, other children, and professionals
- Pain
- Problems with self-esteem
- Restriction of activities
- Sadness
- School absences
- School difficulties
- Sense of powerlessness
- Social isolation
- Stress

steroids), or congenital conditions or injuries—children may retreat from social situations. They may avoid contact even with their former friends.

On the other hand, youngsters with chronic conditions (and their siblings and parents) can experience a sense of pride and accomplishment as they overcome their disabilities and fears, and succeed in their endeavors. Early success in overcoming adversity can yield lifelong inner strength and the ability to master subsequent difficulties.

There are many ways in which children can achieve a strong sense of self-esteem and pride. Try to identify activities that can bring your child pleasure and a feeling of mastery, and then help facilitate his participation in these activities.

Children limited in their ability to take part in certain competitive sports often gain considerable satisfaction from participating in noncompetitive sports. Or they may find a lot of enjoyment—and respect from other children and adults—by becoming knowledgeable about a particular sport, or sports in general.

Many children derive pride and pleasure from various crafts and creative activities such as drawing, painting, writing poetry or fiction, or learning to play a musical instrument. Collecting records, books, stamps, coins, or baseball cards can be great fun and instill feelings of expertise and pleasure. Children may also enjoy and feel pride through reading or academic achievement.

A youngster with a chronic illness is often angry about the restrictions the disorder places on physical activity. You need to help your child accept his limitations, and then find something else in which he can excel. All children need to feel a sense of accomplishment. Explore the options for activities in your community until you find at least one that is attractive to your child and in which he can succeed.

Leading a "Normal" Life

It is best to encourage children with a chronic illness or special health-care needs to lead as normal a life as possible, both at home and at school. Unnecessary restriction of activities can reduce your child's enjoyment of life and interfere with friendships and social activities.

A "normal" life for a child with a chronic health problem means more than controlling the illness and minimizing hospital visits. It also includes developing realistic expectations, keeping up with schoolwork, forming friendships, and participating in the same activities as other children her age whenever possible.

If your daughter has epilepsy, do not discourage her from camping because of your fear that she will have a seizure, but do make arrangements to have her cared for if a seizure should occur. If your son has a heart problem, do not prohibit him from playing Little League baseball if his doctor says it's okay for him to participate; be sure the coach and the team members know about the condition and the precautions appropriate for it.

All parents want to protect their children from pain and disappointment. Parents of children with chronic health conditions may worry about extra risks to their children and may want to protect them from experiencing pain and frustration. On the other hand, all parents want their youngsters to grow up to become self-sufficient and competent adults. To accomplish that in your child, you need to encourage her to be as independent as is reasonably possible during childhood.

As part of this process, continue to give your youngster the information she needs about her illness—both the positives and the negatives. This will permit her to face the condition realistically and begin to master it as fully as possible. Keep in mind, however, that children differ in their ability to understand their health problems and to see ahead toward what they can do in the future. Thus, answer questions fully and try to be certain that your youngster understands your explanations. Expect and encourage more questions as your child's capacity to understand and reason increases.

As children enter school age, they spend an increasing amount of time away from their home and family. A chronic illness, however, can interfere with their widening social networks and activities. The child with diabetes who is embarrassed about dietary restrictions, or the youngster with asthma who becomes upset by her wheezing while playing, may isolate herself from friends.

Other problems can arise. As youngsters mature through middle childhood, they will increasingly seek mastery and control over their activities and social environment. Yet the child with a chronic illness may feel powerless over her own body and well-being. While friends are learning to assert their autonomy and independence, children with chronic conditions may be restricted and unable to keep up with their peers. Some chronic illnesses remain relatively unchanging over time. Others may remit or progress, requiring the child and family to adapt to changing symptoms, altered functional ability, and varying treatment plans. However, even a seemingly stable illness has different meanings for and impacts on the child as she develops. A physical limitation or stigma that had apparently little importance in first grade may become a mortifying problem at puberty.

Children's capacity for independence varies from illness to illness and child to child and will steadily increase with maturity. If your youngster has diabetes, you may have to test her blood sugar level and make sure insulin injections are given regularly during her younger years. If she requires a special diet, you will need to supervise food choices and eating habits closely. At the same time, watch for signals from her that she is able to assume greater responsibility, and help her take on more of the management of the illness little by little as she grows up.

Some children avoid accepting more independence. Families may inadvertently foster dependency because they find it easier to maintain responsibility for their youngster's care, rather than teaching the child to perform certain tasks and relying on her to do so. Also, these children (like most children) may enjoy being the object of their parents' special attention. They may relish having certain tasks' performed for them, and may resist taking responsibility.

It is critical to help your child come to terms with her health condition and accept appropriate responsibility for caring for herself. Do not deprive your child of the important and rewarding experience of mastering day-to-day tasks; it can instill pride and self-confidence that can prepare her for adult life. Praise her efforts at assuming responsibility, and applaud yourself for having the wisdom and courage to let her take these very important steps.

Discuss with your doctor your concerns and the limitations you think are reasonable for your child. Using your physician's input, develop some guidelines for sensible restrictions while also encouraging your child to participate in a diversity of activities. Parents need to recognize their children's changing needs and to plan for them. It is also important for parents to be educated and up-to-date about their child's illness and about new treatments and their effects.

LESSENING FEARS

Some Strategies to Consider

Even with the calming reassurance of a parent or a physician, some children still become terribly anxious about upcoming treatments and surgery. Their hearts may race; they may start to perspire; they may cry frequently and uncontrollably. But while recognizing and accepting how upset your child feels, reassure him about his safety.

During medical procedures, deep breathing exercises sometimes help children to relax. You may also be able to help by encouraging your child to shift his attention away from the therapy, concentrating instead on more pleasant thoughts—perhaps a recent music recital, a hike, or something else he enjoys.

Children can be taught relaxation and self-hypnosis techniques, and can benefit greatly from learning these skills. They take time and practice to learn, and need to be mastered well before a procedure or hospitalization is scheduled. Ask your physician where you and your child can learn these techniques.

What About Pain?

For many children with a chronic condition or special health-care needs, pain is their greatest fear. In your discussions about a procedure, if your child asks, "Is it going to hurt?" you and your doctor should give a direct, honest answer.

When youngsters (as well as adults) hurt—or even when they just anticipate discomfort—they often function less well than usual in their day-to-day lives. Their schoolwork and self-image may suffer. As one youngster said, "When I'm in pain, I don't feel very good about myself or my body."

Children, parents, and even some doctors still believe that pain is unavoidable with a chronic illness. Youngsters are sometimes told: "Pain is just something you're going to have to live with." With some diseases—juvenile rheumatoid arthritis, for instance—some pain may be inevitable. But thanks to new drugs and techniques, pain can often be controlled.

Much of the pain children experience is caused by procedures and treatment, and so part of the treatment plan should be to prevent pain. Anxiety can heighten a child's experience of pain. Whenever possible, parents should be present with their child during painful or frightening procedures. Topical anesthetics applied in advance can reduce and often prevent pain caused by injections or spinal taps. Systemic medicines are available for more severe pain. For children over the age of eight, there are ways to judge the severity of pain, and these measures can be used to help decide when, what, and how much pain medication to use.

In some cases, children can use patient-controlled analgesia (PCA), a system that allows the child to actually control how much medication she receives. The old fear about children with chronic diseases such as cancer or sickle-cell anemia becoming addicted to pain medication is a myth—parents should not worry about this. If your child is in pain, tell your doctor, and jointly develop a plan to manage that discomfort. No child should experience pain unnecessarily.

There are a variety of ways to help control pain. Some treatments using positive imagery, distraction, or hypnosis are quite effective. Some medical centers have pain clinics specializing in pain management. Often they will use a combination of approaches such as medication, relaxation techniques, and electrical stimulation. Monitor your child's pain, and ensure that she is receiving adequate pain management. None of the common chronic health problems of childhood should be accompanied by worsening pain. If your child's pain is increasing, there is the possibility that the disease is progressing or the child is developing a complication. Inform her physician promptly about such changes.

DEALING WITH EMOTIONAL PROBLEMS AND DEPRESSION

Feelings of sadness, depression, or being overwhelmed may come and go for both you and your child. This is normal and healthy. As tumultuous as these times can be, most youngsters and their families emerge with few if any long-term behavioral problems or lasting psychological scars. In fact, the majority of children really do manage their situation well, despite riding an emotional roller coaster on occasion. Researchers believe that the likelihood of emotional and behavioral problems associated with chronic illness has been decreasing recently because parents, school staffs, and health-care providers are learning more effective ways to help children and their parents meet their psychological needs.

Nevertheless, children who have a chronic illness or condition often feel "different," socially isolated, and restricted in their activities. They may have school problems and feel overprotected. They may experience recurrent fear and pain. When these emotional difficulties are not dealt with, they can lead to anxiety, sadness, withdrawal, rebelliousness, or a decreased interest in school.

School-age children rarely state that they are sad or depressed. Instead, they may withdraw from friends and family or exhibit rebellious or angry behavior. They may do poorly in school. They may interfere with their medical treatments, perhaps by refusing to take medication as scheduled. They might experiment with alcohol, drugs, or early sexual activity. Or they may run away from home or contemplate suicide.

Make an ongoing effort to discuss with your child what he is experiencing. Do you think he is displaying signs of despair and hopelessness related to his illness and future? Encourage him to talk about these feelings with you or with another trusted adult. Because your child may not even be aware of his feelings, try beginning these conversations with statements like "If I were you, I think I would be feeling . . ." or "I have read that many kids with this condition feel lonely and sad. How do you feel?"

Some parents are hesitant to discuss feelings about the disease with their child, in an effort to protect the youngster from emotional hurt. Most experts, however, disagree with that point of view. Children can usually adjust much better to an unpleasant truth than to the perception that their parents are upset and hiding something from them. If parents and children do not talk openly, the opportunities for misinterpretation are high. A youngster's imagination can run wild, and fears may emerge or be exaggerated.

Thus, it is best to make a commitment to be as communicative as possible. Remind your child that he is not going through this alone and that you will remain a constant source of love and support. Many studies show that the key to a child's resilience is a relationship with a caring, loving, accessible adult— someone the child can count on and trust.

If you are concerned about your child's coping with these stresses, talk to your physician. If your youngster is exhibiting destructive or unusual behavior, if he refuses to take his medication, if he is severely withdrawn or if his schoolwork has deteriorated, your doctor might recommend some counseling for the child or the entire family. (For more information, see Chapter 23, "Depression.")

SCHOOL ISSUES FOR CHILDREN WITH CHRONIC ILLNESSES

School is more than a place to acquire knowledge and skills. It is also a place where children meet new friends, discover how to interact with other children and adults, experience success and failure, and learn about themselves. Youngsters acquire many important social skills, expectations, and behavior in school, including sharing, empathy, understanding rules, and dealing with peer pressure.

During the school years, children yearn to be accepted by their peers. They want to look and behave like their classmates and participate in the same activities. Their self-image and self-confidence are influenced by whether they are accepted by others of the same age.

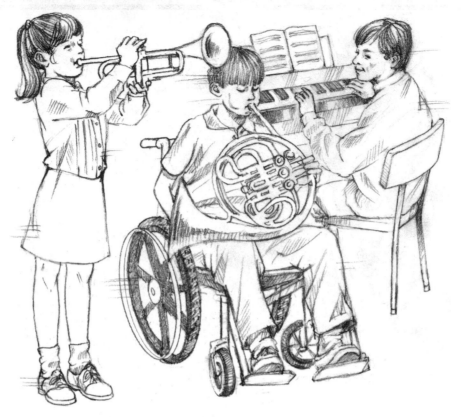

Children with chronic illnesses and disabilities, like all children, yearn to be accepted by their peers.

SOCIAL DIFFICULTIES

A chronic illness can present a special challenge for your child as she relates to other children. Youngsters constantly scrutinize one another. A child with a visible disability or one who receives special treatment may be singled out by classmates because of those differences. Middle childhood is a hard time of life for children to feel that they are different in their appearance or their capacity to keep up with classmates. A condition that requires medication, frequent absences from school, rest periods, or special equipment, such as braces or eye patches, can cause embarrassment and make children feel like outsiders.

However, children who differ in health, race, religion, family, and a myriad of other circumstances can discover that they have more similarities than differences. One of the goals for your child's school experience is that she learn to accept and be accepted by others, regardless of differences. Bear in mind that while feeling different can be traumatic, most youngsters are quite resilient.

They and their families not only usually learn to accept their limitations, but also find creative alternatives to problems that initially may have seemed overwhelming. These children—when assisted and supported by family, friends, and professionals—can develop into stronger individuals, despite their extra burdens.

On the academic side, children with chronic illnesses and normal intelligence should demonstrate classroom achievement just as high as that of their peers. Yet studies show that many of these youngsters underachieve at school. This may occur for a number of reasons. Their stamina may be lower, or their medication may impair their alertness or make them irritable. If their illness causes them frustration, they may have emotional or behavioral problems that can interfere with schoolwork.

With diseases like sickle-cell anemia, asthma, cystic fibrosis, and diabetes, youngsters may frequently miss several days of school at a time, a period that may not be long enough to qualify for a home teacher. Hospitalizations may also keep them away from the classroom. In situations like this, your child could be at a disadvantage. If she falls behind her classmates because she is absent from school too much, she may become frustrated and her motivation may falter. She might also become anxious about having to catch up on missed assignments. This anxiety can lead her to avoid school, even when she is physically able to attend. (See Chapter 24, "School Avoidance.")

Most of these issues, however, can be dealt with successfully by working with the teacher, the pediatrician, and/or a child psychologist. If your child has a health problem that is likely to interrupt her regular attendance at school, plan ahead. Meet with her teacher at the start of each school year to discuss how best to keep your child up to date on her work. Plan how homework will be sent home and thereby prevent your child from slipping too far behind. Since your child may have frequent doctor's appointments, discuss with your child's physician the importance of scheduling them after school hours whenever possible so as to avoid missing class.

Also, by keeping your youngster's teacher updated about her health condition, you and your pediatrician can work with the teacher to prevent unnecessary disruptions of your youngster's academic progress. However, be cautious about requesting preferential treatment for your youngster at school. If her teacher frequently excuses her from homework or exams, your child may become overly dependent on this kind of special attention. The teacher may also underestimate the child's real capacity for learning and therefore have lower expectations. Most schools provide home teaching for long or intermittent, frequent absences; this usually requires a statement of necessity from your child's pediatrician or primary physician and should be based on a careful assessment of the benefits and risks for your child.

SERVING AS A CHILD ADVOCATE

Your child's school should be a place where both his academic and his health-related needs can be met. Federal statutes (such as Public Law 105-17 and Section 540 of the Rehabilitation Act) mandate that every child is entitled to an appropriate public education in the least restrictive environment possible. They require local school systems to develop and implement programs to evaluate and place children with special health-care needs or disabilities into appropriate programs, aimed at providing them with "full educational opportunities." Special classes or schools are acceptable only when the severity and nature of the handicap prevent youngsters from attending a regular class or school.

Many chronic illnesses, such as cancer, sickle-cell anemia, HIV, and severe lung or heart disease, or their treatment, may produce long-term cognitive and learning problems. These biological effects can interfere with a child's ability to be successful in school. Parents need to be aware of their potential problems, inform the school, and advocate to have a child-study team convened to evaluate the need for special education services. For children with chronic illnesses, the special-education category is "physical impairment or other health impairment." This classification allows children to have individual educational plans developed that address the specific needs associated with their illness. It is critical to address this issue because many of the cognitive impairments are subtle, and children's test performance on standardized assessments do not follow patterns typical of children with other types of learning problems. School personnel will need to be provided information about these issues in order to make appropriate plans for your child.

As a parent of a child with a chronic disease, familiarize yourself with these laws so you can be sure that your child is receiving all the routine and special services he is entitled to. If your child needs speech therapy, psychological counseling, or physical therapy, for instance, the school must make them available. He also may be eligible for home tutoring. You should monitor your child's educational experience to be sure that it is allowing him to make the most of his potential, providing appropriate programs without overprotecting or overrestricting him. School personnel should also be careful not to push your child too hard, making school more frustrating than fulfilling.

Your child's teacher and/or school nurse should be prepared to manage any health problems your youngster may encounter during the school day. It may be advisable for you or your child's doctor to speak with the school nurse and/or other school personnel to give them specific information about your youngster's disorder and what to do in the event of a problem during the school day. They should know how to respond to a seizure or an asthma attack, for example, and what activities may lead to a complication of an existing condition.

What Does the School Need to Know?

If you have a school-age child with special health needs, make sure the school has a written document outlining a health-care and emergency plan. This document should contain the following information:

- A brief medical history
- The child's special needs
- Medication or procedures required during school
- Special dietary requirements
- Transportation needs
- Possible problems, special precautions
- Important personnel (e.g., pediatrician, hospital)
- Emergency plans and procedures (including whom to contact)

Some parents are hesitant to give school personnel information about their child's medical condition. But in fact, the school staff will work with you and your child more effectively if they have complete information. Teachers often can identify problems early and help solve them and recognize your child's achievements in managing the illness. Thus, work toward assisting the teacher in becoming an advocate for your youngster, and keep the lines of communication open. If school personnel do not have accurate information to work with, they may start making erroneous assumptions, which can lead to mismanagement of your child's condition or inappropriate academic expectations.

Classmates should also be told about your child's health condition in order to avoid their exaggerating or misinterpreting the severity and danger of the illness and the limits it places on your youngster. Some children may be frightened about a diagnosis like leukemia or diabetes. They may not know how to relate to your youngster; they may be concerned that they will "catch" the disease. If those anxieties are not dealt with effectively, your child may find himself isolated from his classmates.

To avoid this kind of problem, you might suggest that your pediatrician or school nurse visit your child's classroom. Also, some families have become involved in school curriculum committees and PTAs to help educate both parents and students about their youngster's chronic condition. A number of school systems have created programs in which healthy children are taught about chronic illnesses and disabilities.

Teachers are a valuable source of observations of your child. They can let you know about changes in behavior, signs of anxiety or distractibility, and how your child relates to his classmates, as well as updating you on his academic performance.

IF YOUR CHILD'S EDUCATIONAL RIGHTS ARE DENIED

By law, your child is entitled to an education that will help her develop to her full potential. That means providing her, if indicated, with additional services that will assist in both educational programs and extracurricular events.

Sometimes, however, schools do not meet their legal obligations. There may be insufficient sensitivity to your child's special needs in the classroom, or too little flexibility in school policies. Your youngster may be excluded from activities like field trips, or denied help in making up assignments after periods of absence.

Here are some steps you can take if you feel your child's needs are not being met:

- Ask that the teacher and other school staff meet with your child's pediatrician to create guidelines to help your child succeed at school, taking into account health-related and other handicaps. These guidelines should specify the obligations of the school toward your youngster.

- If the school does not cooperate, there are procedures—spelled out by every school district—through which you can appeal and try to rectify the situation. Ask the school for a written copy of these guidelines for resolving complaints.

- If you still are not satisfied, contact the local board of education, or the regional office of the United States Department of Education.

RETURNING TO SCHOOL

When a child begins a new school year, or is about to return to the classroom after a prolonged absence, he might be anxious and fabricate reasons or exhibit behavior to postpone that return. "What are my friends going to think?" he may ask tearfully. "Why do I have to go to school at all?"

You cannot make all your child's anxieties vanish, but you can help ease the transition. Try preparing him for what he might encounter at school with some rehearsal or role-playing, deciding together how to respond to insensitive or embarrassing questions.

For instance, you might pose the following questions to your youngster:

"If your friends ask why you're wearing a wig, what are you going to say?"

Or: "What if kids tease you if you start to wheeze during recess? What are you going to tell them?" Help your child develop some appropriate responses to what he is likely to encounter. This type of preparation will help him deal with these situations more confidently.

Physicians, psychologists, and social workers can provide assistance in this process. Other youngsters with long-term illnesses who have made successful transitions back to school after a prolonged absence can also be a useful resource, as can their parents. Child and parent support groups (see page 572) are available in many communities.

HIDING OR REVEALING THE CONDITION

Some parents urge their youngsters to hide their illness or medication from friends, believing this will protect them from ridicule or insensitive questions. That advice, however, gives a child the message that she has a shameful problem that has to be kept secret.

Ultimately, circumstances often arise that make it apparent to other youngsters that a child has special health needs. Try gently to encourage your child to disclose information to her peers in settings she finds comfortable. A best friend—even just one of them—can greatly ease the isolation felt by a child with a chronic illness.

As your youngster becomes more comfortable and secure with close friends and important school personnel, encourage her to talk with them about her illness. She should go into as much detail as she feels comfortable with; remind her that it is not necessary (or beneficial) to share every personal piece of information indiscriminately. A school nurse or a favorite teacher might be able to assist in this process.

THE FAMILY'S ADJUSTMENT

DEALING WITH YOUR OWN FEELINGS

"When I found out my child had a chronic illness, it seemed like the end of the world. I ached so bad and I felt so angry."

Parents often experience an array of emotions as they come to terms with their youngster's illness. Immediately after the diagnosis, many mothers and fathers enter a mourning period, grieving over the "loss" of their healthy child. They must cope with the shock and the pain and try to accept the new reality of having a youngster with a chronic illness. Parents often deny this reality and tell themselves things like "This can't be happening.... The laboratory must have gotten our test results mixed up with someone else's.... When am I going to wake up from this nightmare?" Eventually, parents usually begin to find ways to accept their child's illness, despite periodically feeling sad, resentful, anxious, and angry.

Common Feelings of Parents of Children with Chronic Illnesses

Negative	Positive
anger	achievement
anxiety	closeness
embarrassment	joy
frustration	love
grief	mastery
guilt	pride
isolation	self-confidence
powerlessness	self-esteem
resentment	strength
sadness	usefulness

Guilt is common among parents, often feeling that they somehow caused the illness. Self-blame is particularly prevalent when the condition was present at birth, has a genetic basis, and/or when the cause is not known. Guilt can be an excruciating and disabling emotion, adding to the stress within the family and sometimes making it difficult for parents to be supportive of their children and each other. If guilt or other emotional difficulties are interfering with your parenting abilities or the quality of your family life, you may benefit from some professional counseling.

Other adjustments may be necessary as well. There can be considerable financial cost associated with a child's chronic illness. As medical bills mount— with frequent doctors' visits, medications, hospitalizations, and other outpatient services—worry over finances can intensify.

Many parents find it to be very difficult to discipline their chronically ill child. However, all children need and benefit from having clear limits and consistent expectations. In their absence, children may become overly dependent, have lower self-esteem, and begin to have behavioral and social problems. Parents should establish a consistent set of expectations, adjusting them as needed for acute episodes as the child's health fluctuates. They should provide an environment that encourages independence and self-confidence.

Sometimes a parent may have to give up a career or education to become the primary caretaker at home; this is particularly true when the child requires a great deal of assistance with daily activities. A parent may have to change jobs, or take on a second job, to increase the family income. These adjustments are sometimes complicated when a new job necessitates switching health insurance policies, causing a situation in which medical bills associated with the child's chronic illness (referred to as a *pre-existing condition*) are not covered. The family might also have to move, relocating closer to the medical services the child needs.

Several state and federal programs are available to help families with the costs of chronic health care. Recent changes in the eligibility criteria for Supplemental Security Income (SSI) for children, for example, now provide cash benefits to many families with children with chronic illnesses. Eligible youngsters generally include those with significant psychiatric conditions and severe chronic illnesses, such as cystic fibrosis, congenital heart disease, malignancies, and many others. Your physician or the social worker at your local hospital should be able to refer you to the proper agencies for help.

STRAINS ON THE MARRIAGE

Every family is a balanced system. After learning of a child's chronic illness, families understandably experience some loss of equilibrium that threatens their stability. The stress of a serious illness can cause severe disruptions, particularly if each parent attempts to deal with his or her own fears and frustrations alone.

In some instances mothers and fathers may become consumed with the care of their ill child, at the expense of nearly everything else in their lives. In these situations parents may find themselves almost constantly investigating new options, reading about alternative treatments, and pondering the future: Is there a better medication for my child? Is it worth getting another doctor's opinion? Can I be doing more?

As a parent, you might sometimes feel that the demands upon you are unending, from trips to the doctor's office to the preparation of special meals. You may feel constantly fatigued, never able to recoup your energy. If anything gets sacrificed, it is often time spent with your spouse, or time for your own personal interests and pursuits.

On the other hand, a child's chronic illness often has some positive effects on families. A child with health problems may bring parents and other family members closer. Families—especially those who communicate openly—may be strengthened by experiences associated with managing their child's health impairment. In many cases, the family's management of a child's chronic illness may provide them with a sense of cohesiveness, mission, mastery, and pride.

Physicians, psychologists, social workers, family therapists, and parents of other children with chronic illnesses are invaluable resources for working through family difficulties. Ask for help. You should not expect or attempt to solve all family problems associated with your child's illness by yourself. Isolation is a preventable side effect of caring for a child with a chronic health condition.

AVOID BURNOUT

For your own physical and psychological health, you need to take some time away from the day-to-day routine now and then. That means finding time to devote to your spouse and to yourself, including recreational activities. To maintain your own health, you need to achieve balance by pursuing activities that are not strictly child-oriented.

Some mothers and fathers, however, have difficulty taking time off. "My child is so vulnerable. I just don't feel comfortable going out of town for even a weekend," said one mother. But if you do not get away, the tasks of parenting can become oppressive, and your child's chronic illness may come to feel like an enormous burden in your life.

If you need to find someone with medical sophistication to watch your child while you are gone, ask your doctor or local hospital staff for suggestions. Many parents work out arrangements with other families who have children with the same disorder. Enlist the help of relatives and friends. Teach family members to participate in the care-giving, and then use their assistance to acquire some time for yourself.

The local social services agency or public health department may provide respite services to families caring at home for children with very severe and demanding illnesses. These agencies often supply other types of support as well, such as loans of medical equipment or transportation to doctors' appointments. Your doctor may be able to help you make the proper connections with social workers who are aware of available services and resources in the community.

It is not a sign of weakness or lack of love if you need to take time off, or if you let doctors, friends, or family know that you are depressed, anxious, or worried about becoming burned out.

WHAT ABOUT YOUR OTHER CHILDREN?

Parents are not the only ones who must adjust to a child's illness. Life changes for the entire family.

Parents have to pay extra attention to an ill child, and brothers and sisters often feel neglected. They might also have difficulty learning to live with the stresses of having a sibling with a chronic health problem.

Are Your Other Children Having Trouble?

When there is a child with a chronic illness in your family, your other youngsters may experience negative repercussions. Here are some warning signs indicating that the siblings of your ill child may need some extra attention. Is a sibling:

- anxious?
- depressed?
- withdrawn?
- angry?
- losing interest in friends?
- doing poorly in school?
- pushing herself too hard to achieve?
- rebellious?
- losing interest in activities that once brought pleasure, such as sports or music lessons?
- blaming herself for her sibling's illness?
- acting in ways to draw attention to herself?

Some children experience guilt that *they* are not sick ("Why him and not me?"). As part of the magical thinking of young childhood, they may wonder whether an evil thought they have had about a sibling might have caused his illness. They may feel anxious about becoming sick themselves, or they may sometimes wish they were sick, too, so they could become the center of the family's attention. They might feel angry if they are asked to assume more household chores than their ill sibling, or guilty when they resent the additional responsibility. They may become embarrassed when strangers stare at their brother or sister in a wheelchair, or when other children tease their sibling because she looks different.

Be aware that while attending to the needs of your child with a chronic illness, you may be neglecting—or creating unfair expectations for—your healthy children. Too often, siblings become invisible unless they demand attention. On the other hand, siblings can participate in the family and feel pride and love in helping their brother or sister with his or her health problem. The presence of a family member with a chronic illness provides opportunities for increased empathy, responsibility, adaptability, problem-solving, and creativity.

Try to establish some balance between the needs of your ill child and those of your other children. Spending time with each child individually may help. Develop a special relationship with each one of your youngsters. Also, keep in mind that siblings need to have honest information about the illness and to have their questions listened to and answered. (See "How to Have a Family Meeting" on page 336.)

DEVELOPING RESILIENCE

No one would choose to have a child with a chronic illness. However, living with a chronic illness can teach adults and children a lot about themselves and those around them. Adults and children can learn about their strengths and limitations, and they can learn new ways to solve problems and to be resilient. These are lessons that can serve them well for the rest of their lives.

In the months and years ahead, continue to reassess your goals for your child and your family. Be willing to make changes that serve both the youngster with the chronic health problem and everyone else in the family. As much as possible, involve your child in these decisions, particularly when they affect him. Stay informed and give yourself credit for all the hard work you have done.

No family knows from the outset how it will adapt to the reality of a child with a chronic health problem. There is no right way or wrong way to adjust; rather, every family should strive for its own balance. Many factors will influence this process, including the course of the disease and the resources available to the family. While all families with chronic health problems struggle through times of fear and despair, many also develop a resilience, a creativity, and a closeness they did not always have.

FAMILY SUPPORT AND ADVOCACY GROUPS

Social isolation is common in families who have a child with a chronic condition. Children with chronic illnesses may try to shelter themselves from other youngsters, or the condition itself may limit or alter their social interactions. Parents may also have fewer social contacts than in the past because of the time required to care for the child, because friends and relatives sometimes find it hard to cope with a childhood cancer or other serious illness, or because of the parents' own sadness about the illness.

This kind of seclusion can be emotionally painful. You need contact with

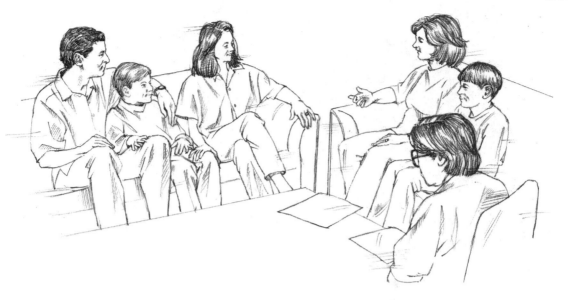

Support groups for parents of children with chronic health problems can help eliminate feelings of social isolation and seclusion.

other adults, including those undergoing similar experiences. Ask your child's physician, a social worker, and/or the staff at your child's school if they can put you in touch with parents of other children with chronic health problems. There are hundreds of organizations across the country that help parents create support networks.

Especially in smaller communities, you may have difficulty locating families or groups dealing specifically with the particular illness your child has. In this case, a more broadly constituted group of parents whose children have a range of chronic health problems can be quite helpful.

These meetings will provide opportunities to share information and emotional comfort. Parents often find it useful to discuss their common concerns—for example, locating good health-care professionals, identifying competent babysitters, and solving the problems of school success.

One mother said, "It's such a relief to find other people like me and to know that I'm not alone. The feelings I've had—even those that I'm not particularly proud of—are the same ones that other parents are having. In the beginning, these people were complete strangers, but after just a meeting or two, I felt closer to them than I do to some of my longtime friends. They've been through it."

Your child with a chronic health problem can also benefit from participation in a support group for children with chronic disorders. If a group like this is not available in your community, work with other parents to put one together. Some communities also have support groups for siblings and grandparents, who can also benefit from information-sharing and emotional support.

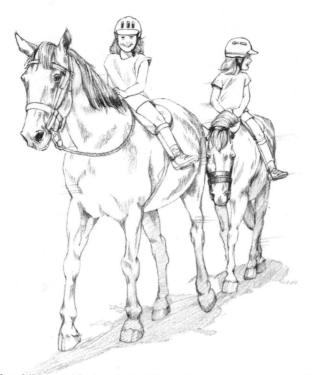

Summer camps for children with chronic health problems can be very beneficial for children who feel isolated by their disease.

Summer camps, some run by nonprofit organizations, are available for children with chronic health problems. They can be enormously beneficial for children who feel isolated by their disease. These camps can also help youngsters increase their ability to care for themselves and their medical needs.

If you need help finding out about these kinds of groups, the parent advocacy groups listed below can provide information and direction.

INFORMATION AND RESOURCES

The following organizations can give parents information about chronic illnesses in children. Many also serve as advocacy groups for these youngsters. Some may be able to supply referrals to support groups in your community.

There are also numerous condition-specific groups like the Cystic Fibrosis Foundation and the Juvenile Diabetes Association, or more broad-based groups like the American Heart Association and the American Lung Association. Many have local chapters, or their national offices may be able to refer you to valuable resources in your community.

Alliance of Genetic Support Groups
4301 Connecticut Ave NW
Suite 404
Washington, D.C. 20008
(800) 336-GENE
Promotes the health and well-being of individuals and families affected by genetic disorders

Association for the Care of Children's Health
19 Mantina Road
Mount Royal, New Jersey 08061
(609) 224-1742
Promotes the better understanding of the emotional needs of children

Beach Center on Families and Disability
University of Kansas
3111 Haworth Hall
Lawrence, Kansas 66045
(785) 864-7600
Encourages the development of methods for the care of retarded and handicapped children

Federation for Children with Special Needs
95 Berkeley St.
Suite 104
Boston, Massachusetts 02116
(617) 482-2915
Acts on behalf of children with developmental disabilities

National Easter Seal Society
230 West Monroe
Suite 1800
Chicago, Illinois 60606
(800) 221-6827
Conducts programs that serve people with disabilities

National Information Center for Children and Youth with Disabilities
P.O. Box 1492
Washington, D.C. 20013
(800) 695-0285
Provides information on educational rights and special services for children with physical, mental, and emotional handicaps

National Organization for Rare Disorders
P.O. Box 8923
New Fairfield, Connecticut 06812
(800) 999-NORD
A clearinghouse of information on rare disorders

READING MATERIAL

Most of the organizations listed above can provide parents with publications, including books and brochures. Here is a sampling of some of the titles that can be ordered from just two of the groups.

The Federation for Children with Special Needs offers publications such as:

- *Becoming Informed About Your Child's Special Health Care Needs*

- *Preparing Children for Medical Tests*

- *Questions When Surgery Is Recommended for Your Child*

- *Checklist of Items for Considering in Developing Individual Educational Plans*

The Association for the Care of Children's Health can provide the following books and booklets for both parents and children. Some of these titles are available in bookstores, too.

- *Your Child with Special Needs at Home and in the Community*

- *Our Brother Has Down's Syndrome* by S. Cairo

PART IX

COMMON MEDICAL PROBLEMS

COMMON MEDICAL DISORDERS

Most school-age children are in excellent health most of the time. By middle childhood, children should be playing a more active role in maintaining their health and staying fit.

Even with the best health habits and preventive care, however, all children experience occasional illness. From time to time they have colds, sore throats, and stomach pains. Parents naturally find these illnesses worrisome. With a little information, and sometimes professional advice, you can sort out most of these common health problems.

This chapter will examine some of the most common medical disorders of middle childhood, with a general look at causes, symptoms, and treatments. These pages cover the information most commonly asked of pediatricians about these problems. If you have specific concerns about your own child's illness, be sure to talk directly to your doctor.

Colds

The common cold is really an upper respiratory infection that inflames the lining of the nose and throat. For five to ten days your child's nose may be runny or stuffy, and his eyes may be red and watery. He may sneeze, cough, experience aches and pains, and have a mild fever.

There is a lot of misunderstanding about how colds are transmitted from child to child. For example, despite myths to the contrary, you *cannot* catch colds from drafts, or from failing to wear a scarf or a heavy jacket in cool wet weather. Instead, colds are caused by viruses and are passed from one individual to another, usually through direct contact or by sharing objects such as utensils or handkerchiefs, as well as by coughs and sneezes. Colds are extremely contagious, particularly during the first day or two of the infection, when many of the symptoms may not yet be evident. Also, colds tend to be more prevalent in the fall and winter, when children are in school and are in closer contact with each other and the cold viruses.

There is no cure for the common cold. But until the symptoms disappear, here is how to keep your child as comfortable as possible.

- When your child has a cold and stuffy nose, he will tend to breathe through his mouth. This will dry his mouth and throat and also cause some increased loss of body water. Give him plenty of fluids, such as fruit juices and water.

- Your child's appetite will probably decrease during the illness. Make sure he eats nutritious meals, even if they are small.

- Use a clean, cool-mist humidifier or vaporizer to ease his stuffy nose.

- Monitor his temperature and how he is feeling.

- Give lots of tender loving care.

Colds do not respond to penicillin or other antibiotics, nor do they respond to most of the advertised cold medications. If your child is running a fever, see the following section on fever; although it may be appropriate to treat a fever, aspirin should *never* be given to a child with a fever because of its association with Reye's syndrome, a serious liver and neurological disease.

Also, take steps to keep your child's cold from spreading to others in your household. Teach your youngsters to wash their hands before meals. Encourage them to cover the mouth with a tissue when they sneeze or cough, and then dispose of the tissue immediately. Keep them from sharing eating utensils and drinking glasses.

Generally, colds are self-limiting and disappear on their own without complications. However, contact your pediatrician if your youngster develops ear pain or a severe sore throat, or has trouble breathing, or if the cold persists for more than ten days, or if a fever lasts longer than forty-eight hours. Children with colds may attend school as long as they feel well enough to participate.

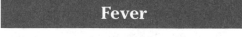

Fever

A fever is usually a symptom of an illness, often a bacterial or viral infection, ranging from urinary tract infections and ear infections to chicken pox and sore throats. Even though you may become concerned about your child's fever, it is usually a positive sign that her body is fighting the infection.

When your youngster feels warm to the touch, check her temperature. In middle childhood most youngsters can hold the thermometer between their lips and under their tongue for the time necessary for a proper reading; however, for a child who still has difficulty keeping the thermometer in place this way, her temperature can be taken rectally. A rectal measurement is also advisable if your child cannot keep her mouth closed with the thermometer in place because her nose is congested.

For a correct measurement, use a digital thermometer. Although temperature strips are popular and convenient—providing a reading when placed across the forehead for several seconds—they can be inaccurate. Before placing the thermometer in your child's mouth, place a clean plastic cover on it. Your youngster should keep it under her tongue for two minutes. Glass thermometers are difficult to read and break easily.

Follow your doctor's advice about treatment of the fever. Your pediatrician may advise that medications for fever are unnecessary.

In children, the use of aspirin has been associated with a rare but serious brain disorder called Reye's syndrome. For that reason, *fevers in children should be treated with acetaminophen or ibuprofen and not aspirin*. Dosages should follow the guidelines on the package or the recommendations of your pediatrician.

(On occasion, seizures occur when a child has a high or rapidly rising fever. For more information, see page 598.)

Sore Throat

Like colds, most sore throats are caused by viruses. Sore throats are often a companion to the common cold.

When sore throats occur, your child may experience swelling and redness of the tissues in his throat and sometimes enlarged tonsils. He may also feel fatigued and run a fever. The pain in the throat can range from mild to burning, and swallowing can be very uncomfortable.

To ease your child's sore throat, have him drink warm liquids and gargle several times a day with warm salt water ($^1/_2$ teaspoon of salt mixed with 8 ounces of water). Sucking on hard candy or throat lozenges can also help sometimes and is usually just as effective as more expensive over-the-counter throat sprays. A clean, cool-mist humidifier or vaporizer can keep the throat moist and more comfortable.

Contact your pediatrician if your child has difficulty swallowing because of severe throat pain or if he is having trouble breathing. Your physician may suggest acetaminophen for pain relief and controlling any accompanying fever.

Even though sore throats are caused primarily by viruses, a minority are caused by streptococcal bacteria. If your doctor suspects strep throat, he or she will recommend performing a rapid strep test or a throat culture, a painless procedure in which mucus is swabbed from the throat and analyzed in the laboratory. If, in fact, the infection involves strep, antibiotics will be prescribed to prevent any complications (most seriously, rheumatic fever). These same antibiotics, however, are *not* effective for viral sore throats. When youngsters have a strep infection, they can return to school twenty-four hours after treatment has started, as long as they are free of a fever.

Children who sleep with their mouths open often awaken with a sore throat. This discomfort usually disappears in a short time, particularly after the youngsters have had something to drink. Using a humidifier while children sleep can reduce this problem.

Vomiting and Diarrhea

At one time or another, nearly all children experience vomiting and diarrhea. While usually not serious, these symptoms can make the child quite uncomfortable. Most often, a viral infection of the stomach (gastritis), intestines (enteritis), or both (gastroenteritis) is to blame.

These symptoms can last from a few days to a week. Because it is usually a viral illness, antibiotics are generally not effective as a treatment. In fact, medication given by mouth can sometimes aggravate an already upset stomach.

What, then, is the most appropriate treatment? Much of the care should be directed at preventing dehydration (excessive fluid loss) due to diarrhea and vomiting. As long as your child takes in somewhat more than she puts out, she will not be at any risk. Make sure she drinks adequate fluids—in small quantities, but frequently. It is usually safe to allow the child to select the liquids she would prefer. Commercially prepared hydration solutions such as Pedialyte, or a mixture of 50 percent Gatorade and 50 percent water, are a good choice for the child in the middle years if only one liquid is preferred.

If drinking liquids aggravates vomiting, reduce the intake to frequent spoonfuls or have the child suck on small ice chips. Children of this age are usually good judges of whether they can tolerate eating and drinking. Notify your doctor if the vomiting continues for longer than six hours, or if abdominal pain and fever are present.

Your child's appetite will probably be decreased. Allow the child to eat whatever she wants. Good choices include toast, bananas, oatmeal, cooked rice, and crackers. A normal diet can be reintroduced as soon as your child is hungry, usually about twenty-four hours after the last vomiting episode.

Sometimes, severe abdominal pain accompanies viral infections of the stomach and intestines. Call your pediatrician at once if this discomfort occurs, so that other, more serious problems, particularly appendicitis, can be ruled out.

Diarrhea can have a number of other causes, including parasites, dietary changes, and antibiotic drugs. If you have questions about your child's loose stools, call your doctor. Be sure to contact a physician if the diarrhea involves a large loss of fluids, contains blood, or lasts more than three days, or if your child appears dehydrated or especially ill. Keep your youngster home from school for as long as the vomiting continues and until she is able to control her bowels without the risk of an accident. Avoid giving your child drugs that interfere with bowel motility. Antidiarrheal medication can make symptoms worse if the illness is caused by a bacteria.

Ear Infections

Middle-ear infections, which doctors call *otitis media,* are less common during middle childhood than at younger ages.

When an ear is infected, the eustachian tube—the narrow passage connecting the middle ear (the small chamber behind the eardrum) to the back of the throat—becomes blocked. During healthy periods this tube is filled with air and keeps the space behind the eardrum free of fluid; during a cold or other respiratory infection, or in children with allergies, this tube can become blocked, fluid begins to accumulate in the middle ear, and bacteria start to grow there. As this occurs, pressure on the eardrum increases and it can no longer vibrate properly. Hearing is temporarily reduced, and at the same time the pressure on the eardrum can cause pain.

Your pediatrician should examine your youngster's ears with an instrument called an otoscope, with which inflammation and

fluid behind the eardrums can be detected. If an infection is present, your physician may prescribe antibiotics to destroy the bacteria and diminish the buildup of fluids. Antibiotics are not always necessary. Acetaminophen can help ease the pain. Heat—using a heating pad or a warm towel over the ear—can also make your child feel better.

Occasionally, when a child has repeated ear infections, and when fluid in the ears tends to persist despite medication, the doctor may suggest inserting small drainage tubes through the eardrum to help remove the trapped fluid. To date, however, the research examining the potential benefits of these tubes is inconclusive, and there are clearly some drawbacks to them—namely, anesthesia is required for insertion, and the tubes can sometimes come out by themselves.

With recurrent ear infections (more frequent than one a month for two to three months), your doctor may decide to place your child on low doses of antibiotics on a long-term basis to prevent infections. This therapy has been shown to decrease the frequency of ear infections. However, this therapy can increase the risk of resistant infections. Some doctors may also suggest surgical removal of the adenoids (adenoidectomy) if they are blocking the child's eustachian tube.

Ear infections are not contagious. Your child can safely return to school after the pain and fever subside. However, he should continue taking the antibiotics as prescribed until the pills or liquid are used up.

Swimmer's Ear

Swimmer's ear, which doctors call *otitis externa,* is an inflammation of the external ear canal. It occurs when water gets into the ear—usually during swimming or bathing—and does not properly drain.

Ear Piercing

Ears may be pierced for cosmetic reasons at any age, and during the middle years of childhood, some youngsters will ask to have their ears pierced. If the piercing is performed carefully and cared for conscientiously, there is little risk, no matter what the age of the child. However, as a general guideline, postpone the piercing until your child is mature enough to take care of the pierced site herself.

For the actual piercing procedure, have a doctor, nurse, or experienced technician perform it. Rubbing alcohol or other disinfectants should be used to minimize the chances of an infection. At the time of the piercing, a round, gold-post earring should be inserted; in fact, some piercing instruments themselves can put the gold posts in place at the same time, thus avoiding any additional probing that can increase the chance of infection. The gold in the posts will reduce the risk of an allergic reaction and inflammation in the area.

After the piercing, apply rubbing alcohol or an antibiotic ointment to the area two times a day for a few days; these applications will cut down the chances of infection and hasten the healing process. The earring should not be removed for four to six weeks, but should be gently rotated each day. If the area of piercing becomes red or tender, an infection may be developing, and you should seek medical attention promptly.

When that happens, the canal can become irritated and infected.

Youngsters with this condition will complain of itching or pain in the ear, the latter particularly when the head or the ear itself is moved. As the canal swells, hearing will decrease. The infected ear may ooze yellowish pus.

Your doctor will diagnose otitis externa after examining the ear canal with an otoscope. He or she may treat it with prescription eardrops. Sometimes you will need to insert a gauze wick into your child's ear to make sure the drops reach the site of the swelling. If it is needed, your physician will demonstrate this procedure. Also, try keeping your child's ear canal as dry as possible during the healing process; that means delaying washing and shampooing until the inflammation has disappeared.

Once a child has had a swimmer's ear infection, you should try to prevent future episodes. To help avoid them, your youngster should place drops in the ears after swimming—either a 70 percent alcohol solution or a mixture of one-half alcohol, one-half white vinegar. Also, dry the ears with a towel immediately after swimming or bathing.

Poison Ivy

Skin reactions to poison ivy or poison oak are very uncomfortable, itchy, and unsightly. They can make a child miserable.

About half of the children who come in contact with either poison ivy or poison oak have an allergic reaction. Typically, the skin becomes reddened, swollen, and blistered, with the rash shaped like streaks or in patches. The children experience severe itching and burning sensations. The rash usually appears one to four days after your child is exposed. Then blisters form and soon rupture, fluid oozes out of them, and they eventually become crusty.

As with all allergies, preventing exposure to the offending agent is most important. Particularly if your child spends time in forests and fields, make sure she knows what the poison ivy and poison oak plants look like. Poison ivy is a red-stemmed, three-leafed plant whose shiny green leaves turn bright red in the fall. Poison oak has green shiny leaves that also grow three to a stem. You might teach your child the poem: "Leaves of three, let them be." Particularly when you have younger children, inspect the parks they play in for any poison ivy or oak, and have the plants removed.

The skin reactions to poison ivy and poison oak are not contagious and cannot be transmitted from one child to another. But if your youngster comes in contact with the plants themselves, she should wash immediately with soap and water to remove as much of the sap or oil as possible. This will keep its absorption—and the ensuing inflammation—to a minimum. Pets playing in yards with poison ivy and poison oak can be a source of exposure to family members.

The rash will heal within about two weeks, although your doctor may suggest some treatment to relieve the symptoms. For instance, to ease both the itching and oozing, have your child soak the affected area in cool water for a few minutes, or rub it gently for ten to twenty minutes, several times a day, with an ice cube; then let the skin air-dry. A hydrocortisone cream might also be helpful. To discourage scratching and further damage to the skin, keep your child's fingernails trimmed. If your youngster cannot sleep at night because of the itching, you may give her an antihistamine. While mild cases can be treated at home, consult a doctor if your child is especially uncomfortable, if the rash is severe, if it has erupted on your child's face or groin, or if it shows signs of infection (fever, redness, and swelling beyond the poison ivy or oak lesions).

Insect Bites and Stings

Stings by bees, wasps, hornets, and yellow jackets will cause pain, swelling, itching, and redness at and near the location of the sting. In some children, allergic reactions to the insects' venom can also trigger other symptoms beyond a local skin reaction; they may become dizzy and weak, or have diarrhea or hives. On occasion, they may have difficulty breathing.

After a bee sting, carefully remove the stinger from your child's skin as quickly as possible, thus minimizing the venom that enters the body. Use the blunt edge of a knife to gently brush away the stinger and the attached venom sac; or, if possible, pull it out with a pair of tweezers. Once the stinger is gone, apply cool, damp compresses or an ice pack to the area in order to minimize swelling and relieve the pain. A solution containing water and a commercial meat tenderizer, wet baking soda, or calamine lotion can also be placed on the bite to reduce the discomfort. Your doctor might also recommend an oral antihistamine or a nonprescription corticosteroid ointment.

Sometimes a bee sting may result in problems that require an emergency response—specifically, if your child is having difficulty breathing or if he is exhibiting signs of shock (such as rapid breathing, dizziness, or cool, clammy skin). In such a case, call 911 or your emergency rescue number. Also, call your doctor if your child has received multiple stings, or if he develops hives in a part of the body away from the sting itself (for example, if he gets stung on the arm but gets hives on the legs).

Children who tend to have severe reactions to stings should take special precautions. When outdoors, they should wear shoes, socks, long trousers, and long-sleeved shirts. Doctors might also suggest allergy shots (*hyposensitization*) for these youngsters, intentionally exposing them to small amounts of the insect's venom. Families can also have an emergency kit available at home, in the car, and with them when they travel; the kit should be equipped with a syringe filled with lifesaving adrenaline that should be administered if a sting occurs that causes difficulty breathing or signs of shock. (A child in shock will appear pale, cold, and clammy and have a weak and rapid pulse; his breathing may be weak and he may be semiconscious or unconscious.)

Snake Bites

Snake bites, although less common than stings, can cause just as many problems. Your immediate task is to determine whether your child has been bitten by a poisonous snake. Call your doctor, poison center, or local emergency room and be prepared to describe what the snake looked like. Your child may need an injection of antivenom serum as quickly as possible. Until you can get her to a hospital emergency room, don't give her anything to eat or drink, and try to keep the bitten region of her body lower than the heart. Constricting bands may be placed two inches above and below the bite site, or only above the bite if it is located near the end of a limb; the bands should not cut off the pulse or the blood flow through the arteries. On your way to the emergency room, keep the area cool by placing ice on it.

Lyme Disease

Lyme disease was first identified in the mid-1970s in children and adults in and around Old Lyme, Connecticut. They developed an unusual circular rash and, in some cases, joint pain. Researchers eventually traced the symptoms to the bites of deer ticks, tiny black-brown creatures no larger than a poppy seed. These ticks carry and transmit the bacteria that cause the disease. Infections are most often acquired in the summer and fall months.

The circular rash, which is the most recognizable symptom of Lyme disease, usually appears shortly after the tick bite has occurred. It has a red border and may feel warm to the touch. After about a week, the rash may be joined by other symptoms, such as headache, fever, chills, sore throat, fatigue, swollen glands, and muscular aches and pains.

If your child develops these symptoms, contact your pediatrician. Parents sometimes believe that their child has merely come down with the flu, although a blood test can help diagnose Lyme disease. It can be successfully treated with oral antibiotics, usually penicillin or tetracycline (tetracycline is not recommended for younger school-age children). If untreated, the symptoms can worsen and become quite severe, occasionally causing heart palpitations, visual disturbances, dizziness, and facial paralysis. Sometimes years after the bite has occurred, joint pain and arthritis can develop. Later-stage Lyme disease is usually treated with intravenous antibiotic therapy.

For prevention of Lyme disease, be sure your child dresses to keep his risk of infection low when he walks through wooded areas. To protect his extremities, he should wear a hat and a long-sleeved shirt, and his pants should be tucked into his socks. If he wears light-colored clothing, it will be easier to spot ticks that land upon him.

Once you return from the outdoors, take a couple of minutes to check for ticks. They often hide behind the ears or along the hairline. Since they need at least twenty-four hours to infect an individual, you can greatly reduce the chances of the disease being transmitted by removing the ticks soon after they've attached themselves to your child's skin.

To get rid of a tick, clean the area gently with a cotton ball soaked in alcohol. Then, using tweezers or fingers (protected with a cloth or tissue), grasp the tick as close to the skin as possible and gently pull it up and out. As an alternative, you can encase the tick in petroleum jelly, thus blocking its airway. It will unhook itself in about twenty minutes. Wipe away the tick and destroy it. Clean the area again and call your pediatrician.

Impetigo

Unlike eczema or other allergic skin conditions, impetigo is a contagious skin infection caused by bacteria (streptococcus and/or staphylococcus). These bacteria enter the skin through a scratch, a small cut, or an insect bite. They cause local irritation and red bumps that develop into small, pus-filled blisters. With time, these blisters tend to rupture, turning into soft yellowish-brown scabs or crusts.

For children in the middle years, impetigo is usually not a serious condition, even though it may be unsightly and uncomfortable. On rare occasions, however, it can lead to complications, including a serious kidney disorder called glomerulonephritis. When treated appropriately, the infection usually heals in about a week.

To get rid of the bacteria that live beneath the scabs, your pediatrician may suggest that you remove these crusts after first softening them. Soak the sores in warm water—or use a clean, wet, warm washcloth—for ten to fifteen minutes, four times a day, followed by washing with a mild soap. Don't scrub, since rubbing away the scabs can be painful. Once the scabs

are gone, antibiotic ointment should be applied to the area several times a day. In particularly troublesome or widespread infections, your doctor may prescribe an oral antibiotic as well.

Because impetigo is contagious, epidemics of this skin disorder sometimes occur in schools and within families. Keep your infected child home until she has been on treatment for a day.

Warts

Viruses in the skin are responsible for the abnormal growth of skin cells that we call warts. While warts may not be visually appealing, they are quite harmless. However, depending on where they develop, they can sometimes be uncomfortable, particularly on the soles of the feet.

Warts usually disappear on their own without any treatment, although this may take as long as a couple of years. If the warts are uncomfortable, if they become infected or bleed, or if your child is self-conscious about them, talk to your doctor about treating and removing them. The pediatrician might recommend daily applications of a nonprescription salicylic-and-lactic acid solution on the wart; after a few months the wart might fall off. However, this kind of treatment is time-consuming and unpredictable. Warts can also be removed by surgery, freezing, or electrical cauterization.

Scabies

Scabies is a skin condition caused by mites, which are tiny insects. These mites burrow into the upper layer of the skin and release a substance that causes severe itching, red bumps, and in some cases, pus-filled sores. Scabies is contagious, as the mites themselves are transferred by skin-to-skin or clothing-to-skin contact.

The irritation associated with scabies tends to develop in places like the knee and elbow creases, the armpits, and the webbing between the toes and fingers. When it occurs, however, it is more irritating than worrisome, although it should be treated. The itching might be eased through cool baths or compresses. Your pediatrician will recommend a prescription medication, or a nonprescription one that contains benzyl benzoate (actually an insecticide), which can eradicate the mite, often with just one application.

Scabies is often discovered in school, but it is not usually spread there because prolonged contact is required. As soon as treatment has been completed, the child may return to school.

Cold Sores

Cold sores are oozing blisters that can erupt on any part of the body, although they tend to occur most often on or near the lips or inside the mouth. The herpes simplex virus, which can be transmitted from child to child or parent to child, often through saliva, is responsible for these sores.

The first time your child has a herpes simplex infection, the lesions will typically spread throughout his mouth. Thereafter, the virus itself changes character and lies dormant within the nerve, occasionally reactivating in response to any of a number of triggers, including sunlight, cold, heat, fever, and stress. Just before these new blisters emerge, your child may feel an itching or tingling sensation in the region.

There are antiviral drugs that are effective against herpes simplex virus; these drugs are used for severe infections and for infections in children whose immune systems are not normal. Although these drugs can relieve symptoms and shorten the duration of the illness, they are not cures and do not prevent recurrences. Most children do not need antiviral therapy; topical therapy is not very helpful, and oral therapy must be started very early to be effective. The only therapy needed in most cases of cold sores is symptomatic relief: Many doctors recommend that children keep cold sores moist with lip balm in order to help relieve discomfort. These sores will eventually form scabs and heal, disappearing after seven to fourteen days. Until they are gone, discourage your child from scratching or picking at them. In general, however, there is no need to keep him home from school.

Conjunctivitis

Most parents call it pinkeye, but when doctors talk about it, they use the term *conjunctivitis*. It is an inflammation of the mucous membrane on the inner side of the eyelids. Although it is common and usually not a serious condition, parents understandably become anxious when their child develops symptoms such as bright pink eyes and yellow-green pus that can make the eyelids stick together, particularly upon awakening in the morning.

A number of different bacteria—including staphylococcus and streptococcus—can cause conjunctivitis. Viruses and allergies also may be responsible for pinkeye. Both the bacterial and viral infections are contagious, so make sure your child does not share towels, washcloths, and pillows with other family members. Careful handwashing is the most important preventive measure.

These viral infections tend to clear up on their own in a few days. Your doctor may prescribe an antibiotic either eyedrops or an ointment—for bacterial conjunctivitis; make sure your child uses the antibiotic for the prescribed time period, even if the symptoms disappear. Two adults may be needed to administer the drops: one to hold the eye open and reassure the child while the other adult actually puts the drops in the eye. Also, periodically wash the eyelids, using a cotton ball soaked in warm water, to keep them from sticking together. Keep your child home until her eyes no longer have a discharge.

Vision Problems

Middle childhood is a common time for the recognition of vision problems, especially when children first have assigned seats in classrooms. Your child may tell you that he cannot read the blackboard unless he squints or moves to a front-row seat. Or you may notice that when he watches television, he sits close to the set. Less commonly, your child may complain that the words on the pages of books are blurry. All of these suggest a focusing problem and call for an examination by an eye doctor.

Myopia, or nearsightedness, is the most common vision problem among school-age children, often developing between age six and adolescence. With this condition the eyeball has an elongated shape, and thus light passing through the lens of the eye is focused in front of the retina rather than on it. As a result the child cannot clearly see distant objects.

Children with hyperopia, or farsightedness, have the opposite problem. Because of the shorter shape of their eyeballs, images are focused behind the retina, causing them to be blurry. These children cannot clearly see objects that are close to them without making an effort to focus, although this effort may not be a conscious one.

Both of these conditions can be inherited. Myopia and hyperopia may require eyeglasses to correct the poor vision. Most doctors recommend that active children wear shatter-resistant plastic lenses to minimize the chances of serious accidents. Some children prefer contact lenses, but because the lenses require diligent care, doctors often discourage their use prior to adolescence. Laser surgery to correct myopia is not done until adulthood, when the eye has finished growing.

Some children also have an astigmatism, in which the front of the eye is shaped more like a football than a basketball. As a result, the vision may be similar to that seen when looking in a mirror with a wavy surface, like a fun-house mirror that makes you seem too tall, too wide, or too thin. Astigmatism is usually inherited, may be present at birth, and may remain little changed throughout life. Normally, the blur from astigmatism is corrected with glasses or contact lenses. Small amounts of astigmatism are common and do not require correction.

Here are some other points to remember about your child's vision:

- Even though visual difficulties can sometimes cause headaches, this pain is most often associated with problems unrelated to the eyes.

- If your child wears glasses and participates in competitive sports, the glasses should be secured in place by attaching a strap that connects the two earpieces and stretches behind the head. Also, special sports glasses are available.

- Some optometrists recommend eye exercises to help treat learning disorders like dyslexia. However, carefully controlled studies have failed to demonstrate any benefits from these eye exercises—or from wearing colored lenses—to treat these disorders.

Urinary Tract Infections

Has your child complained of pain, burning, or stinging when she urinates? Does she seem to go to the bathroom more frequently than normal? Is her urine discolored?

If so, she may have a urinary tract infection (UTI). These infections occur much more often in girls than boys, and they increase in frequency in middle childhood.

Urinary tract infections are caused by bacteria from the child's own body. Normally, these bacteria are present on the skin or in the intestinal tract and can make their way to the urethra (the tube that carries off the urine from the bladder). However, when the bacteria travel along the urethra into the bladder, rather than being washed away during urination, they may attach to the bladder wall and infect the bladder or perhaps the kidney. Because the urethra in girls is much shorter than the urethra in boys, the bacteria have a shorter distance to go to reach the female bladder, and girls get more bladder and kidney infections.

When your pediatrician suspects a urinary tract infection, he or she will examine the child's urine and should have the involved bacteria identified at a laboratory. If a urinary tract infection is diagnosed, your youngster should be placed on an antibiotic. Be sure she takes the full course of medication, even if her symptoms disappear before it is used up. Following a UTI, your doctor may suggest additional evaluations—including frequent urine examinations, ultrasound visualization of the kidneys, or X-ray examination of urinary voiding.

In order to prevent urinary tract infections, children should be encouraged to drink plenty of liquids—six or more glasses of water a day. After going to the bathroom, children—especially girls—should wipe from front to back to keep from contaminating the urethra with more bacteria. Also, girls should wear 100 percent cotton underpants (the moisture that accumulates with nylon panties can promote the growth of bacteria and cause UTIs). Do not use bubble baths, since their chemicals can be irritating and lead to urinary tract infections. Use a bland soap for bathing.

COMMON CHRONIC
HEALTH PROBLEMS

Allergies

The air we breathe is filled with pollen, pollutants, and dust. Most children and adults are unaffected by these intruders. For a large number of children, however, these simple contaminants can make life miserable. Sometimes ingredients in foods or contact with pets trigger a reaction in these hypersensitive children.

Many youngsters react to so-called allergens (dust, pollen, mold, foods, or animal dander) with sneezing, runny noses, itching eyes, skin rashes, wheezing, and other symptoms. Some may feel as if they have a cold that never seems to go away.

These children suffer from allergic symptoms, which affect as many as one in every six youngsters and disrupt day-to-day activities at home, school, and play.

The immune system of allergic children overreacts to substances that are normally quite harmless. When an allergic child comes in contact with an allergen—dust, for instance—his body produces an antibody to it. This antibody sets off a series of bodily processes that ultimately trigger the allergic response.

There are many things to which children may be allergic. An animal's dander (skin), not its hair, can cause allergic symptoms in some children. So can foods like cow's milk, peanuts, fish, shellfish, nuts, and eggs, which can trigger symptoms like hives, diarrhea, severe vomiting, wheezing, or even shock. Some specific allergic symptoms (such as asthma, hay fever, and eczema) will be discussed later.

If your child has allergic symptoms that are particularly bothersome or difficult to control, your pediatrician may refer him to a medical specialist called an allergist. As well as examining your child, the allergist will want to know when symptoms began, what medications have been tried, and the potential allergens (such as pets or pollen) that may exist in or around your home.

The most effective component of treatment is for your child to avoid the substances to which he is allergic. For many children, dust mites (microscopic insects that live in house dust) are the source of their allergic symptoms. If dust mites are the problem, you should thoroughly clean your child's bedroom and the rest of your home. Here are some suggestions to help your youngster avoid the most common allergens:

- If your home has a forced-air heating system, replace the furnace filters frequently, or install an electrostatic filter in the system. A less expensive alternative is to use a room air purifier.

- Vacuum and clean more often than you might otherwise do, especially the child's bedroom, as this is where he spends the most time. If possible, vacuum floors and furniture daily, with a thorough house-cleaning scheduled at least once a week. Use a damp mop to clean up dust rather than push it around. If possible, avoid wall-to-wall carpeting in your home.

- Keep animals with fur or feathers out of the house, even if your child has tested negative on scratch tests for animal allergies. Youngsters can easily develop sensitivity to animal danders.

- Avoid products with strong odors like perfume, mothballs, tar, paints, and camphor.

- Do not smoke cigarettes in the house, the car, or near your child—for the sake of your child's allergies *and* your own health.

- Keep the doors and windows of your child's bedroom closed as much as possible, especially when the room is not being used.

- Place plastic covers over mattresses and box springs. Use foam, not feather, pillows. Avoid fuzzy, dust-catching wool blankets or wool comforters. Choose a smooth-finished cotton or synthetic fabric bedspread.

- Remove stuffed animals from your child's room.

- Read the labels on medications, looking for ingredients that may have caused allergic reactions in the past.

Frequently, allergic symptoms can be relieved, at least partially, by the use of medication. The most common medications to treat nasal symptoms are antihistamines. Sometimes a decongestant may also be recommended. More troublesome or persistent nasal symptoms can be helped by other medications prescribed by your pediatrician or allergist.

Allergists may also conduct skin or scratch tests to determine the particular allergen to which your child is reacting. In this test, the doctor will scratch your child's skin and then place a small amount of the suspected substance onto the scratched surface. The doctor may test several substances at the same time, and if your child is allergic to one or more of them, antibodies will trigger a reaction in the skin, causing red patches to appear.

After the allergen has been identified, the allergist might recommend allergy shots if the symptoms are sufficiently troublesome. These injections carefully and gradually *in*crease your child's exposure and resistance to the allergens to which he is sensitive. As that happens, the immune system's sensitivity to the allergen may slowly subside. Eventually, when your child routinely encounters the allergen in his day-to-day life, he will respond with fewer symptoms.

Allergies tend to run in families. Some children seem to outgrow their allergies as they become older; for others, however, allergies are a lifelong problem. There is no way to predict which pattern your child will follow.

Asthma

For as many as 8 million children in the United States, the simple, usually unconscious process of breathing is a daily concern and problem. These youngsters have asthma, a respiratory condition in which the air passages of the lungs (the bronchioles) tighten up, making breathing difficult.

During an asthmatic episode the membranes lining the airways become inflamed; they swell, and thick mucus builds up within the air passages, and the bronchial

The Signs of Asthma

The following symptoms are those that your child may experience during an asthma attack.

Tightness. Your child may describe a tight feeling in his chest.

Cough. A repeated short cough may be the first symptom that a parent notices. This occurs most often during the night and early morning hours.

Rapid breathing. As your child attempts to move more air in and out of the lungs through the narrowed airway, he will breathe faster than normal.

Wheezing. This is a whistling sound that occurs during obstructed breathing.

Extended exhalation. Because air tends to encounter more obstruction leaving the lungs rather than entering, exhaling usually takes more time than inhaling.

Retraction. During episodes of difficult breathing, the ribs and clavicle may be more visible as the skin is stretched by the greater effort it takes to inhale and exhale.

---

muscles surrounding the airways go into spasm. With every breath the air must struggle through the narrowed breathing tubes to make its way into and out of the lungs. Each time the child exhales, she may make the high-pitched wheezing sound so often identified with asthma.

What causes asthma? In those children whose airways are susceptible, it is usually an overreaction to infections, allergens, cold air, exercise, or something in the air that the child breathes. For instance, viral respiratory infections (colds, influenza) are responsible for many asthma attacks, and some children experience asthma only when they have such an infection.

Inhaled pollens can also provoke an episode, as can other allergens like animal dander, dust mites, and irritating fumes. A sudden change in temperature—for instance, exposure to very cold air—can trigger an episode too. Emotional distress can sometimes bring on an asthma attack, as can some medications.

Children with asthma often miss more school than their friends and sometimes are restricted from playground activities that could worsen their condition. Asthma can be a frightening disorder for both parent and child. Although it is not a common event, hundreds of children do die from asthma attacks every year in the United States. However, keep in mind that most asthma is treatable, and newer medications are capable of preventing attacks and reducing symptoms, with minimal side effects.

When a child has an asthma attack, she needs immediate treatment to relieve bronchial muscle-tightening. If possible, the first treatment involves removing the child from the situation that has triggered the symptoms: stop exercising, come in from the cold, get away from the cat, and so on.

The front line of therapy for a child who is experiencing wheezing from asthma is a hand-held inhaler (metered dose inhaler) or nebulizer. Most children over four years of age can use these devices on their own very successfully, particularly when the instruments are equipped with a chamber or "spacer" that makes it easier for the child to coordinate her breathing with the release of the drug, and ensures that the desired dosage is inhaled. Be sure your child understands and follows the instructions of the doctor carefully when using an inhaler, to maximize its effect in controlling asthma symptoms. The most common problem when these inhalers fail to work is the lack of proper administration.

If your child does not respond to her medication, contact your doctor promptly. Sometimes your youngster's asthma episode may warrant an immediate call to the doctor's office. Call your physician if your child's wheezing is severe and her breathing becomes very difficult. Also, contact your doctor immediately if your child's lips turn blue, if she cannot speak, or if she vomits asthma medication that she took by mouth.

During exercise some children develop shortness of breath and other symptoms of asthma. The child who wheezes during exercise does not necessarily need to limit her participation in most sports. Instead, your doctor may recommend that your youngster use an inhaler about ten minutes before exercising as a way to prevent symptoms from occurring. In certain sports like swimming, children with asthma actually do quite well.

Schools vary in their rules about asthma medication. Some insist that *all* medication be kept in the principal's office and that it be administered only by the school nurse. This may be a problem for children who require medication but feel embarrassed about leaving class to take it. These youngsters may need encouragement and support to recognize that the medicine is preferable to having a serious, disruptive asthma attack.

Whenever possible, youngsters should stay away from those things that tend to trigger their asthma. In some children, that may mean avoiding certain foods. Others need to keep away from cigarette smoke, feather pillows, or flowers, or remain indoors on particularly smoggy days.

Hay Fever

If your child is sneezing and has a clear nasal discharge and swollen nasal membranes, he may have hay fever. Also called *seasonal allergic rhinitis,* hay fever is an allergic condition affecting the upper respiratory tract. While the offending allergen may be hay or other pollen-producing plants, this disorder has nothing to do with fever, despite its name.

A youngster with this condition may have dark circles under red, teary eyes, and he may itch in places he cannot easily scratch, like inside the nose and ears, or on the roof of the mouth. As a result, he might wrinkle or rub his nose a lot to try to relieve the discomfort.

For each child there tends to be a hay fever season that depends on the geographical location; usually it starts in the early spring and continues through the fall. Symptoms may appear when the air contains high levels of pollen from ragweed, grass, weeds, and trees, as well as from mold spores.

Hay fever is actually the most common of all allergic conditions, and the tendency to develop it is frequently inherited. Since the allergens that cause hay fever are in the air, they are very difficult to avoid. Nonetheless, as with other types of allergies, the best defense against hay fever is for your child to stay away from the allergens that trigger the attacks. For example, if possible, your child should sleep with the windows closed and the air conditioner on.

When symptoms occur, your doctor may recommend an antihistamine to help control the runny nose, sneezing, and itchiness. As a general rule, begin giving the antihistamine when symptoms first appear; your doctor may recommend that it be taken preventively throughout the hay fever season. Your doctor should personalize and adjust the dosage of the antihistamine and try different types to find the best one for your child. The newer prescription antihistamines on the market do not cause drowsiness.

For more severe cases, special nasal sprays—such as cromolyn or corticosteroid sprays—might be prescribed. Allergy shots can also help create an immunity to the offending allergen.

Hay fever—or *seasonal* allergic rhinitis—is a different condition than *perennial* allergic rhinitis. The perennial type occurs throughout the year in response to ever-present allergens such as the house mite, a microscopic insect that is present in dust. Mites may be more plentiful during some seasons and may thus also be a cause of seasonal allergies. The treatment options are the same for both symptom patterns but must be applied year-round for perennial allergies.

Eczema

Eczema is a chronic, noncontagious skin condition, usually beginning early in life. Occasionally, eczema develops later in life or fails to resolve as the child gets older. It is a red, very itchy rash that develops in the creases of the fingers, knees, wrists, or elbows. If your child scratches the rash, it may ooze, and the skin can become raw and scaly. After a while the affected skin becomes darker and thickens.

There are many types of eczema. Some are caused by an allergic reaction to something consumed (medication, food) or touched (plants, certain types of clothing). Most often, however, the cause is unknown.

To treat the condition, your doctor should suggest a lubricating ointment to help combat dry skin. Your child should use this ointment at least once a day, twice a day is better. If she applies it after her bath, it can keep some of the moisture in the skin. Doctors often recommend that the cream be used just after applying a corticosteroid ointment.

When the eczema flares up, your doctor might recommend a corticosteroid cream. Some of these ointments are nonprescription ($\frac{1}{2}$% or 1% hydrocortisone ointment). Your child should apply some at the first sign of an outbreak. Discourage her from scratching, which will only make the condition worse. Antihistamine medication may be taken to reduce itching, although the older types of these drugs can make children sleepy.

To keep eczema flare-ups to a minimum, your child should avoid blankets and clothes made of wool and other itchy materials. Cotton is a much better choice. Also, keep your child away from other potential triggers of eczema, such as extreme temperatures (heat or cold), dry air, and chemicals. Avoid harsh soaps and bubble baths too.

One other warning: In children with eczema, the herpes virus can cause a serious skin infection. For that reason, keep children and adults with active herpes-related cold sores away from a youngster with eczema. These children are also at greater risk of bacterial skin infections, such as impetigo.

Hives

Hives (also called *urticaria*) are a common skin reaction in children, characterized by a raised, flat pink rash called wheals. The shape of these bumps can vary, and their size can range from about one-half inch to several inches in diameter. The larger wheals often have pale centers.

In most cases, hives are caused by allergies. Foods like shellfish, milk, peanuts, or chocolate can trigger them. So can insect bites or drugs like penicillin. In winter some children develop hives when they are exposed to cold air. Occasionally, children with a strep throat will have hives. In most cases, however, doctors are unable to identify the specific cause of an outbreak.

Unlike most allergic conditions, hives often occur only once in a child. The first symptom may be itching sensations, followed by the appearance of wheals. Although these raised bumps usually disappear within a few hours, they often resurface on a different part of the body. Eventually, the spots disappear completely, with the entire cycle usually taking only three or four days, and rarely longer than ten days.

In mild cases of hives, your doctor may determine that no treatment is required. However, to make your child less itchy and more comfortable, the doctor might suggest an oral antihistamine. Your youngster also might find that a cool bath or cold compresses can further relieve the itching. In the most severe cases, your child may have trouble speaking and even breathing because of swelling in the mouth and throat; if that happens, contact your doctor and go to an emergency room immediately. Also, let your physician know if your youngster with hives is feeling any joint pain or if he develops a fever, since this could suggest another complication called serum sickness.

Diabetes

Diabetes is a very serious metabolic disorder that prevents the normal breakdown and use of food, especially sugars (carbohydrates) by the body. It can damage the heart, blood vessels, kidneys, and neurological system and can cause a progressive loss of vision over many years.

In children, diabetes is caused by inadequate production of the hormone insulin by the pancreas. When that happens, the body is unable to properly metabolize sugars, which build up in the bloodstream; these sugars cannot be used by the body and are excreted in the urine. This leads to the major symptoms of diabetes: increased urination, thirst, and increased appetite, as well as weight loss.

While diabetes can begin at any age, there are peak periods at about ages five to six and then again at ages eleven to thirteen. The first sign is often an increase in the frequency and amount of urination. However, the other cardinal symptoms must be present as well for the diagnosis of diabetes: Your child will complain of being thirsty and tired, she will begin to lose weight, and her appetite will increase. If these symptoms are not noticed early in their course, some children may require hospitalization by the time a diagnosis is made in order to receive treatment with intravenous insulin and fluids to stabilize their condition.

Although there is no cure for diabetes, children with this disease can lead a nearly normal childhood and adolescence if their disorder is kept under control. *It is essential to control diabetes properly in order to avoid complications.* Regular insulin injections—usually two per day, just before breakfast and dinner—can keep blood sugar levels within a normal range and reduce the likelihood of symptoms. A diet high in complex carbohydrates with restrictions on refined sugar is important too. A child with diabetes may need to be reminded that insulin shots alone cannot control diabetes; she also has to pay attention to her diet, following the doctor's nutritional guidelines. At least thirty minutes of exercise a day can help your child manage her disease as well.

By working with your children in their middle years, you can help them gradually begin to take responsibility for caring for their disorder. They can start giving themselves insulin injections. They can also check the sugar in their blood at least twice a day, using simple, chemically treated test strips. By attending summer camps for diabetic children, they can see how other children with this illness have become more self-reliant in caring for the disease.

However, you need to oversee these self-care tasks to make certain your child is following your doctor's guidelines. If your child takes too *much* insulin, she can experience insulin shock, with symptoms that include clammy or tingling sensations, trembling, a rapid heartbeat, and a loss of consciousness. Conversely, if she takes too *little* insulin, the major symptoms of diabetes (weight loss, increased urination, thirst, and appetite) can return.

When a youngster does not assume self-care responsibilities in the middle years, you may find it even more difficult to introduce this concept during adolescence, when the desire for independence often overrules common sense. If your youngster develops good habits *before* her teenage years arrive, however, she has a much better chance of an easier young adulthood.

For more information about childhood diabetes, ask your doctor or contact the Juvenile Diabetes Foundation, 432 Park Avenue South, New York, New York 10016. In many communities, parent groups are available in which the parents of children with diabetes can meet to discuss their common concerns. Ask your pediatrician to recommend a book or two that can further familiarize you with diabetes; one of the best, which can be read by both parents and children, is *An Instructional Aid on Insulin-Dependent Diabetes Mellitus* by Luther B. Travis, M.D. (American Diabetes Association, Texas Affiliate, 8140 North Mopac, Austin, Texas 78759).

Stomachaches

Some children have frequent recurrent abdominal pain. Overeating can cause stomach discomfort. So can gas, constipation, food intolerance, intestinal infections and food poisoning, urinary tract infections, appendicitis, and many other serious medical conditions, the majority of which are quite rare. Some (perhaps most) stomachaches have no known physical basis.

Most stomachaches disappear on their own, usually within an hour or two. But in some cases the discomfort can last much longer.

When should you contact a physician? If your child's pain is severe, let your pediatrician know. Also, call the doctor if your youngster's discomfort is continuous for more than two hours, if the pain ebbs and flows over a period longer than twelve hours, or if the stomachaches are recurrent. Other things that should prompt you to call your physician include vomiting blood or green bile, an associated high fever, blood in the stool, and pain that awakens your child from sleep.

Over the short term your child may feel better if he lies down quietly for ten to fifteen minutes. Sometimes it helps to place a heating pad on his stomach. Although you can give him clear fluids, avoid solid foods. Do not administer laxatives or an enema without your doctor's approval.

When acute appendicitis—an inflammation of the appendix of the intestine—is the cause of a stomachache, the first symptom is usually pain in the area of the navel. The discomfort may eventually move to the lower right part of the abdomen, which can be tender to the touch. Usually, a slight fever develops, and your child may become nauseous and vomit. Call your doctor immediately if you suspect appendicitis. Delays in seeking care for children with appendicitis are the most common reason for complications and prolonged hospitalization.

Stomachaches can be stress-related, associated with emotional turmoil at home or at school. The stress does not have to be extraordinary, just the usual stresses of childhood. It can also be caused by a divorce or other major dissension in the family, or a poor relationship with other children or a teacher. Some children develop anxiety-related stomach pains when it is time to leave for school in the morning, only to have the discomfort subside once they are allowed to stay home for the day. Try to get to the underlying cause of this emotional agitation, and resolve it as soon as possible. (See Chapter 24, "School Avoidance.")

Headaches

At one time or another, almost all children complain of a headache. In fact, the three most common recurring pain symptoms that pediatricians see are abdominal pain, chest pain, and headaches.

While a sudden severe headache may suggest a serious problem within the head or central nervous system and require prompt evaluation, headaches are most often a symptom of other medical or emotional problems. Your child may be feeling stress and tension. Or she may have a cold, the flu, or a strep throat. Sometimes fevers and headaches occur at the same time, so if your child complains of head pain, check her temperature.

Some children experience a recurrent headache called migraine, which can begin in childhood. Unlike headaches caused by tension, these are often accompanied by other symptoms. Children may have a pre-

monition that they will occur. Often, the headache occurs along with nausea, vomiting, or visual disturbances. The head pain itself is typically throbbing or stabbing and may affect one or both sides of the front part of the head. There may also be other unpleasant sensations in the head, including burning, tingling, aching, or squeezing. The child may prefer a darkened room. Migraines tend to run in families.

Migraine pain is caused by chemicals produced in the brain that alter blood vessels in the brain. (By comparison, stress headaches are characterized by a contraction of the muscles at the back of the head.) The head pain typically lasts for several hours or even overnight.

In diagnosing your child's headache, your pediatrician will look for an underlying disease or condition. For most types of headaches, rest and some pain medication like acetaminophen or nonsteroidal anti-inflammatory drugs may be all that is necessary, along with treatment of the primary disorder. Depending on the type of headache, your doctor might also recommend prescription drugs or stress-management techniques. If migraines occur more than two to three times a month—and particularly if they interfere with attending or functioning well in school—your doctor may prescribe medication as a preventive measure. A number of oral and nasal drugs that can control the attack are now available for older children. The doctor may also suggest some counseling to explore whether emotional factors may be contributing to the headaches. Headaches should not be allowed to control home or school activities.

Seizures and Convulsions

Seizures are a symptom of disordered inhibitory functioning of the brain. They are caused by abnormal electrochemical activity within the nerve pathways in the brain. They become obvious when they cause stiffening or movement—jerky, sometimes repetitive or occasionally violent shaking of the body's muscles.

Seizures take many forms. Some are much more subtle and appear as loss of muscle tone or periods of staring, unintelligible noise-making, odd sensations, or altered thought processes.

Most seizures are single, unique events in the lives of children. They are caused by high fevers, or a variety of illnesses or traumas, and are unlikely to recur. When they do happen in children, parents are understandably frightened. Any child having a seizure requires prompt medical attention to determine the cause.

Febrile Seizures

In preschool children, seizures most commonly occur in conjunction with a high or rapidly rising fever. Called febrile seizures, these convulsions typically last less than five minutes. They rarely take place before age six months or after six years. There is no evidence that such febrile seizures cause brain damage or have any negative consequences, such as a greater likelihood of developing recurrent convulsions, or epilepsy, later in life. In general, no treatment is required, but the cause of the fever should be determined.

Nonfebrile Seizures

Seizures that occur without a fever are not uncommon, but most are single, isolated events, perhaps caused by a temporary interruption in the normal pattern of brain functioning. Recurrent seizures (epilepsy) affect perhaps one in every one hundred to two hundred children and may be a chronic problem.

If your youngster has two or more seizures, your doctor may conduct tests to determine if the chronic, recurrent form of seizure disorder (epilepsy) is present. Epilepsy is generally treated with anticonvulsant medications, which are selected based on the pattern of the seizures.

Generalized Seizures

In most cases, when a generalized seizure occurs, this is what you can expect: Your child will lose consciousness and fall to the floor. His body will stiffen. His arms and legs will jerk violently. His eyes will roll back in his head. The child may temporarily lose bowel or bladder control.

During the seizure, try to stay calm. Leave your child on a flat surface like the floor, unless he is in a place where his thrashing may cause injury. Loosen any restrictive clothing, particularly a tight collar. Turn his head to the side to drain vomit or saliva and to ease his breathing. *Never* put any object, including your finger, between his teeth, throw water on his face, or give him something to drink.

Let the seizure run its course; do not try to restrain your youngster's convulsions. After the seizure, your child may feel confused and quite tired; if he wants to sleep, let him do so.

Once the seizure is over, call your physician. Describe as completely as possible what the convulsion was like. The doctor may ask how your child was behaving before the seizure, whether anything seemed to trigger it, and how long it lasted. The doctor may want to examine and evaluate your child right away or within the next day or two.

There are other types of seizures that may be less evident and dramatic than those described above. Some children have only a stare, peculiar hand or face movements, or altered awareness.

Fortunately, in about 80 percent of children with recurrent seizure disorders, the convulsions can usually be controlled with medication that suppresses the abnormal activity of the brain cells. Once started, anticonvulsant medication is usually taken for a long time. These drugs may control symptoms, but are not a cure. Be sure your youngster takes this medication regularly and as directed; if he stops taking it abruptly, he is likely to experience a seizure. For this reason, be sure to refill the prescription *before* he runs out of the drug.

Every seizure medication has potential side effects that your pediatrician considers when deciding which to prescribe. Each drug is different, but the more common symptoms include dizziness, insomnia, sleepiness, unsteadiness, imbalance, and nausea. Some drugs can impair the liver, blood, and other body functions, and so to assure that the medication dosage is correct and that no damage is being done, children taking anticonvulsants have to undergo regular blood tests.

If the seizures are *not* well controlled, your doctor may suggest some limitations on your child's physical activity, particularly in those sports in which a seizure could cause a serious fall—that is, activities like high-diving and rope climbing. Head-contact sports should be avoided. If he swims, make sure he is closely supervised by someone in the water with him.

Some children have to take anticonvulsant medication indefinitely. However, for many children who have been seizure-free for a year or two, the doctor may gradually decrease and eventually stop their medication. The majority of these youngsters continue to be free of seizures.

If a child experiences a seizure for the first time, promptly call 911 or your pediatrician. Of course, during any subsequent convulsion, call 911 immediately if the child seems in greater distress than usual. Also, call for help if the seizures last longer than fifteen minutes.

For additional information about epilepsy, contact the Epilepsy Foundation of America, 4351 Garden City Drive, Landover, Maryland 20785.

COMMON EMERGENCIES

Before an emergency ever occurs, make sure you are prepared. Have emergency phone numbers—including your doctor's office and 911 (if that is the emergency number in your area)—by your telephone. Most communities have a poison control center, whose number should also be handy. Find out where the closest hospital emergency room is located and the quickest route to get there. Also, ask your pediatrician how he or she would like you to respond to emergencies, both during and after office hours.

When an emergency occurs, quickly assess the situation, use some common sense, and decide whether to implement life-saving procedures (such as CPR) immediately, call for an ambulance, or phone your pediatrician for advice. When dialing 911, explain your child's condition or injury as calmly as possible. Your youngster will need immediate attention if he has stopped breathing, or if he has no pulse. He will also require emergency help if he has lost consciousness. The box on the following page contains a list of situations that typically warrant emergency care.

Some emergency situations are described in the previous chapter—for example, severe asthma (see page 592) and seizures (page 598). In the remainder of this chapter you will find descriptions of other common childhood emergencies. This information will be of most value if you read it in advance of any emergency. The chart on page 606 reviews basic first aid and CPR guidelines.

Acute Bleeding

Cuts and Lacerations

Nearly all youngsters scrape their knees or elbows from time to time, often causing mild bleeding. However, when children suffer a serious cut or laceration, or profuse bleeding, this should be treated as an emergency.

First, clean the wound with soap and water, even placing it under running water, which will allow you to examine the wound closely and gauge the intensity of the bleeding. Next, your immediate task is to stop the bleeding. Apply a sterile gauze pad over the cut. (If gauze is not available, use a clean handkerchief, towel, or shirt.) Press forcefully with the palm of the hand until the bleeding subsides, and then keep the dressing on for a few extra minutes. If the gauze becomes saturated, put a new layer over the one that is there. Seek medical attention to determine if the laceration

When Is Your Child in an Emergency Situation?

A parent's instincts can help decide whether a child needs emergency attention. Here are some situations that generally require immediate attention.

- severe cuts or lacerations

- a head injury accompanied by loss of consciousness or vomiting

- a very high fever in a child who is excessively sleepy or not normally responsive and has a headache, vomiting, or a stiff neck

- severe burns of all types, including chemical and electrical burns, especially on the face

- poisoning, caused by ingesting dangerous chemicals or medications

- convulsions lasting more than fifteen minutes, or any unexpected convulsions

- a serious animal bite, particularly one that has caused a break in the skin

- difficulty in breathing, or a cessation of breathing, including airway obstructions and choking

- the cessation of a heartbeat and pulse

- sudden onset of a severe headache

- signs of shock, including pale, cold, clammy skin and a weak and rapid pulse

- an altered mental state: either a decrease in the level of consciousness or, conversely, uncontrollable agitated behavior

- a fracture (broken bone)

---

requires suturing in order to be closed and heal well.

If the bleeding is pulsating or spurting and continues this way for several minutes, it may be harder to stop. In that case, apply direct pressure and call 911 or your emergency number. Large amounts of blood loss can cause a lapse into a state of shock. You can minimize the chances of shock, however, by having your child lie down and elevate her feet a few inches until the emergency team arrives. If the cut is deep or its edges are rough, take your child to the emergency room. Wounds such as this almost always need emergency care.

Nosebleeds

Nosebleeds can have a variety of causes, including a child's picking his nose, a blow to the nose, allergies, and sinus infections. As with other types of bleeding, the primary treatment for nosebleeds is to apply pressure. Have your child sit down and, if he is old enough, use his thumb and index finger to squeeze *firmly* just behind the tip of the nose while continuing to breathe through the mouth. Parents of a younger child will have to apply the pressure themselves. After five to ten minutes the bleeding should stop.

In most cases you do not need to become overly concerned about blood loss

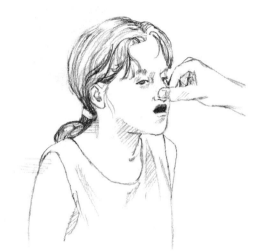

from a nosebleed. However, if the bleeding continues for more than ten minutes or recurs, call your pediatrician, who might suggest that your child be seen by a doctor, perhaps in an emergency room.

Sudden Loss of Consciousness

Head Injuries

When a child loses consciousness, you need to take the situation very seriously. Although unconsciousness can have several causes, head injuries are responsible for many cases. Quite often the child will regain consciousness just seconds after a blow to the head, but even so, she should still be examined by a doctor.

While most head injuries are relatively minor, contact your doctor if blood or clear fluid is draining from the ears or nose. Immediate examination by your physician is also necessary if your youngster fits any of the following descriptions: She complains of a headache or dizziness; acts agitated, irritable, or incoherent, or exhibits a decrease in mental alertness; breathes oddly or noisily; has convulsions; has difficulty seeing or walking; looks sweaty and pale; or vomits more than twice or after several hours have passed.

If your child wants to sleep after a minor head injury, your doctor may advise you to let her do so. During the first night, awaken the child every two hours to make sure she can be aroused and recognizes you. Check that her breathing is normal, her color is fine, the pupils of her eyes are of equal size, and she is not vomiting. If she cannot be aroused, or if any of these other signs are present, call 911 immediately.

If the head injury appears to be a serious one, call for emergency help at once. Do not move the child except to prevent additional injury. If she is bleeding severely, apply pressure with gauze or a clean handkerchief or towel to stop the flow. Monitor her breathing and pulse until emergency help arrives.

Fainting

All fainting spells require consultation with your doctor, although brief periods of unconsciousness are usually not serious. Prior to fainting, a child may feel lightheaded and nauseated; then she will become limp and fall to the floor. These episodes typically take place when there is temporarily an inadequate supply of blood and oxygen to the brain, often related to stress, fear, or overexertion. Hot weather, pain, an empty stomach, or a peculiar odor can also sometimes cause a child to faint.

Generally, fainting spells last for just a minute or less, after which normal blood flow returns and the child regains consciousness. Until then, keep your child lying down with her feet slightly elevated.

Some fainting episodes require immediate attention. Call 911 if your child remains unconscious for over two minutes, has difficulty breathing, or if she shakes or jerks while unconscious. A weak pulse or shallow breathing requires emergency care.

Seizures

Seizures are sudden, temporary changes in physical movement, caused by abnormal electrical impulses in the brain. In some instances the affected child's body may experience violent convulsions. Or it may stiffen suddenly, or completely relax.

Most seizures are not medical emergencies, but the child should be seen by a physician to determine the course of treatment. Your immediate attention should be directed toward protecting your child from injuring himself during the seizure. Lay him on his side with his hips higher than his head, or place him in a semi-sitting position, so that he will not choke if he vomits.

If the seizure continues for more than two to three minutes, if it seems unusually severe, or if one attack rapidly follows another, call 911 or your local emergency number for help. Do *not* leave your child unattended.

(For more information about seizures, see page 598.)

Breathing Emergencies

Although children under age four are most at risk for choking on food and small objects, youngsters in their middle years can choke too. A number of foods or other items (for instance, hot dogs, poorly chewed pieces of meat, grapes, raw carrots, hard candy, balloons, small toy parts) can become lodged in the child's airway (or trachea), keeping oxygen from reaching the lungs and the rest of the body as well. When the brain does not receive oxygen for more than four minutes, permanent brain damage and death can result.

If your child is having some breathing difficulties—but is still able to speak or has a strong cough—do nothing yourself; the child's cough is better than any back blows or abdominal thrusts (Heimlich maneuver) you can administer. But call 911 so that she can be transported to an emergency department, since a partial blockage of the airway could turn into a complete one.

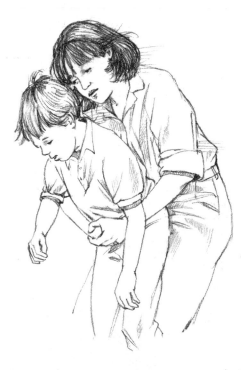

Heimlich Maneuver

However, if your youngster cannot breathe at all, or if she appears pale or her cough is very weak, then she needs immediate attention. First, have someone call 911 for emergency services. Perform the Heimlich maneuver on your youngster. For the middle-years child, this technique can be used while the youngster is lying down, sitting, or standing.

For a conscious child who is sitting or standing, position yourself behind her and wrap your arms around her waist. Place the thumb side of your fist on the middle of her abdomen, well below the lower tip of the breastbone. Then grab that fist with your free hand, press inward with rapid, upward thrusts. Repeat the thrusts until the object is coughed up or the youngster begins to breathe or cough.

Tongue-Jaw Lift

If the child is unconscious, lower her to the floor on her back and try using the tongue-jaw lift. Open the youngster's mouth, with your thumb held over her tongue, and your fingers wrapped around the lower jaw; as this draws the tongue away from the back of the throat, you may be able to clear the airway. If you can see the foreign object, try removing it with a sideways sweep of a finger; use this approach carefully, however, since it could push the object even farther down the airway, causing additional blockage.

If breathing still has not resumed, tilt the child's head back gently and lift her chin. Then place your own mouth over her mouth and, pinching her nose shut, give two slow breaths, each lasting one and a half to two seconds. If this technique is not successful, return to the Heimlich maneuver. Kneeling at the child's feet, place the heel of one of your hands in the midline between the navel and rib cage. Then place your other hand on top of the first one. Next, press firmly but gently into the abdomen, using six to ten rapid inward and upward thrusts.

Repeat the steps above—the finger sweep, the slow breaths, and the abdominal thrusts—until the child begins breathing or emergency help arrives.

CPR

Cardiopulmonary resuscitation (CPR) is another first-aid procedure, to be used only when a youngster has no pulse, indicating that his heart has stopped beating. CPR involves compression of the chest, using the heel of the hand applied to the lower half of the breastbone. These compressions should be administered over an approximately four-second period in groups of five, followed by a gentle mouth-to-mouth breath, after which the cycle is repeated. This technique can keep a child breathing and his blood circulating until emergency help arrives. It should be performed by an individual who has received specific training in this approach.

CPR is even more important if you have a

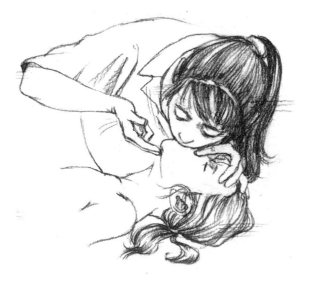

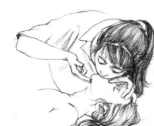

Cardiopulmonary Resuscitation (For Children Over One Year)

To be used when child is unresponsive or when breathing or heart beat stops.

1. Tilt head back. Seal your lips tightly around child's mouth, pinch nose shut.
2. Give 2 slow breaths until chest gently rises.

If air goes in:
3. Briefly check for a pulse

If there's a pulse:
4. Give 1 slow breath every 4 seconds for about 1 minute (15 breaths).
5. Recheck pulse about every minute.
Continue rescue breathing as long as pulse is present but child is not breathing.

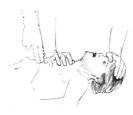

If no pulse:
4. Find hand position near center of breastbone.
5. Position shoulders over hands.
6. Compress chest 5 times.

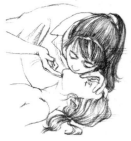

7. Give 1 slow breath.
8. Repeat cycles of 5 compressions to 1 breath until you feel a pulse or help arrives.

If air won't go in:
3. Retilt head back. Try to give 2 breaths again.

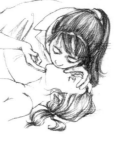

4. Place heel of 1 hand on child's abdomen above middle of navel and below rib cage.
5. Give up to 5 abdominal thrusts.

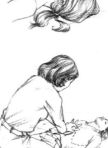

6. Lift jaw and tongue. If foreign object is seen, sweep it out with finger.
Repeat steps 3-6 until breaths go in or child starts to breathe on own.

swimming pool or a hot tub at home, or live near a lake or other body of water. Prevention, of course, is the first line of defense against drownings: No matter what their age, children should never be left unsupervised in or near a pool or body of water, even if they appear to be good swimmers. Swimming pools should be completely fenced in to prevent unsupervised access and use.

If a youngster is drowning, her breathing must be restored promptly to prevent asphyxia (lack of oxygen). Here are some guidelines to keep in mind:

- Remove your child from the water as soon as possible. Unless you are a strong swimmer yourself, try to avoid jumping into the water to pull out a drowning youngster. Instead, attempt to grab her with an outstretched arm, a long pole, or a life ring.

- Call 911 for emergency assistance.

- If the youngster has stopped breathing, administer mouth-to-mouth resuscitation, using about fifteen slow, steady breaths per minute. If she also has no pulse, then chest compressions and full CPR must be performed.

Although this book's descriptions of lifesaving techniques can familiarize you with standard procedures, they are NOT a substitute for your completion of a certified first-aid course in which you learn mouth-to-mouth resuscitation and CPR. All parents should have this training. Contact your local American Red Cross or American Heart Association office for information on where these classes are offered in your community.

Cold and Heat Emergencies

If your child is exposed to extreme temperatures—usually for an extended period of time and without appropriate clothing or other protection—he could find himself in a life-threatening situation.

Hypothermia

Hypothermia develops when a child's temperature falls below normal due to exposure to cold. This condition often occurs when a youngster is playing outdoors in extremely cold weather without wearing proper clothing. As hypothermia sets in, the child may shiver and become lethargic and clumsy; his speech may become slurred and his body temperature will decline.

Call 911 at once. Until help arrives, take the youngster indoors, remove any wet clothing, and wrap him in blankets or warm clothes. If his breathing or pulse stops, he will need mouth-to-mouth resuscitation or CPR.

Frostbite

Frostbite takes place when the skin and outer tissues become frozen. This condition tends to occur on extremities like the fingers, toes, ears, and nose, which may become pale, gray, and blistered. At the same time, the youngster may complain that his skin burns or has become numb. Bring the child indoors, where you should place the frostbitten parts of his body in warm (not hot) water; warm washcloths may be applied to frostbitten nose, ears, and lips. Do not rub the frozen areas. After a few minutes, dry and cover him with clothing or blankets. Give him something warm to drink. If the numbness continues for more than a few minutes, call your doctor.

Heatstroke

Heatstroke can occur when a child overexerts himself in very hot weather and becomes dehydrated. The mechanisms in the brain that control body temperature can stop working, and he may run a fever of 105 degrees or higher. His skin will become hot, *dry* (not perspiring), and flushed. He may feel dizzy and nauseous, and experience stomach cramps and rapid breathing.

You should move a child with heatstroke out of the sun, and call for emergency help (911) at once. Take off his clothing and place him in a cool (not cold) bathtub. To help restore circulation, massage his arms, legs, and other body parts.

Your child should always increase his fluid intake in hot weather, especially while exercising. Encourage him to drink readily available liquids regularly. When your child participates in organized sports in the hot months of summer, he should dress in a minimal amount of loose-fitting clothing.

Burns

Fires occur in the United States about every twenty seconds, and in many instances they result in burns to both children and adults. In addition to fires, children suffer burns in a variety of other ways, ranging from hot-water scalds and sun exposure to chemical agents and electrical burns. Thermal burns from sun exposure are the most common types of burns, and while most cause only temporary inconvenience, in the long term they have been found to be related to developing skin cancer. Children also suffer burns when they are using fireworks or playing with wires that are not properly covered.

There are three types of burns: *First-degree burns* are the least serious, causing redness and, in some cases, mild swelling of the skin; they usually heal in a week or two with no scarring. *Second-degree burns* result in redness, blistering, and a lot of swelling; the burn can ooze fluid, the pain can be severe, and some scarring may result. *Third-degree burns* are the most serious, injuring not only the surface skin but the deeper layers as well, with the skin often having a dry, leathery appearance and a color that can range from black to pearly white.

Immediately after a burn has occurred, immerse the affected area in cool water. Do *not* use ice, but rather run the water over the burn, relieving the pain and cooling the area. Also, remove all clothing from the burned area, except for clothing stuck to the skin.

Cover the injured area with a sterile gauze pad, applying it lightly if the burn is oozing. Do not apply grease, butter, or powder to the burn.

For chemical burns, flush the burned area immediately with large amounts of water, using a shower or a garden hose. Do not even take the time to remove the child's clothing before this flushing process begins; however, the clothing can be removed once flushing has started. Call 911 for emergency services while continuing to soak the child with water for ten to twenty minutes.

Contact your doctor at once for all serious burns, as well as for any burns to the mouth, hands, or genitals. Your child may have to be hospitalized if she has suffered third-degree burns, or if more than 10 percent of her body has been burned.

You can help prevent burns by installing smoke detectors in your home in all rooms in which people sleep, as well as in the hallways outside the bedrooms. Also place detectors in the kitchen and the living room.

Your family should practice fire drills regularly. Remind your children to crawl to the exits if there is smoke in the room, thus staying below the smoke, where there is more oxygen. Also teach your youngsters to stop, drop, and roll on the ground if their clothing catches fire.

Animal Bites

If your child is bitten or scratched by a pet or other animal, do not ignore the wound.

Most animal bites are by cats and dogs, but serious infections can come from the bites of many animals, domestic and wild. Human bites can also be serious.

Whether the wound is a puncture or just a scratch, clean it with soap and water and keep it under running water for several minutes. Then wrap it in sterile gauze and call your pediatrician. The doctor will monitor the wound for infection and, in some cases, may suggest an antibiotic or a tetanus vaccination. In some instances, such as puncture wounds to the hands that have a high risk of infection, prophylactic antibiotics may be indicated. You also need to locate the animal who inflicted the wound; the animal may need to be quarantined to make sure it does not develop rabies.

The psychological harm associated with an animal bite may be as serious as the physical wound itself. Once bitten—or even snapped at or growled at by a dog—a child may develop a lifetime fear of all dogs and other animals. (For more information, see Chapter 39, "Pets.")

Poisoning

Most accidental poisonings occur in children younger than their middle years. However, the consumption of household pesticides, chemicals, cosmetics, outdoor plants, or medications can happen at any age, causing serious reactions. These poisonings need to be treated rapidly.

Immediately call your doctor or local poison control center (keep the numbers by your phone). Have the container of the ingested substance nearby. Explain what your child has swallowed, when, and how much, as well as any symptoms (such as flushing, drowsiness, vomiting, seizures) that have already developed.

Vomiting is often the best and quickest way to deal with the immediate problem. If the poison center or your doctor advises using syrup of ipecac, follow the instructions on the bottle. Vomiting will generally occur in a few minutes. If vomiting does not take place within fifteen minutes, the same dosage of ipecac should be taken again, followed by another glass of water.

Always call the poison center or your doctor before inducing vomiting. They may advise *against* inducing vomiting if your child has swallowed certain lyes, acids, or mineral spirits, since they might burn the tissues in the throat and mouth—or be breathed into the lungs—as they are brought up.

As a preventive measure, keep all medications and chemicals securely locked away from curious children. Also, have syrup of ipecac in the house for emergency use.

Meningitis

Meningitis is a life-threatening emergency but fortunately not a common infection. Although most of its victims are younger children, it can occur during middle childhood as well.

Meningitis is an inflammation of the meninges, which are the membranes that enclose the brain and spinal cord. Symptoms can develop suddenly, and include fever, chills, vomiting, neck stiffness, headache, and sleepiness, as well as seizures. Upon diagnosis, a child is immediately hospitalized. Doctors will perform a spinal tap—withdrawing fluid from the spinal canal for analysis—in order to confirm the diagnosis.

Meningitis is contagious, so if you know that your child has been exposed to it, keep a careful eye on him. Speed is of the essence, so call your doctor *immediately* if any of the symptoms listed above occur. Full recovery depends on *early* diagnosis and hospitalization. Children who have been exposed to meningitis caused by bacteria may need to receive antibiotics to prevent them from becoming ill.

Treatment for meningitis varies, depending on whether it is caused by a virus or bacteria. It is important to find out which of these is the cause, and many of the tests that will be done are to make this determination. Generally, viral meningitis tends to be the less serious form of the disease and may require little more than observation and bed rest. For bacterial meningitis, the treatment is much more vigorous, including immediate hospitalization and antibiotic therapy. The majority of children with bacterial meningitis recover fully. Bear in mind, however, that early and proper treatment is critical; without it, children may die, and those who survive are vulnerable to serious complications, which can range from deafness to mental retardation.

The occurrence of one of the more common types of meningitis (*Haemophilus influenzae B*) has now been nearly eliminated through immunization; check with your pediatrician for the recommended schedule for these shots.

Other Emergency/First-Aid Guidelines

Here is what you need to keep in mind to deal with other common emergency situations:

Eye Injuries

If a foreign substance is splashed in your child's eye, flush it gently with water for at least fifteen minutes. Call your pediatrician or local poison center for additional recommendations. If your child's eye is injured or if it hurts, do not touch or rub the injured eye; do not apply medication. Gently place a soft eyepatch over the painful eye (do not apply pressure) and go to your doctor's office promptly. If an object becomes stuck in the eye, do not try to remove it; take your child to an emergency room immediately.

Fractures and Sprains

If your child has a neck or back injury, do *not* move her, since this can cause serious additional harm. If an injured part of the body hurts or is swollen or deformed, or if moving it causes pain, there might be a fracture. Splint the injured limb, perhaps using a rolled-up newspaper or magazine to keep further movement to a minimum. Apply a cold compress, and call an ambulance or your pediatrician. (See "Sports Injuries" on page 119.)

Fingertip Injuries

Children's fingers sometimes get caught in closing doors or banged by hammers. If there is bleeding from the fingertips, wash gently with soap and water and cover the injury with a soft, sterile dressing. Apply an ice pack to keep down the swelling. Call your doctor at once if there is excessive swelling or a deep cut. Over the ensuing hours, contact a doctor if the swelling and pain worsen, if there is drainage from the injury, or if a fever develops. Pain from blood under a fingernail can be relieved by your physician.

Teeth

If a baby (primary) tooth is knocked out or broken, apply clean gauze to the gum to control the bleeding and call your dentist. If a permanent tooth is dislodged, rinse the tooth gently without handling the root. Then insert the tooth into its socket and hold it there on the way to the dentist's office; or transport the tooth in a glass of cold cow's milk. Time is important, so get your child into the dentist's chair as soon as possible.

If the tooth is broken, save the pieces, and gently clean the injured area with warm water. Apply a cold compress to reduce swelling, and go to the dentist at once.

Index